Radiation Medicine Rounds

Charles R. Thomas, Jr., MD

Editor-in-Chief

Professor and Chair
Department of Radiation Medicine
Professor, Division of Hematology/Oncology
Department of Medicine
Knight Cancer Institute
Oregon Health & Science University Cancer Institute
Portland, Oregon

Editorial Board

Forthcoming Issues

Head and Neck Cancer
Dwight E. Heron, MD, and Roy Tishler, MD, PhD
Guest Editors

Gynecologic Cancer
A. J. Mundt, Catheryn Yashar, and Loren Mell
Guest Editors

Radiation Medicine Rounds

VOLUME 2, ISSUE 1

Prostate Cancer

Guest Editors

Allen M. Chen, MD
Assistant Professor
Department of Radiation Oncology
Davis Cancer Center
University of California
Sacramento, California

Srinivasan Vijayakumar, MD, DMRT, FACR
Professor and Chair
Department of Radiation Oncology
University of Mississippi Medical Center
Jackson, Mississippi

demosMEDICAL
New York

Acquisitions Editor: Richard Winters
Cover Design: Joe Tenerelli
Compositor: Newgen Imaging
Printer: Hamilton Printing

Visit our website at www.demosmedpub.com

Radiation Medicine Rounds is published three times a year by Demos Medical Publishing.

Business Office. All business correspondence including subscriptions, renewals, and address changes should be sent to Demos Medical Publishing, 11 West 42nd Street, 15th Floor, New York, NY, 10036.

The ideas and opinions expressed in *Radiation Medicine Rounds* do not necessarily reflect those of the Publisher. The Publisher does not assume any responsibility for any injury and/or damage to persons or property arising out of or related to any use of the material contained in this periodical. The reader is advised to check the appropriate medical literature and the product information currently provided by the manufacturer of each drug to be administered to verify the dosage, the method and duration of administration, or contraindications. It is the responsibility of the treating physician or other health care professional relying on independent experience and knowledge of the patient, to determine drug dosages and the best treatment for the patient. Mention of any product in this issue should not be construed as endorsement by the contributors, editors, or the Publisher of the product or manufacturer's claims.

ISSN: 2151-4208
ISBN: 978-1-936287-33-8

Library of Congress Cataloging-in-Publication Data

Prostate cancer / guest editors, Srinivasan Vijayakumar, Allen Chen.
    p. ; cm. — (Radiation medicine rounds; v. 2, issue 1)
  Includes bibliographical references and index.
  ISBN 978-1-936287-33-8
  1. Prostate—Cancer—Radiotherapy. I. Vijayakumar, Srinivasan. II. Chen, Allen. III. Series: Radiation medicine rounds ; v. 2, issue 1.
    [DNLM: 1. Prostatic Neoplasms—radiotherapy. 2. Disease Progression. 3. Tumor Markers, Biological—therapeutic use.
W1 RA162HD v. 2 issue 1 2011 /WJ 762]
  RC280.P7P742224 2011
  616.99′463—dc22
                                                                                            2011004858

Reprints. For copies of 100 or more of articles in this publication, please contact Reina Santana, Special Sales Manager.

Special discounts on bulk quantities of Demos Medical Publishing books are available to corporations, professional associations, pharmaceutical companies, health care organizations, and other qualifying groups. For details, please contact:

Reina Santana, Special Sales Manager
Demos Medical Publishing
11 W. 42nd Street
New York, NY 10036
Phone: 800–532–8663 or 212–683–0072
Fax: 212–941–7842
E-mail: rsantana@demosmedpub.com

Made in the United States of America
11 12 13   14   15   5 4 3 2 1

Contents

Foreword

■ FROM THE EDITOR-IN-CHIEF

Radiation Medicine Rounds is a quarterly, hard cover, periodical series that is designed to provide an up-to-date review of a dedicated radiation medicine topic of interest to clinicians and scientists who are involved in the care of patients receiving radiotherapy. It is intended to serve as both a reference and instructional tool by students, housestaff, fellows, practicing clinicians, medical physicists, cancer/radiobiologists, and interdisciplinary colleagues throughout the oncology spectrum.

The current issue, *Prostate Cancer*, is a successful attempt to concisely summarize one of the diseases that has served as a paradigm for implementation of emerging technology and understanding of cancer biology over the past two decades. Our volume editors, Drs. Allen M. Chen and Srinivasan Vijayakumar, have assembled a dedicated group of investigators who have authored a compilation of succinct and timely reviews addressing high-priority aspects of radiotherapy for this very common tumor in men. On behalf of the editorial board, I congratulate Allen and Vijay for putting together a state-of-the-art, easy-to-read, and valuable resource in the field of prostate cancer radiation medicine.

Dr. Charles R. Thomas, Jr.
Series Editor-in-Chief
Radiation Medicine Rounds
Portland, Oregon

Preface

Clinical treatment decisions for prostate cancer are more complicated than ever, and technological advances in the field of radiation oncology continue to revolutionize the management of this disease at a breathtaking pace. This volume of *Radiation Medicine Rounds* was designed with the intention of providing the practicing radiation oncologist with a broad and well-balanced synopsis of many of the relevant issues surrounding the management of prostate cancer with radiation therapy. Particular attention is focused not only on many of the current controversies, but also on future strategies, which may play an increasingly significant role in the future.

The opening articles consider the principles of the sciences underlying the presentation of prostate cancer. Accordingly, controversies regarding diagnostic stratification and how they may affect treatment are emphasized. Along these lines, specialized clinical scenarios detailing the utility of postoperative radiation therapy, brachytherapy, and androgen deprivation are illustrated given the widespread utilization of these modalities. The middle articles focus heavily on the emergence of advanced technologies such as stereotactic body radiotherapy, proton beam radiotherapy, and image-guided radiotherapy, and how they may potentially affect the therapeutic ratio. Lastly, articles surrounding the all-important issues of prevention and quality of life bring this volume to a close.

We hope this volume serves as an instructive reference for the radiation oncology community and thank the many contributors for their time and expertise in helping to bring this project to fruition.

Allen M. Chen, MD
Srinivasan Vijayakumar, MD, DMRT, FACR

Contributors

Al Barqawi, MD
Associate Professor of Urology
Division of Urology
University of Colorado School of Medicine
   Aurora, Colorado

Thomas P. Boike, MD
Assistant Professor of Radiation Oncology
University of Texas Southwestern
   Medical Center
Dalla, Texas

Ronald C. Chen, MD, MPH
Assistant Professor
Department of Radiation Oncology
University of North Carolina
Chapel Hill, North Carolina

Sravana K. Chennupati, MD
Senior Resident
Department of Radiation Medicine
Knight Cancer Institute
Oregon Health & Science University
Portland, Oregon

Seungtaek Choi, MD
Department of Radiation Oncology
The University of Texas MD Anderson
   Cancer Center
Houston, Texas

Anthony V. D'Amico, MD, PhD
Professor
Chief of Genitourinary Radiation
   Oncology
Department of Radiation Oncology
Dana-Farber Cancer Institute/Brigham and
   Women's Hospital
Boston, Massachusetts

Anees H. Dhabaan, PhD
Department of Radiation Oncology
Emory University and Winship
   Cancer Institute
Atlanta, Georgia

Steven J. Frank, MD
Assistant Professor
Department of Radiation Oncology
The University of Texas MD Anderson
   Cancer Center
Houston, Texas

Michel Ghilezan, MD, PhD
Associate Professor
Oakland University William Beaumont
   School of Medicine
William Beaumont Hospitals
Rose Cancer Center
Royal Oak, Michigan

Daniel A. Hamstra, MD, PhD
Assistant Professor
Department of Radiation Oncology
The University of Michigan
   Medical Center
Ann Arbor, Michigan

Jordan A. Holmes, BS
Doris Duke Clinical Research Fellow
Department of Radiation Oncology
University of North Carolina
Chapel Hill, North Carolina

Arthur Y. Hung, MD
Assistant Professor
Department of Radiation Medicine
Knight Cancer Institute
Oregon Health & Science University
Portland, Oregon

Ashesh B. Jani, MD, MSEE
Associate Professor and Residency
    Program Director
Georgia Cancer Coalition (GCC) Distinguished
    Cancer Clinician/Scientist
Department of Radiation Oncology
Emory University
Atlanta, Georgia

John A. Kalapurakal, MD
Professor
Radiation Oncology
Northwestern University Feinberg
    School of Medicine
Chicago, Illinois

Irving D. Kaplan, MD
Assistant Professor
Department of Radiation Oncology
Beth-Israel Deaconess
    Medical Center
Harvard Medical School
Boston, Massachusetts

Mariam Korah, MD
Department of Radiation
    Oncology
Emory University and Winship
    Cancer Institute
Atlanta, Georgia

Patrick Kupelian, MD
Professor and Vice Chair
Department of Radiation
    Oncology
UCLA Health System
Los Angeles, California

Andrew K. Lee, MD, MPH
Department of Radiation Oncology
The University of Texas MD Anderson
    Cancer Center
Houston, Texas

Brandon Mancini
Wayne State University
    School of Medicine
Detroit, Michigan

Alvaro Martinez, MD
Professor and Chairman of Radiation Oncology
Oakland University William Beaumont
    School of Medicine
William Beaumont Hospitals
Rose Cancer Center
Royal Oak, Michigan 48073

Sean M. McBride
Resident
Harvard Radiation Oncology Program
Boston, Massachusetts

Nasiruddin Mohammed, MD, MBA
Resident
Department of Radiation Oncology
William Beaumont Hospitals
Rose Cancer Center
Royal Oak, Michigan

Quynh-Nhu Nguyen, MD
Department of Radiation Oncology
The University of Texas MD Anderson Cancer Center
Houston, Texas

Richard E. Peschel, MD, PhD
Professor
Department of Therapeutic Radiology
Yale University School of Medicine
New Haven, Connecticut

Jason M. Phillips, MD, MBA
Resident, Urology
Division of Urology
University of Colorado School of Medicine
Aurora, Colorado

Thomas J. Pugh, MD
Assistant Professor
Department of Radiation Oncology
The University of Texas MD Anderson Cancer Center
Houston, Texas

Peter J. Rossi, MD
Assistant Professor
Department of Radiation Oncology
The Winship Cancer Institute of
    Emory University
Atlanta, Georgia

Matthew H. Stenmark, MD
Department of Radiation Oncology
The University of Michigan Medical Center
Ann Arbor, Michigan

Chirag Shah, MD
Resident
Department of Radiation Oncology
William Beaumont Hospitals
Rose Cancer Center
Royal Oak, Michigan

Robert D. Timmerman, MD
Professor of Radiation Oncology
Professor of Neurosurgery
University of Texas Southwestern Medical Center
Dalla, Texas

Javier F. Torres-Roca, MD
Department of Radiation Oncology and
    Experimental Therapeutics
H. Lee Moffitt Cancer Center and Research
    Institute
Tampa, Florida

demos
MEDICAL

RMR
RADIATION
MEDICINE ROUNDS

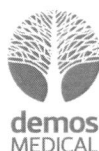

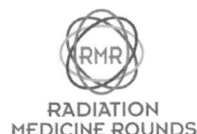

New Biomarkers in Prostate Cancer: A Radiation Oncology Perspective

Javier F. Torres-Roca*

H. Lee Moffitt Cancer Center and Research Institute, Tampa, FL

■ ABSTRACT

A fundamental aim of clinical medicine is to develop methods to assess the health risks posed by a specific disease to an individual. This risk classification is central in clinical decision-making, influencing treatment choices, and patient counseling. In oncology, the clinical stage has been the cornerstone in assessing clinical prognoses in virtually every disease site. Recently, the development of novel biomarkers has promised clinicians the ability to more accurately predict clinical outcomes and potential treatment benefits. At its most basic, a biomarker is an objectively measured analyte that indicates a particular biological state with correlation to disease progression or response to a specific treatment. This study will focus reviewing recent progress in biomarker development for prostate cancer from the perspective of radiation oncology.

Keywords: prostate cancer, predictive/prognostic biomarkers, RTOG, systems biology

Prostate cancer is the most commonly diagnosed malignancy and the second most common cause of cancer-related mortality among men in the United States (1). Treatments for patients with clinically localized disease (surgery, external beam radiation therapy [RT], brachytherapy) are generally highly effective; however, a randomized trial has shown that surgically treated patients show a slight improvement in prostate cancer mortality at 10 years when compared with conservatively managed patients (observation) (2). Thus, there is a significant need for the

development of biomarkers that can identify patients with a higher risk of disease progression. This review focuses on novel prognostic/predictive biomarkers in the field of prostate cancer and radiation oncology.

■ BIOMARKERS IN RADIOTHERAPY COLLABORATIVE TRIALS—RTOG TRANSLATIONAL RESEARCH PROGRAM

The RTOG GenitoUrinary Translational Research Program has played a central role in evaluating novel biomarkers in patients treated with RT in RTOG collaborative phase 3 clinical trials (Table 1). All biomarkers were evaluated in RTOG 86–10 and/or 92–02 using immunohistochemistry techniques. The

*Corresponding author, Department of Radiation Oncology and Experimental Therapeutics, H. Lee Moffitt Cancer Center and Research Institute, 12902 Magnolia Dr, Tampa, FL 33612

E-mail address: Javier.Torresroca@moffitt.org

Radiation Medicine Rounds 2:1 (2011) 1–10.
DOI: 10.5003/2151–4208.2.1.1

TABLE 1 Biomarkers evaluated in RTOG clinical trials

Marker	Distant Metastases	Cause-Specific Survival	Overall Survival	References
p53	RR = 2.15, P = .04	RR = 2.45, P = .003	RR = 2.34, P = .02	(3)
	HR = 1.72, P = .013	HR = 1.89, P = .014	NS	(4)
P16	RR = 2.15, P = .02	RR = 2.98, P = .007	RR = 1.79, P = .07	(5)
	HR = 0.61, P = .04			(6)
Ki-67	5 year = 13.5% vs. 50.8%, P = 0.005	5 year = 97.3% vs. 67.7%, P = 0.0039	NS	(7)
	RR = 2.39, P = 0.0008	RR = 2.07, P = 0.0174	NS	(8)
MDM2	RR = 1.85, P = 0.06	NS	NS	(9)
	HR = 1.84, P = 0.004	HR = 1.65, P = 0.032	HR = 1.42, P = 0.007	(10)
PKA	HR = 2.27, P = 0.018	NS	NS	(11)
	HR = 2.21, P = 0.006	HR = 1.83, P = 0.05	NS	(12)
DNA ploidy	NS	NS	RR = 1.55, P = 0.03	(13)
Bcl-2	NS	NS	NS	(14,15)
Bax	NS	NS	NS	(14,15)
Androgen receptor CAG repeats	NS	NS	NS	(16)
Cox-2	HR = 1.18, P = 0.004	NS	NS	(17)
Stat3	RR = 0.79, P = 0.04	NS	NS	(18)
Cyp3A4	NS	NS	NS	(19)

RR, relative risk; HR, hazard ratio; NS, not significant.

general strategy has been to initially screen biomarkers using RTOG 86–10 and then performing confirmatory analyses in RTOG 92–02, although this has not been performed in every instance. This body of work is unique in that markers were exclusively evaluated in RT-treated patients using high quality clinical datasets. Initially, the RTOG evaluated p53 as a prognostic biomarker in a subset of patients from RTOG 86–10. This initial analysis consisted of 129 patients and abnormal p53 protein expression was correlated with clinical outcome as determined by an increased risk of distant metastases (relative risk [RR] = 2.15, P = .04), worse progression-free survival (RR = 2.45, P = .003), and poorer overall survival (RR = 2.34, P= .02) (3). These observations were further confirmed in a second larger dataset consisting of 777 patients from RTOG 92–02. An association between clinical outcome and abnormal p53 expression was confirmed in this study as patients with high p53 expression had a worse cause-specific survival (hazard ratio [HR] = 1.89, P = .014) and a higher risk of distant metastasis (HR = 1.72, P = .013) (4).

Ki-67, a proliferation marker was also evaluated in both RTOG 86–10 and 92–02. Ki-67 staining was generated in 108 patients from RTOG 86–10, 60 of which received external beam radiation therapy alone. Using a cut-point at a staining index of 3.5%, Ki-67-high patients had an increased risk of distant metastasis (Ki-67-low vs. Ki-67-high, 13.5% vs. 50.8%, P = .0005) as well as a worse 5-year disease-specific survival rate (Ki-67-low vs. Ki-67-high, 97.3% vs. 67.7%, P = .0039) However, the 5-year overall survival rate was not different in this initial analysis (Ki-67-low vs. Ki-67-high, 70% vs. 55%, P = .17) (7). This marker was further evaluated in RTOG 92–02 in a total of 537 patients. When treated as a categorical variable, Ki-67 was associated with the risk of distant metastases (RR = 2.39, P = .0008) and disease-specific survival (RR = 2.07, P = .0039). Importantly, Ki-67 was the strongest predictor of distant metastases, and disease-specific survival, over the Gleason score, prostate-specific antigen (PSA) evaluation, and the clinical stage. However, it should be noted that the cut-point first reported in RTOG

86–10 (Ki-67-Staining Index >3.5%) was not found significant (8).

Given the success of p53 as a biomarker in these trials, the RTOG evaluated murine double-minute p53 binding protein (MDM2), an oncoprotein that promotes p53 degradation as a biomarker in RT-treated patients. An initial analysis was conducted in 108 patients from RTOG 86–10. A trend toward an increased risk in distant metastasis ($P = .06$) was observed in this cohort (9). In a follow-up study, MDM2 was evaluated in conjunction with Ki-67 as prognostic of the outcome in 478 patients from RTOG 92–02. In addition, p53 was also evaluated in the same cohort. Multivariate analysis demonstrated that high expression of both MDM2 and Ki-67 were associated with distant metastasis, cause-specific mortality and overall mortality, and they were both superior to p53 (10). In addition, a model combining both proteins was the most effective prognostic device, suggesting that it could be used for patient stratification in clinical trials. However, it should be noted that the numerous cut-points and approaches for analysis (manual, automated) were explored in this study, increasing the possibility of chance playing a role in the findings. For example, cut-points utilized for Ki-67 include a staining index of 7.7%, 4.5%, and 12.8%, as well as mean intensity score cut-points of 182.95, 167.1, and 195.25, none of which are the same as seen in previous studies (Staining Index, 3.5% and 7.1%).

Protein kinase A type 1 ($PKA_{RI\alpha}$), which belongs to a family of cyclic AMP-dependent holoenzymes related to cellular proliferation and transformation, is another marker that was evaluated in both subject trials. In 86–10, the analysis was limited to 80 patients; however, on multivariate analysis there was a correlation between PKA overexpression and a higher risk of biochemical failure ($P = .03$) and distant metastasis ($P = .018$) (10). These observations were further confirmed in RTOG 92–02 where 313 patients were analyzed. $PKA_{RI\alpha}$ overexpression was confirmed to be associated with the risk of clinical failure after RT and AD, as determined by distant metastasis ($P < .01$), local failure ($P < .05$), and biochemical failure ($P \leq .01$) (12).

Loss of p16 expression is the last biomarker with data from both studies. The initial analysis in RTOG 86–10 revealed an association between loss of p16 expression and an increased risk of local failure, distant metastasis, and disease-specific survival (5). The correlation with metastatic risk ($P < .04$) was confirmed in an analysis that included 612 patients

treated on RTOG 92–02. Interestingly, in patients with high levels of p16 staining, the use of long-term androgen suppression therapy was associated with an improved cause-specific survival as well as a lower risk of distant metastasis, suggesting that p16 expression could be a marker of hormone sensitivity (6).

Table 1 also includes a number of biomarkers that have been evaluated in only one of the studies (RTOG 86–10 or 92–02) but have not been confirmed.

In conclusion, these studies have shown a number of promising biomarkers that may significantly impact clinical practice in the future. However, at this time, none of them are ready to be used in routine clinical practice. A central issue has been the standardization of methods, including image analysis and selection of cut-points. Combining several of these promising biomarkers in a biologic model is a strategy currently being pursued in the RTOG, and initial preliminary evidence is encouraging.

■ NEW GENETIC MARKERS: *TMPRSS2-ETS* FUSION GENE

The observation that a significant proportion (40%–80%) of prostate cancer patients experience a chromosomal rearrangement that leads to the fusion of the androgen-responsive promoter of the *TMPRSS2* gene (21q22) to ETS transcription factors family members (ERG, ETV1, and ETV4) is one of the most important discoveries in prostate cancer research of the last decade (20,21). However, the prognostic role of these rearrangements remains controversial (22–26). Thus, it is unclear at this time whether this genetic marker could serve clinically as a prognostic marker. However, a potentially diagnostic application has been suggested in a recent study of 78 patients where TMPRSS2-ERG fusion transcripts were shown to be detectable in urine after DRE in prostate cancer patients, providing a sensitivity and specificity of 37% and 93%, respectively, in prostate cancer diagnoses (27). These same authors proved that combining this urine-based test along with PCA3 improved sensitivity to 73%. An independent group also showed that a multiplex biomarker in a urine-based approach including PCA3, TMPRSS2-ERG, GOLPH2, AMACR, ERG, SPINK1, and TFF3 had a sensitivity and specificity of 65.9% and 76%, respectively, suggesting that this approach could lead to a more accurate diagnostic test for prostate cancer (28).

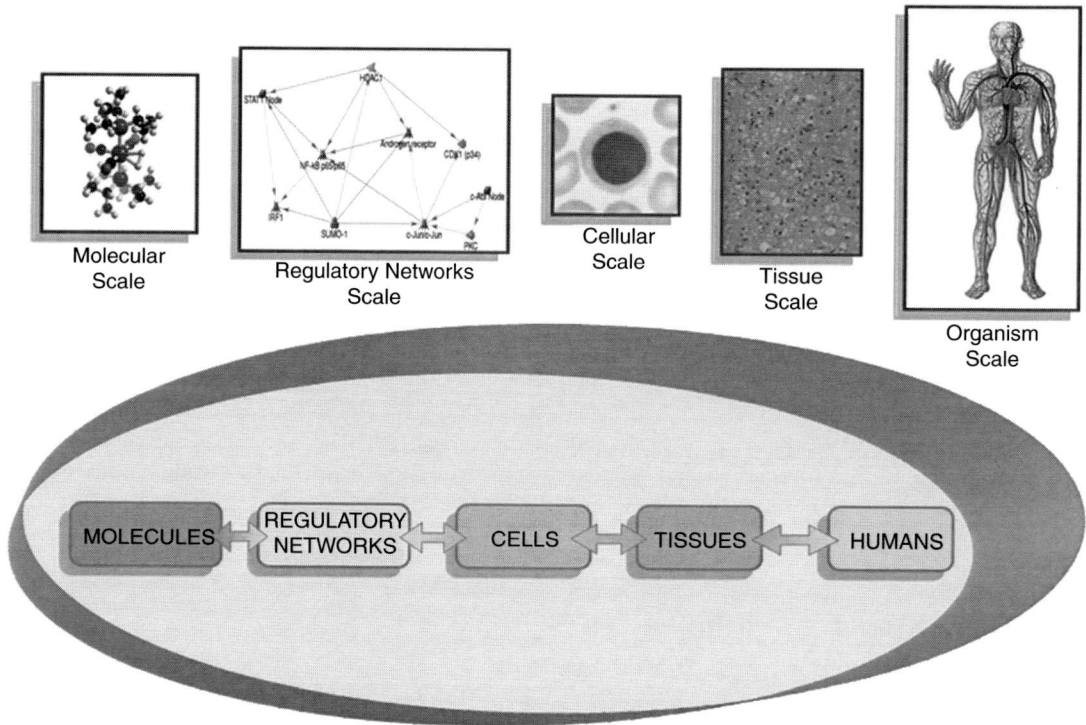

FIGURE 1   Systems biology approaches to modeling disease. Adapted from Ref. (40).

■ SYSTEMS BIOLOGY: A NOVEL APPROACH TO MODEL BIOLOGY AND DISEASE

The generation of high-throughput datasets in the "omics" era has provided an opportunity to address the identification of biomarkers from a different perspective. For example, gene expression signatures have been shown to be prognostic in cancer of the prostate, breast, lung, head and neck, and colon (29–35). In addition, these high-throughput technologies have been central to the development of a systems-view of complex biological systems (36,37). In systems biology, it is proposed that regulatory pathways be organized as complex interacting networks similar to the World Wide Web (36–39). Thus, a central concept in systems biology is that biological networks are multidimensional and highly complex, and thus strategies to elucidate central features of a biological system must incorporate information at multiple levels or scales. This contrasts with the single analyte approach that has been the main strategy pursued in biomarker development.

Figure 1 shows a systems biology approach to modeling disease. One important feature of systems

biology is that it integrates biological scales (molecular, regulatory network, cellular, tissue, and organism) when modeling disease, thus representing a more global approach to modeling. An advantage of systems modeling is that it may provide insights into the central function of a biological system by considering all the scales involved. A classic example to explain the advantages of systems modeling involves the respiratory system. In respiration, a person breathes (organism level) the lung exchanges gases (tissue level) but the type one pneumocyte (cellular level) does neither. This means that if we focused our study of the system to one of the most abundant components at the cellular level, we would probably miss its main function. Thus, integrating information from different biological scales is central to systems biology.

■ MATHEMATICAL MODELS: BRIDGING SCALES WITHIN BIOLOGY AND/OR DISEASE

A central feature of systems modeling is the application of mathematical models in bridging biological scales. Figure 2 shows a general experimental

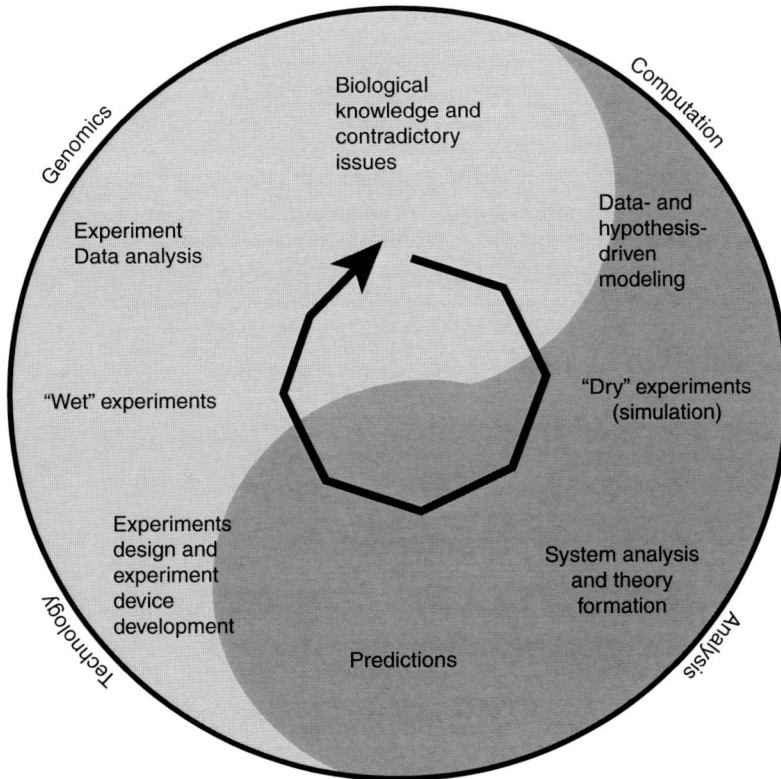

FIGURE 2 Experimental approaches to systems biology. Data and hypothesis-driven models are developed to explain a question of interest. The models can be used to simulate experiments (computationally based) and generate predictions. These predictions can then be tested in "wet" experiments. If the model is validated then it can be further mined for additional predictions, and if the model is not validated then alternative models may be pursued. Adapted from Ref. (39).

approach in systems modeling where "dry" models are developed in an effort to understand a question of interest (38). The model can be queried for predictions that can then be experimentally tested in "wet" experiments in the laboratory and/or clinic. This approach can lead to significant insights into biology and/or disease. Furthermore, mathematical modeling has played a central role in the development of central clinical concepts in radiation oncology. The linear quadratic model, even with its imperfections, has been key to the development of fractionation schemes in radiotherapy delivery, as well as understanding the concept of early and late responding tissues. Thus, mathematical modeling can lead to important mechanistic insights into biology and disease.

■ SYSTEMS PATHOLOGY

In recent work, Donovan et al. have proposed an integrated approach to advancing standard tissue-based pathology (41). They integrate information within multiple scales, including standard histopathology, molecular imaging data, and clinical history, to develop a prognostic model of clinical outcome in patients with prostate cancer. They have developed models to predict outcome after radical prostatectomy based on surgical specimen (42) as well as the results of diagnostic needle biopsies (41). The latter model has also been tested on 52 patients treated with RT, with results reported in abstract form (43).

The general approach to model development identifies potential clinicopathological, imaging and immunofluorescence features in an initial training set of patients. Individual features that are found most informative in predicting clinical outcomes are then combined in a comprehensive model which is then tested in a validating set from the same initial cohort but different from the training cohort. In their initial study, features were identified and the model was initially developed on a training set of 373 patients that included 33 patients that had experienced clinical failure. The features identified involved all three scales evaluated including AR levels (immunofluorescence), primary Gleason grade (clinicopathological), lymph node involvement (clinicopathological), and three quantitative characteristics from H&E staining (molecular imaging). The resulting model was then validated in 385 patients with encouraging results (Concordance Index: 0.84, sensitivity: 84%, and specificity: 85%) (42).

Since most treatment decisions are based on needle biopsies prior to definitive treatment, the same investigators utilized the same approach to develop a model based on tissue obtained at the time of diagnostic biopsy (44). This was performed in a cohort of 1,027 patients with cT1-T3 prostate cancer treated with radical prostatectomy. A model was developed in a training cohort of 686 patients that included 87 patients with clinical progression. Interestingly, the features selected in model development were different from what was used in the previous model, but once again all scales evaluated were represented by at least one feature. Model features in this approach included three: clinicopathological (preoperative PSA, Gleason score, and primary Gleason grade), immunofluorescence (AR dynamic range at low Gleason grade + total Ki-67 at high Gleason grade), and molecular imaging features (mean distance between epithelial tumor cells and isolated tumor epithelial cell area/total tumor area). The resulting model was then validated in 341 patients derived from the same cohort of 1,027 patients. Once again, results were encouraging, although inferior to the first model, based on the surgical specimen (Concordance Index: 0.73, sensitivity: 76%, and specificity: 73%).

In summary, this group shows that it is possible to develop comprehensive models to predict outcomes, that perform better than standard clinicopathological features. An important issue is that the analytical parameters of the features within the test are objective and not prone to inter/intraobserver variability. However, it could be argued that additional validation in additional datasets would be important before this test is advocated in routine practice, as the improvement over standard nomogram-based models is not large. In addition, a central therapeutic issue in prostate cancer is identifying patients that do not require treatment. However, this model is developed exclusively in patients that were treated with prostatectomy and thus it is

unclear whether their findings of a favorable outcome would apply in the setting of active surveillance. Finally, although the preliminary data of the model in RT-treated patients is interesting (44), it is unclear if the model is applicable to patients that choose RT as their definitive treatment.

■ SYSTEMS BIOLOGY APPROACHES TO RADIATION-SPECIFIC BIOMARKERS

It could be argued that most biomarkers that have been studied in RT-based clinical trials have not been developed specifically as markers of intrinsic radiosensitivity. For example, of those studied by RTOG, p53 and p16 are tumor suppressor proteins which regulate cell cycle (45,46), Ki-67 is a marker for cellular proliferation (47,48), and MDM2 is a negative regulator of p53 (49–51). Although their mechanistic role in radiation response has also been studied (52–56), these studies have been secondary to their primary biological function. In addition, the prognostic value of these biomarkers is not specific to RT. For example, Ki-67 has been shown to be prognostic in patients that undergo radical prostatectomy (57,58). However, when counseling patients, clinicians would be much better served if they had biomarkers that predicted outcomes specific to the treatment chosen.

A reasonable criticism of the biomarker development field in radiation oncology is the lack of a strategy in the discovery of novel biomarkers that are specific to intrinsic radiosensitivity. In an effort to fulfill this research goal, our group has developed a systems biology-based strategy for the discovery of radiation-specific biomarkers (59,60). In a radiation-specific approach, the biological strategy is focused on identifying biomarkers using cellular radiosensitivity as the main biological endpoint.

In recent studies, we identified a 10-gene network that we propose plays a central role in determining radiophenotype (Figure 3). The systems biology-based strategy used a biologically validated linear regression algorithm to identify genes that were associated with cellular radiosensitivity in a dataset of 48 cancer cell lines of mainly epithelial origin. A specific model was then developed to predict an index of cellular radiosensitivity based on the 10 genes identified. The radiosensitivity index (RSI) is modeled on the survival after 2 Gy (SF2) for the

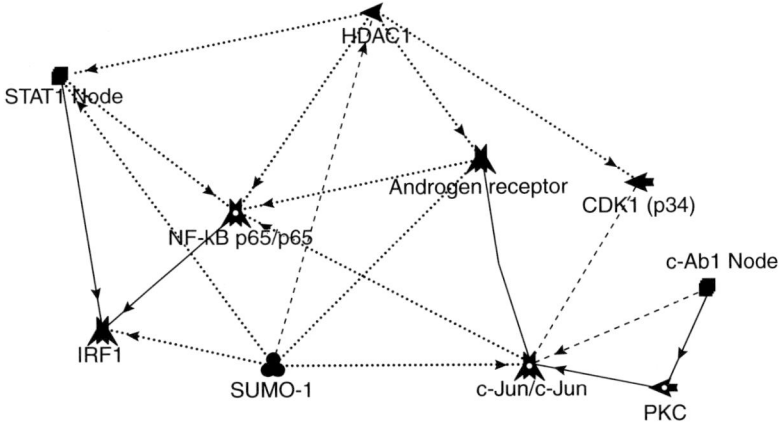

FIGURE 3 Radiosensitivity network hubs: 10 hubs were identified from an original analysis that had identified a 500-gene network. Known biological interactions were used to interconnect the network and hubs were identified as those having more than five connections within the network. A clinical assay to predict intrinsic radiosensitivity was developed based on gene expression of the 10 hubs. This test has been validated in three independent datasets totaling 118 patients with rectal, esophageal and head and neck cancer. Currently an NCI-sponsored clinical trial is underway to prospectively validate the radiosensitivity test.

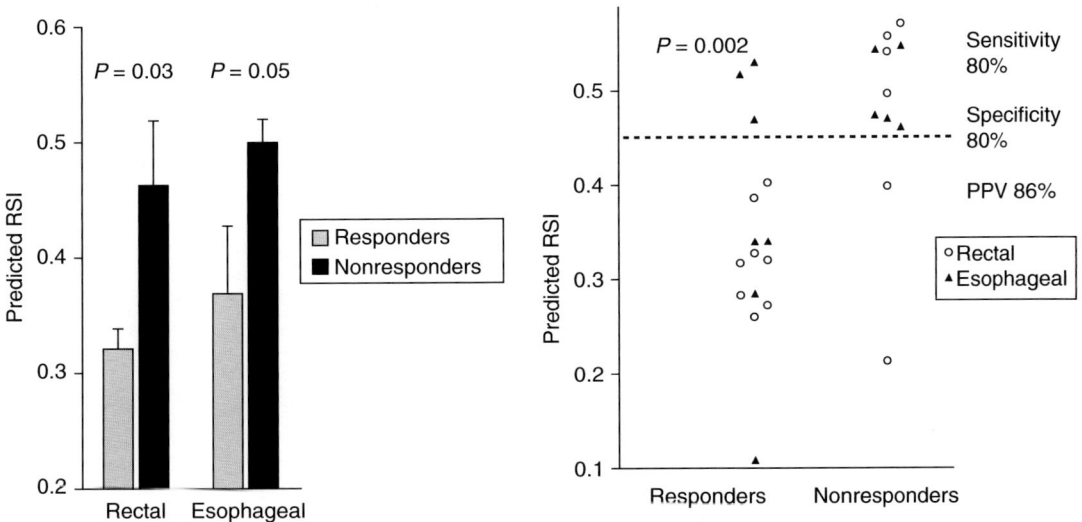

FIGURE 4 Radiosensitivity Index (RSI) is correlated with clinical response to concurrent radiochemotherapy in rectal and esophageal cancer patients. (Left) The mean predicted RSI of responders is significantly lower than in nonresponders in both clinical cohorts. (Right) Predicted RSI of each individual patients in the cohorts.

48 cell lines. This model was then tested as a predictor of clinical response to preoperative concurrent radiochemotherapy in two independent datasets of rectal and esophageal cancer patients. Responders in both datasets had a lower radiosensitivity index (radiosensitive) when compared to nonresponders (0.34 vs. 0.48, $P = .002$). An ROC analysis revealed a cut-point (RSI = 0.46) where the sensitivity, specificity, and positive predictive value are 80%, 82%, and 86%, respectively (Figure 4) (61).

Time to Locoregional Recurrence

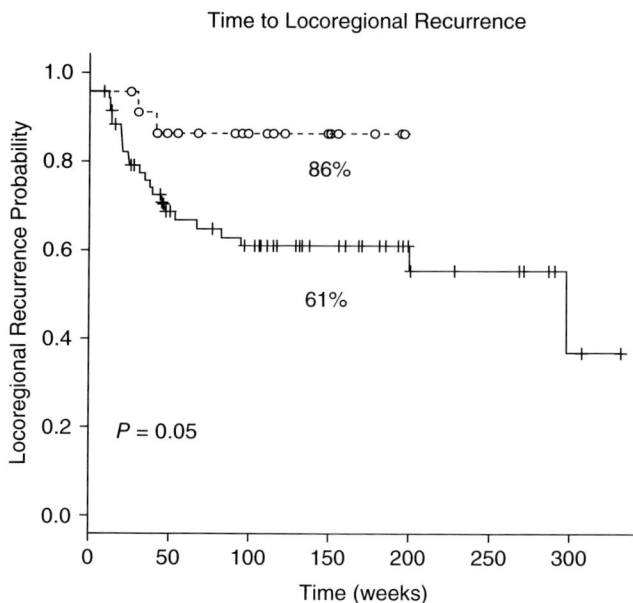

FIGURE 5 Radiosensitivity Index (RSI) distinguishes clinical populations with different disease-related outcomes in an HNC cohort of 92 patients treated with definitive concurrent radiochemotherapy. Using the 25th percentile (RSI < 0.023), there is a superior 2-year LRC in the predicted radiosensitive group (86% vs. 61%, P = .05).

We further tested the model in a dataset of 92 patients with locally advanced head and neck cancer that had been treated with concurrent radiochemotherapy. Tissue biopsies were frozen and gene expression was obtained using the NKI microarray. We generated RSIs for all patients in the dataset using the same model previously generated in cell lines and validated in rectal and esophageal cancer patients. Interestingly, the radiosensitive patients had an improved 2-year locoregional recurrence-free survival rate when compared to the radioresistant patients (2-year LRFS 86% vs. 61%, P = .05, Figure 5), also confirming the clinical validity of the gene expression model.

Although not yet tested in prostate cancer, the data above support the idea that developing biomarkers specifically for cellular radiosensitivity might provide an interesting approach to the development of predictive biomarkers that are associated with a specific therapeutic strategy. A central problem with prognostic biomarkers, as those described in the prior sections, is that they provide outcome risks that are independent of treatment. For example, risk classification using Gleason score, clinical stage, and pretreatment PSA predicts outcomes, regardless of received treatment. However, it is likely that there are patients that stand to benefit more from one definitive treatment than another. If the systems biology strategy described in this section is successful, it might possibly lead us to the identification of a specific subpopulation that derives a large therapeutic benefit from RT.

■ REFERENCES

1. American Cancer Society. *Cancer Facts and Figures 2010.* Atlanta, GA: American Cancer Society; 2010.
2. Bill-Axelson A, Holmberg L, Ruutu M, et al. Radical prostatectomy versus watchful waiting in early prostate cancer. *N Engl J Med.* 2005;352(19):1977–1984.
3. Grignon DJ, Caplan R, Sarkar FH, et al. p53 status and prognosis of locally advanced prostatic adenocarcinoma: a study based on RTOG 8610. *J Natl Cancer Inst.* 1997;89(2):158–165.
4. Che M, DeSilvio M, Pollack A, et al. Prognostic value of abnormal p53 expression in locally advanced prostate cancer treated with androgen deprivation and radiotherapy: a study based on RTOG 9202. *Int J Radiat Oncol Biol Phys.* 2007;69(4):1117–1123.
5. Chakravarti A, Heydon K, Wu CL, et al. Loss of p16 expression is of prognostic significance in locally advanced prostate cancer: an analysis from the Radiation Therapy Oncology Group protocol 86–10. *J Clin Oncol.* 2003;21(17):3328–3334.
6. Chakravarti A, DeSilvio M, Zhang M, et al. Prognostic value of p16 in locally advanced prostate cancer: a study based on Radiation Therapy Oncology Group Protocol 9202. *J Clin Oncol.* 2007;25(21):3082–3089.
7. Li R, Heydon K, Hammond ME, et al. Ki-67 staining index predicts distant metastasis and survival in locally advanced prostate cancer treated with radiotherapy: an analysis of patients in radiation therapy oncology

group protocol 86–10. *Clin Cancer Res.* 2004;10(12 Pt 1):4118–4124.

8. Pollack A, DeSilvio M, Khor LY, et al. Ki-67 staining is a strong predictor of distant metastasis and mortality for men with prostate cancer treated with radiotherapy plus androgen deprivation: Radiation Therapy Oncology Group Trial 92–02. *J Clin Oncol.* 2004;22(11):2133–2140.

9. Khor LY, Desilvio M, Al-Saleem T, et al. MDM2 as a predictor of prostate carcinoma outcome: an analysis of Radiation Therapy Oncology Group Protocol 8610. *Cancer.* 2005;104(5):962–967.

10. Khor LY, Bae K, Paulus R, et al. MDM2 and Ki-67 predict for distant metastasis and mortality in men treated with radiotherapy and androgen deprivation for prostate cancer: RTOG 92–02. *J Clin Oncol.* 2009;27(19):3177–3184.

11. Khor LY, Bae K, Al-Saleem T, et al. Protein kinase A RI-alpha predicts for prostate cancer outcome: analysis of radiation therapy oncology group trial 86–10. *Int J Radiat Oncol Biol Phys.* 2008;71(5):1309–1315.

12. Pollack A, Bae K, Khor LY, et al. The importance of protein kinase A in prostate cancer: relationship to patient outcome in Radiation Therapy Oncology Group trial 92–02. *Clin Cancer Res.* 2009;15(17):5478–5484.

13. Pollack A, Grignon DJ, Heydon KH, et al. Prostate cancer DNA ploidy and response to salvage hormone therapy after radiotherapy with or without short-term total androgen blockade: an analysis of RTOG 8610. *J Clin Oncol.* 2003;21(7):1238–1248.

14. Khor LY, Desilvio M, Li R, et al. Bcl-2 and bax expression and prostate cancer outcome in men treated with radiotherapy in Radiation Therapy Oncology Group protocol 86–10. *Int J Radiat Oncol Biol Phys.* 2006; 66(1):25–30.

15. Khor LY, Moughan J, Al-Saleem T, et al. Bcl-2 and Bax expression predict prostate cancer outcome in men treated with androgen deprivation and radiotherapy on radiation therapy oncology group protocol 92–02. *Clin Cancer Res.* 2007;13(12):3585–3590.

16. Abdel-Wahab M, Berkey BA, Krishan A, et al. Influence of number of CAG repeats on local control in the RTOG 86–10 protocol. *Am J Clin Oncol.* 2006;29(1):14–20.

17. Khor LY, Bae K, Pollack A, et al. COX-2 expression predicts prostate-cancer outcome: analysis of data from the RTOG 92–02 trial. *Lancet Oncol.* 2007;8(10):912–920.

18. Torres-Roca JF, DeSilvio M, Mora LB, et al. Activated STAT3 as a correlate of distant metastasis in prostate cancer: a secondary analysis of Radiation Therapy Oncology Group 86–10. *Urology.* 2007;69(3):505–509.

19. Roach M 3rd, De Silvio M, Rebbick T, et al. Racial differences in CYP3A4 genotype and survival among men treated on Radiation Therapy Oncology Group (RTOG) 9202: a phase III randomized trial. *Int J Radiat Oncol Biol Phys.* 2007;69(1):79–87.

20. Tomlins SA, Rhodes DR, Perner S, et al. Recurrent fusion of TMPRSS2 and ETS transcription factor genes in prostate cancer. *Science.* 2005;310(5748):644–648.

21. Tomlins SA, Mehra R, Rhodes DR, et al. TMPRSS2:ETV4 gene fusions define a third molecular subtype of prostate cancer. *Cancer Res.* 2006;66(7):3396–3400.

22. Demichelis F, Fall K, Perner S, et al. TMPRSS2:ERG gene fusion associated with lethal prostate cancer in a watchful waiting cohort. *Oncogene.* 2007;26(31):4596–4599.

23. Lotan TL, Toubaji A, Albadine R, et al. TMPRSS2-ERG gene fusions are infrequent in prostatic ductal adenocarcinomas. *Mod Pathol.* 2009;22(3):359–365.

24. Yoshimoto M, Joshua AM, Cunha IW, et al. Absence of TMPRSS2:ERG fusions and PTEN losses in prostate cancer is associated with a favorable outcome. *Mod Pathol.* 2008;21(12):1451–1460.

25. FitzGerald LM, Agalliu I, Johnson K, et al. Association of TMPRSS2-ERG gene fusion with clinical characteristics and outcomes: results from a population-based study of prostate cancer. *BMC Cancer.* 2008;8:230.

26. Saramäki OR, Harjula AE, Martikainen PM, Vessella RL, Tammela TL, Visakorpi T. TMPRSS2:ERG fusion identifies a subgroup of prostate cancers with a favorable prognosis. *Clin Cancer Res.* 2008;14(11):3395–3400.

27. Hessels D, Smit FP, Verhaegh GW, Witjes JA, Cornel EB, Schalken JA. Detection of TMPRSS2-ERG fusion transcripts and prostate cancer antigen 3 in urinary sediments may improve diagnosis of prostate cancer. *Clin Cancer Res.* 2007;13(17):5103–5108.

28. Laxman B, Morris DS, Yu J, et al. A first-generation multiplex biomarker analysis of urine for the early detection of prostate cancer. *Cancer Res.* 2008;68(3):645–649.

29. Nakagawa T, Kollmeyer TM, Morlan BW, et al. A tissue biomarker panel predicting systemic progression after PSA recurrence post-definitive prostate cancer therapy. *PLoS ONE.* 2008;3(5):e2318.

30. Varambally S, Yu J, Laxman B, et al. Integrative genomic and proteomic analysis of prostate cancer reveals signatures of metastatic progression. *Cancer Cell.* 2005;8(5):393–406.

31. Glinsky GV, Glinskii AB, Stephenson AJ, Hoffman RM, Gerald WL. Gene expression profiling predicts clinical outcome of prostate cancer. *J Clin Invest.* 2004;113(6):913–923.

32. van't Veer LJ, Dai H, van de Vijver MJ, et al. Gene expression profiling predicts clinical outcome of breast cancer. *Nature.* 2002;415(6871):530–536.

33. Beer DG, Kardia SL, Huang CC, et al. Gene-expression profiles predict survival of patients with lung adenocarcinoma. *Nat Med.* 2002;8(8):816–824.

34. Chung CH, Parker JS, Karaca G, et al. Molecular classification of head and neck squamous cell carcinomas using patterns of gene expression. *Cancer Cell.* 2004;5(5):489–500.

35. Eschrich S, Yang I, Bloom G, et al. Molecular staging for survival prediction of colorectal cancer patients. *J Clin Oncol.* 2005;23(15):3526–3535.

36. Hood L, Heath JR, Phelps ME, Lin B. Systems biology and new technologies enable predictive and preventative medicine. *Science.* 2004;306(5696):640–643.

37. Hood L, Perlmutter RM. The impact of systems approaches on biological problems in drug discovery. *Nat Biotechnol.* 2004;22(10):1215–1217.

38. Kitano H. Computational systems biology. *Nature.* 2002;420(6912):206–210.

39. Kitano H. Systems biology: a brief overview. *Science.* 2002;295(5560):1662–1664.

40. Butcher EC, Berg EL, Kunkel EJ. Systems biology in drug discovery. *Nat Biotechnol.* 2004;22(10):1253–1259.

41. Donovan MJ, Costa J, Cordon-Cardo C. Systems pathology: a paradigm shift in the practice of diagnostic and predictive pathology. *Cancer.* 2009;115(13 suppl):3078–3084.

42. Donovan MJ, Hamann S, Clayton M, et al. Systems pathology approach for the prediction of prostate cancer progression after radical prostatectomy. *J Clin Oncol.* 2008;26(24):3923–3929.

43. Donovan MJ, Khan FM, Fernandez G, Bayer-Zubek V, Albertsen P. *A Pre-treatment Systems Pathology Model Predicts the Likelihood of Disease Progression in Patients Treated With Primary Radiotherapy.* ASCO. Chicago, IL; 2010.

44. Donovan MJ, Khan FM, Fernandez G, et al. Personalized prediction of tumor response and cancer progression on prostate needle biopsy. *J Urol.* 2009;182(1):125–132.

45. Kirsch DG, Kastan MB. Tumor-suppressor p53: implications for tumor development and prognosis. *J Clin Oncol.* 1998;16(9):3158–3168.

46. Nevins JR. The Rb/E2F pathway and cancer. *Hum Mol Genet.* 2001;10(7):699–703.

47. Scott RJ, Hall PA, Haldane JS, et al. A comparison of immunohistochemical markers of cell proliferation with experimentally determined growth fraction. *J Pathol.* 1991;165(2):173–178.

48. Cher ML, Chew K, Rosenau W, Carroll PR. Cellular proliferation in prostatic adenocarcinoma as assessed by bromodeoxyuridine uptake and Ki-67 and PCNA expression. *Prostate.* 1995;26(2):87–93.

49. Momand J, Zambetti GP, Olson DC, George D, Levine AJ. The mdm-2 oncogene product forms a complex with the p53 protein and inhibits p53-mediated transactivation. *Cell.* 1992;69(7):1237–1245.

50. Oliner JD, Pietenpol JA, Thiagalingam S, Gyuris J, Kinzler KW, Vogelstein B. Oncoprotein MDM2 conceals the activation domain of tumour suppressor p53. *Nature.* 1993;362(6423):857–860.

51. Chen J, Marechal V, Levine AJ. Mapping of the p53 and mdm-2 interaction domains. *Mol Cell Biol.* 1993;13(7):4107–4114.

52. Gudkov AV, Komarova EA. The role of p53 in determining sensitivity to radiotherapy. *Nat Rev Cancer.* 2003;3(2):117–129.

53. El-Deiry WS. The role of p53 in chemosensitivity and radiosensitivity. *Oncogene.* 2003;22(47):7486–7495.

54. Cuddihy AR, Bristow RG. The p53 protein family and radiation sensitivity: Yes or no? *Cancer Metastasis Rev.* 2004;23(3–4):237–257.

55. Mu Z, Hachem P, Agrawal S, Pollack A. Antisense MDM2 sensitizes prostate cancer cells to androgen deprivation, radiation, and the combination. *Int J Radiat Oncol Biol Phys.* 2004;58(2):336–343.

56. Stoyanova R, Hachem P, Hensley H, et al. Antisense-MDM2 sensitizes LNCaP prostate cancer cells to androgen deprivation, radiation, and the combination in vivo. *Int J Radiat Oncol Biol Phys.* 2007;68(4):1151–1160.

57. Laitinen S, Martikainen PM, Tolonen T, Isola J, Tammela TL, Visakorpi T. EZH2, Ki-67 and MCM7 are prognostic markers in prostatectomy treated patients. *Int J Cancer.* 2008;122(3):595–602.

58. Rubio J, Ramos D, López-Guerrero JA, et al. Immunohistochemical expression of Ki-67 antigen, cox-2 and Bax/Bcl-2 in prostate cancer; prognostic value in biopsies and radical prostatectomy specimens. *Eur Urol.* 2005;48(5):745–751.

59. Torres-Roca JF, Eschrich S, Zhao H, et al. Prediction of radiation sensitivity using a gene expression classifier. *Cancer Res.* 2005;65(16):7169–7176.

60. Eschrich S, Zhang H, Zhao H, et al. Systems biology modeling of the radiation sensitivity network: a biomarker discovery platform. *Int J Radiat Oncol Biol Phys.* 2009;75(2):497–505.

61. Eschrich SA, Pramana J, Zhang H, et al. A gene expression model of intrinsic tumor radiosensitivity: prediction of response and prognosis after chemoradiation. *Int J Radiat Oncol Biol Phys.* 2009;75(2):489–496.

Risk Stratification in Nonmetastatic Prostate Cancer: Implications for Treatment

Richard E. Peschel*

Yale University School of Medicine, New Haven, CT

■ ABSTRACT

A simple classification system using three clinical parameters—clinical T stage, prostate-specific antigen levels, and Gleason score—can be used to define favorable group (FG), intermediate group (IG), and poor group (PG) prostate cancer patients. This classification system defines reproducible clinical outcomes following treatment and can be used to select radiation treatment programs based on a simple use of intensity-modulated radiation therapy principles with (IG and PG) or without hormones (FG). Overall biochemical disease-free survival using these radiation therapy programs is similar or better than surgery.

Keywords: prostate cancer, risk stratification, intensity-modulated radiation therapy

■ INTRODUCTION

In the past decade, enormous progress has been made in the treatment of localized, nonmetastatic prostate cancer. This progress includes new radiation therapy treatment programs such as intensity-modulated radiation therapy (IMRT) and image-guided IMRT (IG-IMRT) (1–3). Scientific prospective randomized clinical trials that prove the efficacy of dose escalation techniques and demonstrate the proper use of hormone therapy with external beam radiation therapy have been completed (1). New surgical techniques such as robotics assisted prostatectomy (da Vinci robotic interface) have dramatically changed the surgical environment as well (4). Along with these innovative new treatment programs, has been the development of a new patient clinical classification system that more clearly defines the prognostic and treatment programs for early prostate cancer. Although many different types of histological tumors can originate in the prostate (small cell, lymphoma, squamous cell, etc.), I shall confine my remarks to the overwhelmingly most important histology: adenocarcinoma (5,6). The grade of an adenocarcinoma involving the prostate is a crucial clinical component and is given by the Gleason score (GS) 2–10 (6). GS 2 is a very low-grade and well-differentiated cancer of the prostate, and GS 10 is a very poorly differentiated and high-grade tumor. In general, the higher the GS, the more aggressive the prostate cancer is, with a worse prognosis (6). The new clinical classification system is now based on the clinical T stage,

*Corresponding author, Department of Therapeutic Radiology, Yale University School of Medicine, PO Box 208040, New Haven, CT 06520

E-mail address: Richard.peschel@yale.edu

Radiation Medicine Rounds 2:1 (2011) 11–16.
DOI: 10.5003/2151–4208.2.1.11

the prostate-specific antigen (PSA—all values are in nanograms per milliliter), and the GS and can be used to define different categories of patients, thus replacing the traditional TNM staging system. One example of a traditional TNM staging system is reviewed in Table 1 (5). Although the TNM staging systems have historically been useful in prostate cancer patients, over the last few decades—due to PSA screening and new urological technology—there has been a tremendous stage migration, such that most prostate cancer patients now are diagnosed with TNM stage I or II disease, and the traditional TNM staging system does not adequately stratify

these early stage patients in order to predict prognosis or to specify treatment programs (7). The newer classification system based on T stage, PSA, and GS is more accurate and much more useful in defining treatment of local prostate cancer. This classification system includes a favorable group (FG), an intermediate group (IG), and a poor-risk group (PG) (1,2). The FG, IG, and PG classification system is used almost universally to publish treatment results and to define radiation therapy treatment programs for individual patients (1,2). The FG, IG, and PG classification system based on clinical variables is defined in Table 2. In general, the 5-year biochemical disease-free

TABLE 1   Summary of TNM staging system

Primary tumor	
T1	Clinically undetectable tumor; not palpable or visible by imaging
T1a	Incidental histological tumor in 5% or less of resected tissue
T1b	Incidental histological tumor in more than 5% of resected tissue
T1c	Tumor identified by needle biopsy, e.g., because of a high PSA level
T2	Tumor confine to the prostate
T2a	Tumor involving one-half of one lobe or less
T2b	Tumor involving more than one-half of one lobe but not both lobes
T2c	Tumor involves both lobes
T3	Tumor extending through the prostatic capsule
T4	Tumor fixed or invading adjacent structures
Regional lymph nodes	
NX	Regional nodes cannot be assessed
N0	No regional node metastasis
N1	Regional node metastatic disease
Distant metastasis	
M0	No distant metastatic disease
M1	Distant metastatic disease
Stage groups	
Stage I	T1a N0 M0, grade 1
Stage II	T1a N0 M0, grade 2,3,4
	T1b N0 M0, any grade
	T1c N0 M0, any grade
	T2 N0 M0, any grade
Stage III	T3 N0 M0, any grade
Stage IV	T4 N0 M0, any grade
	Any T N1 M0, any grade
	Any T any N M1, any grade

From Ref. (5)

TABLE 2 Clinical classification system for local prostate cancer

FG (favorable group)	PSA < 10, Gleason score < 7, clinical T1 or T2 disease
IG (intermediate group)	Any one parameter increased compared to FG (e.g., PSA = 20 or Gleason score > 7 or clinical T3 disease
PG (poor group)	Any two parameters increased compared to FG (e.g., clinical T3 disease and PSA = 20; or PSA = 20 and Gleason score 8

TABLE 3 Five-year biochemical disease-free (bNED) survival by clinical prognostic group following treatment

Clinical Group	5-Year bNED Survival
FG	90%
IG	70%–80%
PG	40%–60%

From Ref. (1).

(bNED) survival rates are amazingly similar for surgery, implant or IMRT in cases of FG, IG, and PG prostate cancer (1,2). The 5-year bNED survival rates for treated patients, separated by prognostic group, are summarized in Table 3.

■ TREATMENT PROGRAMS

In addition to providing consistent clinical outcome data, the FG, IG, and PG clinical classification system allows for easy and clear treatment policies for each individual patient. At Yale Medical School, we have treated thousands of prostate cancer patients with a variety of treatment programs including nonconformal external beam radiation therapy, implant therapy, IMRT, and IG-IMRT with and without hormone therapy. Based on our complication data (discussed below), we have uniformly adopted IMRT and IG-IMRT as our treatments of choice. We also base our treatment policies on the numerous scientific prospective randomized studies proving the efficacy of external beam radiation therapy with or without hormones, completed over the last decade (1). Our treatment policy using IMRT has been described previously in great detail (2). Briefly, a tumor volume is defined by the attending physician and drawn on a CT scan of the pelvis. A planning tumor volume is then defined as the tumor volume plus a margin around the tumor volume. A

total dose of 7,560 cGy at 180 cGy per fraction is specified to the planning tumor volume. An optimization software package plans the treatment (inverse treatment planning) using multiple beams with the shape and intensity modified for each beam but with very specific safety guidelines for the rectum and bladder, that must be adhered to. For example, for the rectum: 1) the D25 (dose allowed for 25% of the rectal volume) is always confined to 7,000 cGy or less, 2) the 50% isodose line cannot cover the entire rectum, and 3) the 90% isodose line can only cover up to 50% of the rectum's width on a slice by slice CT inspection of the entire rectum. For the bladder, D25 must be <6,500 cGy, and 40% of the bladder volume must be treated with <5,000 cGy. In general, only the base of the seminal vesicles are included in the tumor volume when using IMRT for FG, IG, and PG patients. Each IMRT plan for every patient is reviewed by the attending physician. Using these rectal, bladder, and seminal vesicle constraints, we have very low acute and long-term complication rates as discussed below, despite treating the planning tumor volume with 7,560 cGy or higher. Using these general IMRT principles, our treatment policies are as follows (1,2):

For FG, we use IMRT alone at 7,560 cGy. We do not routinely use hormone therapy along with IMRT for FG patients. A short course (6 months) of hormone therapy is sometimes used for patients with enlarged prostates due to benign prostatic hypertrophy or patients with severe urinary symptoms, in order to "down size" the prostate, prior to IMRT. Clearly, not all FG patients need to be treated. Observation is appropriate for patients with very low GS or multiple comorbidities, whose life expectancy is <10 years (1).

For IG, we use 6 months of hormone therapy (Lupron) and IMRT (1,2). All of the IG patients are offered therapy since these patients have a significant cause-specific mortality due to prostate cancer (1).

For PG patients, we use long-term hormone therapy (Lupron) for 1 to 2 years plus IMRT to the prostate (1,2). For patients with a particularly high risk of pelvic lymph node disease, we sometimes use whole pelvic radiation therapy at 4,500 cGy at 180 cGy per fraction followed by an IMRT boost to the prostate at 7,560 cGy. In general, we find only a slight increase in acute toxicity using whole pelvic radiation therapy plus an IMRT boost, compared with local IMRT alone, and no increase in long-term gastro-intestinal or genito-urinary complications (8). All PG patients are offered treatment over observation because the cause-specific mortality of these patients is significant. Using these simple treatment policies, our 5-year bNED survival rates are the same or superior to surgery (2). In particular, for the PG patients, our 5-year bNED survival rate is 62% with IMRT, compared with 38% for surgery alone (2). A summary of our results using IMRT versus surgery is given in Table 4.

Because of multiple side effects that can occur using hormone therapy (cardiac disease, anemia, osteoporosis, diabetes, and metabolic disorders), one must observe caution when using hormone therapy for patients over 50 years of age with active comorbid diseases, and a careful medical history must be an important part of the complete medical history when evaluating patients for IMRT with hormones (9,10). Communication with the patient's primary care physician or cardiologist can be critical.

Other radiation treatment programs can be used to treat localized cases of prostate cancer. For example, we have used implant therapy using iodine-125 or palladium-103 for FG, IG, and PG patients with good bNED survival and low complication rates (11). Implant therapy is a good approach, however, our decision to recommend IMRT is based on our complication data, as discussed later, and on the superior scientific data supporting external beam radiation therapy over other treatment methods (1).

TABLE 4   Five-year bNED survival for IMRT versus surgery at Yale by clinical treatment group

Clinical Group	IMRT (%)	Surgery (%)	P
FG	85.3	92.8	P = 0.2
IG	82.2	86.7	P = 0.46
PG	62.2	38.4	P < 0.001

From Ref. (2).

■ COMPLICATIONS

Our basic treatment recommendations have evolved over time. Our current policies are based on long-term complication data that we have published, on over 1,500 prostate cancer patients, treated for over 30 years, and is summarized in Table 5 (11–14). We define long-term complications as occurring for 6 months or more following radiation and we define grade 3 complications, or higher, as those complications that affect the quality of life. A review of Table 5 shows a dramatic decrease in overall complication rates and a reduction in the complications that affect quality of life using IMRT treatment versus any other radiation treatment modality used at Yale for prostate cancer since 1974. In addition, the acute complication rates with IMRT are very low. This is due to the careful planning of the treatment and the dose restrictions we use for the bladder, rectum and seminal vesicles, as discussed earlier.

■ TREATMENT OF RECURRENT DISEASE

A review of Table 4 indicates that most patients remain free of recurrence following IMRT. For those patients that have a PSA recurrence, careful follow-up is indicated and treatment is usually not necessary immediately since these patients are asymptomatic and have only a rising PSA. Treatment is indicated, usually with hormone therapy, only if the PSA doubling time is <1 year or the patient displays symptoms secondary to prostate cancer, or a positive bone scan or CT scan suggesting progressive clinical disease. Repeated IMRT is not suggested, although local radiation therapy can be given for painful boney metastatic disease.

■ OTHER IMPORTANT CLINICAL PARAMETERS

Age

It has been common practice in the United States to refer younger patients (<60 years) with localized prostate cancer for surgery rather than for radiation therapy (14,15). Such policy is based largely on opinion, theory, and the lay press (16), without much scientific data to support this approach. The

TABLE 5 Long-term radiation therapy complication rates using various treatments for local prostate cancer: a review of over 1,500 patients treated from 1974 to 2009

Treatment Program	Grade 2 (%)	Grade 3 (%)	Grade 4 (%)	Grade 5 (%)	Total (%)
IMRT 1998–2009 N = 700+	0.4	0.8	0.0	0.0	1.2
Implant (11,12) N = 325	4.1	2.8	1.0	0.0	7.9
PD-103 implant 1996–2005	2.0	1.0	1.0	0.0	4
I-125 implant 1992–1998	8.0	6.0	1.0	0.0	15
Nonconformal (13) EB 1974–1998 N = 340	NA	10.2	2.4	0.3	>12.9
Sup-implant (13) 1974–1984 N = 141	NA	8.5	1.4	0.0	>9.9

Key: EB, external beam radiation therapy; implant, transperineal, ultrasound guided prostate implant (I-125, iodine-125 or PD-103, palladium-103); IMRT, intensity modulated radiation therapy; N, number of patients treated; NA, not available; sup-implant, supra-pubic, open I-125 prostate implant.

Grade 2 = rectal or bladder complication that does not affect quality of life.

Grade 3 = rectal or bladder complication that requires treatment or minor surgery that affects quality of life.

Grade 4 = rectal or bladder complication that requires major surgery (colostomy, bladder diversion) and dramatically affects quality of life.

Grade 5 = lethal complication.

radiation therapy literature supports the conclusion that a younger patient population could be referred for radiation therapy and a young age is not an absolute contraindicator for referral to a radiation therapist (2,14,15).

Race

There are reports in the literature that document African Americans with early prostate cancer having an inferior disease-free survival rate when compared with non-Latino white patients, following surgery (17). A similar trend is not seen in IMRT patients and, race is not a contraindicator for IMRT (2).

■ FUTURE DIRECTIONS

We are now using IG-IMRT for dose escalation in all FG, IG, and PG patients. IG-IMRT allows for corrections in daily prostate motions and allows one to use smaller margins around the tumor volume to plan the IMRT treatment. We are using two different systems for IG-IMRT: 1) a Varian Trilogy accelerator that takes a CT scan of the prostate every day and can correct for daily prostate motion and 2) a calypso radiofrequency seed emitter system that can detect prostate motion between treatments and during IMRT (18,19). We have used both of these IG-IMRT systems for dose escalations to a total dose of 7,920 cGy, on over 300 prostate cancer patients. We use hormones for IG and PG patients, as well as IG-IMRT. IG-IMRT is used only by itself for FG patients. Thus far, we have seen no increase in the acute or chronic complication rates, using the same restrictions for the rectum, bladder and seminal vesicles as discussed above. We intend to escalate to a higher dosage but longer follow-up is necessary to determine if these higher doses translate into improved bNED survival rates with similarly low complication rates.

■ SUMMARY

A simple clinical stratification system using three clinical parameters (clinical T stage, PSA, and GS) can be used to define FG, IG, and PG patients. This classification system defines reproducible clinical outcomes following treatment and can be used to select radiation treatment policy based on a simple use of IMRT or IG-IMRT principles, with (IG and PG) or without hormones (FG). Overall, bNED survival with this policy is similar or better than surgery. Complication rates are low. Future dose escalation trials using IG-IMRT are underway.

Finally, it is important to acknowledge that the most recent update (2010) of the American Joint Committee on Cancer (AJCC) TNM staging system now includes arranging the clinical T stage, PSA, and GS into a stratification system that closely parallels the FG, IG, and PG system (20). All prostate cancer patients should be officially staged according to the newest 2010 AJCC TNM staging system.

■ REFERENCES

1. Peschel RE, Colberg JW. Surgery, brachytherapy, and external-beam radiotherapy for early prostate cancer. *Lancet Oncol.* 2003;4(4):233–241.
2. Aizer AA, Yu JB, Colberg JW, McKeon AM, Decker RH, Peschel RE. Radical prostatectomy vs. intensity-modulated radiation therapy in the management of localized prostate adenocarcinoma. *Radiother Oncol.* 2009;93(2):185–191.
3. Pawlowski JM, Yang ES, Malcolm AW, Coffey CW, Ding GX. Reduction of dose delivered to organs at risk in prostate cancer patients via image-guided radiation therapy. *Int J Radiat Oncol Biol Phys.* 2010;76(3):924–934.
4. Akduman B, Barqawi AB, Crawford ED. Minimally invasive surgery in prostate cancer: current and future perspectives. *Cancer J.* 2005;11(5):355–361.
5. Greene FL, Page DL, Fleming ID, Fritz AG, Balch CM, Haller DG, Moorow M, eds. *AJCC Cancer Staging Handbook.* 6th ed. New York: Springer; 2002:337–345.
6. Bostwick DG, Pathology of prostate cancer. In: Ernstoff MS, Heaney JA, Peschel RE, eds. *Prostate Cancer.* Cambridge and Oxford: Blackwell Science, Inc. 1998:15–41.
7. Han M, Partin AW, Piantadosi S, Epstein JI, Walsh PC. Era specific biochemical recurrence-free survival following radical prostatectomy for clinically localized prostate cancer. *J Urol.* 2001;166(2):416–419.
8. Aizer AA, Yu JB, McKeon AM, Decker RH, Colberg JW, Peschel RE. Whole pelvic radiotherapy versus prostate only radiotherapy in the management of locally advanced or aggressive prostate adenocarcinoma. *Int J Radiat Oncol Biol Phys.* 2009;75(5):1344–1349.
9. D'Amico AV, Manola J, Loffredo M, Renshaw AA, DellaCroce A, Kantoff PW. 6-month androgen suppression plus radiation therapy vs radiation therapy alone for patients with clinically localized prostate cancer: a randomized controlled trial. *JAMA.* 2004;292(7):821–827.
10. Kintzel PE, Chase SL, Schultz LM, O'Rourke TJ. Increased risk of metabolic syndrome, diabetes mellitus, and cardiovascular disease in men receiving androgen deprivation therapy for prostate cancer. *Pharmacotherapy.* 2008;28(12):1511–1522.
11. Colberg JW, Decker RH, Khan AM, McKeon A, Wilson LD, Peschel RE. Surgery versus implant for early prostate cancer: results from a single institution, 1992–2005. *Cancer J.* 2007;13(4):229–232.
12. Peschel RE. Prostate implant therapy: iodine-125 versus palladium-103. *Cancer J.* 2005;11(5):383–384.
13. Morton JD, Peschel RE. A detailed analysis of the chronic complications from iodine-125 implant versus external beam irradiation for prostate cancer. *Endocurietherapy/Hyperthermia Oncology.* 1988;4:113–119.
14. Peschel RE, Khan A, Colberg J, Wilson LD. The effect of age on prostate implantation results. *Cancer J.* 2006;12(4):305–308.
15. Burri RJ, Ho AY, Forsythe K, Cesaretti JA, Stone NN, Stock RG. Young men have equivalent biochemical outcomes compared with older men after treatment with brachytherapy for prostate cancer. *Int J Radiat Oncol Biol Phys.* 2010;77(5):1315–1321.
16. Beck M. Weighing options. *The Wall Street Journal.* 2009:B9
17. Latini DM, Elkin EP, Cooperberg MR, Sadetsky N, Duchane J, Carroll PR. Differences in clinical characteristics and disease-free survival for Latino, African American, and non-Latino white men with localized prostate cancer: data from CaPSURE. *Cancer.* 2006;106(4):789–795.
18. Willoughby TR, Kupelian PA, Pouliot J, et al. Target localization and real-time tracking using the Calypso 4D localization system in patients with localized prostate cancer. *Int J Radiat Oncol Biol Phys.* 2006;65(2):528–534.
19. Budiharto T, Haustermans K, Kovacs G. External beam radiotherapy for prostate cancer. *J Endourol.* 2010;24(5):781–789.
20. Edge SB, Byrd PR, Compton CC, Fritz AG, Trotti AD, eds. *AJCC Cancer Staging Manual.* 7th ed. New York, Dordrecht, Heidelberg, London: Springer; 2010:457–464.

Treatment of Favorable-Risk Prostate Cancer

Patrick Kupelian*

UCLA Health System, Los Angeles, CA

■ ABSTRACT

Favorable-risk prostate cancer patients have a multitude of management options to choose from. This chapter focuses on the radiotherapy options, including a variety of external beam radiotherapy or brachytherapy-based techniques. The high cure rates achieved with favorable-risk prostate cancers have to be balanced with the toxicity and inconvenience associated with with these approaches.

Keywords: favorable-risk prostate cancer, radiotherapy, brachytherapy, dose escalation, hypofractionation

■ INTRODUCTION

Prostate cancer is diagnosed in about 190,000 men in the US each year and is the most common cancer diagnosed in men and the second cause of cancer death among men. In the current era, ushered by PSA (prostate-specific antigen) screening in the late 1980s, the majority of patients diagnosed with prostate cancer fall in the favorable-risk group. Favorable-risk prostate cancer, whichever way defined, is characterized by a low potential of progression, few events occurring within the first 15 years after diagnosis, and a low mortality from prostate cancer as the cause of death. Therefore, although facing an overall positive outlook, patients with favorable-risk prostate cancer present a significant management challenge. The most obvious challenge in evaluating different management options is the long timeframe of progression of the majority of prostate cancers, which makes such evaluation often impractical. Given the long natural history of favorable prostate cancer, identifying patients who might not need treatment at all is an imperfect science at this stage, with an ongoing controversy about how to define "insignificant" or "indolent" prostate cancer (1–4). With favorable-risk prostate cancer patients, the disease is typically of small volume and localized to the prostate gland, making a multitude of local modalities as possible options for treatment. Each approach has its champions and advocates amongst researchers, physicians, and patients. In addition, the current cultural, social, and societal pressures of dealing with a disease with such high prevalence make favorable prostate cancer a model of management confusion. This environment renders direct comparisons of different modalities difficult through randomized controlled studies, which are extremely unlikely to demonstrate clinically significant differences between the currently available treatment options within 10 to 15 years (5–7). An important focus, however, should be on ensuring that the best treatment technique is applied for the treatment of an individual patient.

*Corresponding author, Department of Radiation Oncology, UCLA Health System, 200 UCLA Medical Plaza, Ste B265, Los Angeles, CA 90095

E-mail address: pkupelian@mednet.ucla.edu

Radiation Medicine Rounds 2:1 (2011) 17–26.
DOI: 10.5003/2151–4208.2.1.17

■ A DISEASE OF OPTIONS

The spectrum of management options spans active surveillance, hormonal therapy, cryotherapy, high-intensity-focused ultrasound, surgical removal (with multiple surgical techniques), and radiotherapy (with multiple options). This current review concentrates on radiation therapy. The radiotherapeutic options are either implant based (brachytherapy) or external. At this stage, either low-dose- or high-dose-rate brachytherapy options involve relatively mature techniques, whereas external radiotherapy options are still evolving at the level of definition of treatment volumes, treatment schedules (e.g., fractionation), and treatment techniques (e.g., intensity modulation, image guidance).

This review will concentrate on the radiotherapeutic options (brachytherapy and external beam radiotherapy) used in the management of favorable-risk localized prostate cancers. Given that most brachytherapy techniques for favorable-risk prostate cancer are relatively mature, the focus will mostly be on the developments in external beam radiotherapy.

■ DEFINITION OF FAVORABLE RISK

The most important prognosticators of outcome for localized prostate cancer are still defined by clinical stage, pretreatment PSA, and biopsy Gleason score (8). The risk categorization for individual patients has been mostly dependent on these three parameters. The use of nomograms, with a number of other parameters included in the risk assessment, refines the quantification of recurrence risk in different clinical settings. Although imperfect in many ways, risk categorization on the basis of clinical stage, pretreatment PSA, and biopsy Gleason score has remained widely used and has remarkably remained unchanged throughout the PSA era. Favorable-risk prostate cancer is typically defined as clinical stage T1 or T2A, pretreatment PSA 10 ng/mL or less, and a biopsy Gleason score of 6 or less.

■ BRACHYTHERAPY

Brachytherapy is currently performed for favorable-risk prostate cancers either with low-dose-rate permanent seed implants or with high-dose-rate temporary implants. Low-dose-rate brachytherapy is performed with either iodine, palladium, or cesium sources. High-dose-rate brachytherapy is performed with iridium sources.

Patient eligibility: In addition to operative risk, significant pre-existing obstructive uropathy and poor anatomy (large prostate, large median lobe, and large TURP defects) are the most relevant exclusion criteria for brachytherapy.

Brachytherapy—Low-Dose Rate

Technique: Brachytherapy with permanently implanted radioactive seeds matured in the early 1990s into a transperineal ultrasound-guided technique. The seeds are typically peripherally loaded, deployed through either preloaded needles or a Mick applicator. A total of 140 to 160 Gy is typically delivered with an iodine implant, and 110 to 125 Gy with a palladium implant. The typical prescribed dose with cesium is 115 Gy. The recent technical developments have mostly focused on the ability to perform delivery planning or delivery adjustments immediately preoperatively or intraoperatively, mostly to accommodate potential anatomical variations between the time of planning and the time of actual implantation. These modifications have improved the predictability and reproducibility of radioactive seed placements and consequent dosimetric results. Postoperative evaluation of the implant dosimetry is crucial to document quality of individual implants (9,10). The most commonly used metric to assess adequate target coverage is the prostate D90 (minimum dose received by 90% of the target volume as delineated on the postimplant CT) and/or the V100 (% of the target volume delineated on the postimplant CT receiving 100% of the prescribed dose). Particular attention has been paid to limiting urethral and rectal doses. Urethral doses are preferred to remain less than 150% of the prescribed dose. The R100 (the volume of the rectum receiving 100% of the prescription dose) is the metric utilized to assess rectal doses. Future refinements might include increased automation of needle placement and seed deployment, in addition to intraoperative real-time dosimetric evaluations (11–13). Overall, although the technique is relatively mature, significant variability in the quality of implants is seen dependent on the experience of individual brachytherapy teams (14,15).

Results: For favorable-risk prostate cancers, monotherapy with radioactive seeds alone has provided excellent control rates. Long-term results show bio-chemical relapse-free survival (bRFS) rates exceeding 90% to 95% beyond 10 years after treatment for this group of patients (16,17). Recent series of patients comparing permanent radioactive seed implants to radical prostatectomy demonstrate nearly identical bRFS rates beyond 10 years after therapy (18,19). With respect to toxicity, acute toxicity remains lim-ited to urinary obstructive symptoms. Urinary reten-tion rates have been reported in the 5% to 15% range. Such retention is nearly always temporary. Milder urinary obstructive and irritation symptoms can per-sist for periods up to 2 years. Patient-based quality-of-life reports of urinary function indicate a return to near normalcy in the majority of patients within the first 2 years after therapy (20).

Rectal irritation symptoms are relatively rare, with late rectal bleeding rates reported below the 5% range. Finally, best estimates of erectile dysfunction, as reported by patients, are around 30% to 50%, with the main predictors being preimplantation erectile function and comorbidities such as diabetes (21).

Pros: Radioactive seed implants are effective and relatively well tolerated. This approach has also the advantage to be convenient.

Cons: Seed implantation is still invasive, although less so that a prostatectomy. The technique, although mature, is still operator dependent, requir-ing an experienced brachytherapy team.

Brachytherapy—High-Dose Rate

Technique: High-dose-rate (HDR) brachytherapy uses radioactive sources at dose rates of 20 or more cGy per minute to a designated target point or vol-ume. HDR brachytherapy is delivered with dedicated remote afterloading devices that contain a radioactive source or a miniaturized X-ray tube. Special applica-tors are utilized for source delivery. A typical source is iridium-192. Computerized treatment planning is accomplished with specialized hardware and soft-ware. HDR brachytherapy can be used as the only treatment for prostate cancer or it can be used in combination with external beam radiation therapy. However, in the context of favorable prostate cancer, it is delivered as monotherapy. Two separate implant procedures are performed typically 1 or 2 weeks apart. The procedure includes the introduction of plastic hollow catheters transperineally. The catheters are left in place for approximately 2 days each time for the delivery of three treatments per implant. The dose of radiation delivered per treatment is around 6 to 8 Gy. Therefore, a total of 36 to 48 Gy are delivered to the prostate gland. The catheters are then removed.

Results: The published 5- and 8-year outcomes of HDR monotherapy for favorable-risk prostate can-cer are around 95%. The toxicity rates are similar to permanent seed implantation with significant com-plications, such as grade 3 complication rates, being in the 5% to 10% range (22).

Pros: HDR brachytherapy is effective and rela-tively well tolerated. Compared to permanent seed implants, this approach does not leave any radio-active or metallic objects within the patient once the treatment is completed. The technique also allows better control of radiation delivery since the plan is performed and dosimetry checked prior to the actual treatment delivery.

Cons: The implantation is invasive, although less so that a prostatectomy. It is more inconvenient than permanent seeds given the separate implantation ses-sion and the hospital stay required for the delivery of individual treatments. The technique is still operator dependent, requiring an experienced brachytherapy team.

External Beam Radiotherapy

External beam radiotherapy has evolved dramatically over the past decade with increasing ability to shape and aim radiation fields. This has, in turn, enabled dose escalation either through standard or altered fractionation. High-dose external radiotherapy yields cure rates that are similar to either surgery or brachytherapy in favorable-risk patients (Figure 1). Dose escalation through larger fraction sizes has resulted in the recent implementation of short treat-ment courses with high fraction sizes through ste-reotactic body radiotherapy (SBRT). Favorable-risk prostate cancer has been an ideal site to investigate the effectiveness of many of these improvements over the past decade. This evolution has still not yet resulted in an agreed upon optimized method of uti-lizing external beam radiotherapy in the treatment of localized prostate cancers. This section will include discussion, in the context of favorable-risk prostate cancer, of the use of intensity modulation in improv-ing dose-shaping, the use of in-room guidance in improving aiming of radiation fields, and the issues related to dose-escalation and/or hypofractionation.

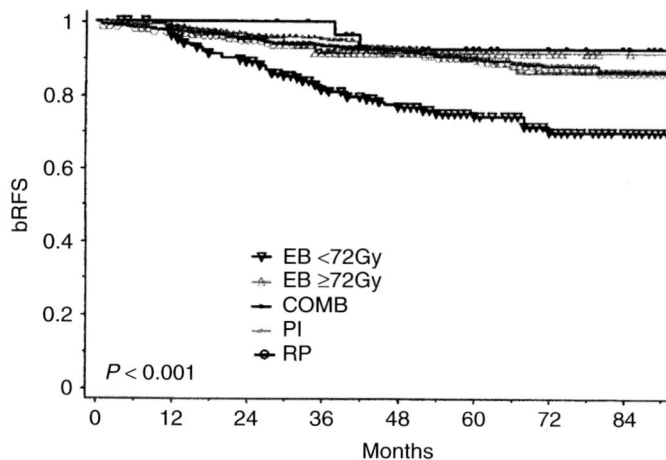

FIGURE 1   Comparison between low-dose external beam <72 Gy (EB < 72 Gy), high-dose external beam ≥72 Gy (EB ≥ 72 Gy), combination external beam and permanent seed implants (COMB), permanent seed implants (PI), and radical prostatectomy (RP) in favorable-risk patients. From Ref. (6).

Patient eligibility: There are only relative contraindications to external beam radiotherapy such as prior radiation therapy to the pelvis.

■ IMPROVED DELIVERY: 3D CONFORMAL RADIOTHERAPY

Intensity-Modulated Radiotherapy

Conformality was introduced with the introduction of CT scans in the treatment planning process versus planning on plain x-rays. This was the transition from 2D to 3D planning. In addition, with the advent of computerized treatment planning systems, 3D planning became a process by which individual structures were defined, and subsequently quantitatively targeted or avoided in the planning process. In the context of favorable-risk prostate cancer, since the target is the prostate gland itself, 3D conformal radiotherapy (3D CRT) enabled significant individualization of treatment fields adjusting for size and position of the prostate gland while avoiding large areas of the rectum and bladder.

A further refinement of 3D CRT was intensity-modulated radiotherapy (IMRT). IMRT enabled even further conformality with two significant changes. IMRT is the combination of computer algorithms that calculate an optimized radiation fluence pattern based on different cost functions that are weighted by the planner, and a delivery system modulating the radiation beam using binary or multileaf collimators. For favorable-risk prostate cancers, this facilitated even further dose escalation through better conformality of delivery fields by adjusting to the posterior convexity of the prostate gland and allowing further decrease in rectal doses. Although not an absolute requirement for dose escalation, IMRT is now documented to be associated with better toxicity rates compared to prior techniques such as 3D CRT. This has made IMRT the standard of care technique for the treatment of localized prostate cancers.

Improved Targeting: In-Room Guidance

Over the past 15 years, with increasing evidence that dose escalation has an important role in the management of prostate cancers, planning target volumes have been shrinking. Current treatment margins for localized prostate cancers are in the 5 to 8 mm range. Given the notable daily positional variations of the prostate gland within the pelvis, daily localization techniques became a necessity (23–27). Although there has been attempts to avoid adopt less than daily target localization, the current consensus is that tight treatment fields require daily localization (28). A multitude of techniques are currently utilized for daily prostate localization such as transabdominal ultrasound, intraprostatic metallic fiducials detected with in-room x-rays or CT scans, and electromagnetic tracking.

These techniques have individual advantages and disadvantages that are important to understand. What has been defined as image-guided radiotherapy therefore is based on imaging techniques that are heterogeneous. For example, inter-user variability is large for transabdominal ultrasound and relatively limited when intraprostatic markers are used (29,30). On the other hand, ultrasound provides some soft tissue imaging and is not associated with any ionizing radiation. Clinical outcomes have not been specifically documented to be different between these techniques in patients with favorable-risk prostate cancer, and they are not necessarily expected to show dramatic differences. However, they have been adopted and implemented on the basis of their technical merits.

In image guidance for favorable-risk prostate cancer, the following are still relevant controversies:

1. Are fiducials necessary?

The use of intraprostatic fiducials was introduced in 1990s and has stood the test of time. Although invasive, transrectal placement of metallic fiducials is a simple procedure with a negligible risk of complications. Typically, three to four markers are implanted. Once within the prostate, migration is very infrequent and the presence of more than one marker mitigates the rare migration event. Therefore, implanted fiducials are a reliable surrogate for the position of the prostate (31). Although there are some minor concerns about prostate deformation confounding the prostate versus marker position, if the markers are implanted close to the prostate/rectal interface, deformation and rotation of the prostate gland becomes a relatively small concern. Ultimately, the overwhelming advantage of using markers is the ease of detection and absence of any significant inter-user variability (32,33). Even when in-room CT scans are obtained, fiducials were demonstrated to significantly decrease inter-user variability.

2. Is soft tissue imaging necessary?

With the advent of in-room CT imaging, documentation of variation of pelvic anatomy is possible. Deformation of the prostate and variations in rectal and bladder filling can be better appreciated. In addition, dosimetric evaluation (such as dose recalculations and adaptive radiotherapy) are facilitated with the availability of soft tissue images throughout a treatment course (33,34). Today, in-room CT scans are utilized to align the prostate gland on the basis of implanted fiducials, and only intervene if there is significant deformation due to extreme bladder or rectal anatomic variation.

3. Is adjusting for intrafraction motion necessary?

Intrafraction motion has mostly been appreciated with the use of repeat in-room KV x-rays, but mostly with MRI-based studies and electromagnetic tracking of implanted transponders (24,27,35–37). Intrafraction motion is clearly variable from patient to patient, and from day to day. If intrafraction monitoring is performed, it is typically done with gating using arbitrary thresholds of 2 to 3 mm. It is still debatable if intrafraction motion correction leads to any clinical benefit. Dosimetric differences are difficult to document when taking into consideration intrafraction motion. These suggest relatively small dosimetric variation due to intrafraction motion when an entire fractionated treatment course is taken into account. However, one study showed decreased acute toxicity with intrafraction motion management using a 2 mm threshold (38).

4. Are there other methods that will decrease prostate motion?

Rather than observing and reacting observed intrafraction motion, strategies to decrease motion have also been suggested. In a randomized study, abdominal compression was shown not to be a factor in decreased interfraction or intrafraction motion (39). Dietary modifications showed little impact on motion (40,41). Placement of intrarectal balloons does reduce intrafraction motion without eliminating it (42). Finally, a more novel approach of proper targeting while sparing normal tissues might be the use of implanted or injected spacers (43). In this case, separation of the prostate and rectum could be achieved by the presence of a physical spacer in the prostate/rectal interface, with the spacer material being absorbed after completion of treatment.

Dose Escalation (Standard Fractionation)

Conformal radiotherapy techniques, including IMRT—which are used in 3D reconstructions of patient and tumor anatomies for designing treatment fields—have been used to deliver higher than standard radiation doses (exceeding 80 Gy) without dramatic increases in toxicity rates. There is a clear radiation dose response with respect to biochemical failures. In a recent publication by Diez et al., a meta-analysis was performed of studies satisfying the following criteria: external beam radiotherapy series with at least 200 patients reported up to 2008, no brachytherapy or hypofractionation, with at least two dosegroups compared (44). A total of five retrospective and four prospective randomized studies were included in the analysis. Looking specifically at the favorable-risk group, there was a clear improvement in outcomes with the higher radiation doses. However, the magnitude of the benefit was somewhat smaller in the randomized studies versus the prospective studies. This was confirmed in a similar analysis by Viani et al. (45). The dose response curve for favorable-risk prostate cancer was demonstrated to be relatively shallow. This indicates that improvements in outcome would only be associated with relatively large increases in dose. In addition, clinically relevant outcomes such as local failure and/or distant failure have been impacted by radiation dose in all risk groups; radiation dose was demonstrated to be associated with less local or distant failure independently from risk groups defined by T stage, pretreatment PSA, and biopsy Gleason score.

With respect to toxicity, dose escalation to the 78 to 80 Gy range has been associated with relatively minimal increases in toxicity rates. A recent report of RTOG 9406 comparing different dose groups from 68.4 to 78.0 Gy observed that a mild increase in rectal and urinary morbidity was observed with the higher radiation doses (46). However, the authors remarked that "The rates of late grade 3 toxicity are not significantly large enough to be modeled." The urinary and gastrointestinal RTOG grade 3 and higher toxicity events were observed in 6% and 7% of the patients who were in the highest dose groups. These are overall relatively low toxicity rates. Although complications, in general, have remained relatively minimal, increasing doses to increasing rectal volumes does result in increased rectal bleeding. The typical limits used to minimize rectal toxicity are: 1) limit >70 Gy to <25% of the rectal volume (more stringently <15%) or 2) limit 78 Gy to <10 mL of the entire rectum. However, changing daily anatomy can result in unexpected low or high cumulative doses within normal structures, particularly the rectum.

Urinary toxicity is more difficult to correlate with bladder dose/volume parameters. However, a limit of <25% of the bladder to receive >65 Gy has been typically used.

Finally, with respect to potency after radiation therapy, the results are highly variable for a multitude of reason. A recent review of the literature revealed 44% to 100% of patients being potent prior to radiotherapy (47). At evaluation times ranging from 12 to 78 months, the potency rates after radiotherapy were 27% to 65%. If patients were potent prior to

radiotherapy, 46% to 65% were still potent after radiotherapy. These ranges indicate the heterogeneity of patient cohorts and the heterogeneity of methods of evaluating and reporting on potency after treatment in localized prostate cancer patients. With respect to treatment planning, there is data emerging that the doses to the penile bulb/crura are important in predicting radiation-induced impotence. Typically, a limit of <50% of the penile bulb to receive >50 Gy is a reasonable guideline with respect to the evaluation of treatment plans. However, there is still controversy about the correlation between penile bulb doses and post-treatment potency status.

Hypofractionation (Including SBRT)

Conventional fractionation in external beam radiotherapy typically consists of doses around 1.8 to 2 Gy delivered daily, 5 days per week, for total doses in the 75 to 80 Gy range. Treatment courses are typically 8 to 9 weeks long. The rationale behind shortening radiation therapy courses in favorable-risk prostate cancers has been the greater sensitivity to dose fractionation, similar to late-reacting normal tissues. The alpha/beta ratio, derived in the linear-quadratic radiobiological model defining tissue responses to radiation, is demonstrated to be low around a value of 1.5 to 2 Gy. This is notably lower than for late-reacting normal tissues, making hypofractionation an attractive approach in the treatment of favorable prostate cancers. In addition, large fraction size would indicate a shorter treatment course, increasing convenience for patients.

Modern high-dose hypofractionated radiotherapy has been performed with a variety of schedules ranging from 2.1 to 10 Gy per fraction, and total radiation doses ranging from around 33 Gy to 75 Gy. The shortest treatment schedules consisted of only five fractions and the treatment has been termed "stereotactic body radiotherapy," which is defined as five fractions or less. However, this definition is somewhat arbitrary and the SBRT is simply at the extreme of hypofractionation schedules.

The largest hypofractionation experience has been reported with a schedule of 70 Gy delivered at 2.5 Gy per fraction (48). With a median follow-up of 45 months, the bRFS rates were 94% at 5 years for favorable-risk patients (Figure 2). For all 770 cases in the series, the grade 3 toxicity rates were relatively infrequent at around 2% for either urinary or rectal

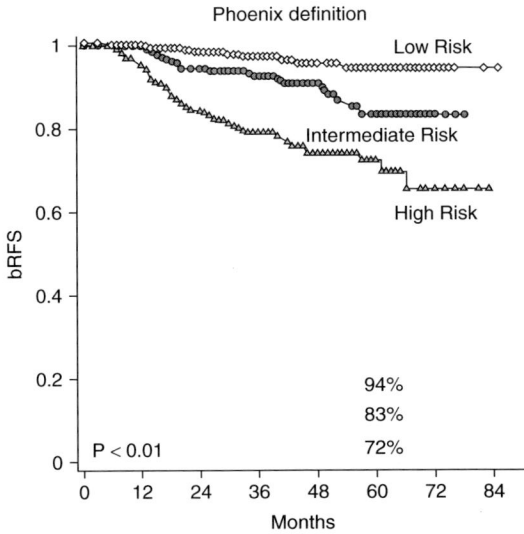

FIGURE 2 Biochemical relapse-free survival with hypofractionated external beam radiotherapy using a regimen of 70 Gy in 28 fractions, 2.5 Gy per fraction. From Ref. (48).

complications. Currently, there are multiple reports on hypofractionated radiotherapy regimens, including multiple prospective Phase II and Phase III trials that have used fraction sizes between 2 and 5 Gy, all of which use IMRT and daily image guidance. Most of these trials have been performed in patients with mostly favorable-risk and some intermediate-risk prostate cancer.

The relevant Phase II studies are the following:

1. The University of Wisconsin Phase I/II Trial, which has tested three dose groups: 2.94 Gy × 22 (total dose 64.68 Gy), 3.63 Gy × 16 (total dose (58.06 Gy), and 4.30 Gy × 12 (total dose 51.60 Gy). The trial has been completed and results are pending. However, the preliminary reports have been encouraging (49,50).
2. The Princess Margaret Hospital Phase II Trial testing 3 Gy × 20 (total dose 60 Gy). The treatment was well tolerated as reported by Martin et al. (51). The grade 3 complication rates have been reported around 1%.

The relevant Phase III studies are the following:

1. M.D. Anderson Cancer Center: testing 77.4 Gy at 1.8 Gy versus 72.0 Gy at 2.4 Gy. A total of 204 patients were accrued. With a median follow-up of 4.7 years, the 5-year bRFS rates were 94% versus 97%, the grade ≥3 rectal toxicity rates were 1% and 3%, and the grade ≥3 urinary toxicity rates were 1% and 0%. There were no statistical differences between the two groups.
2. Fox Chase: testing 76.0 Gy at 2.0 Gy versus 70.2 Gy at 2.7 Gy. A total of 307 patients were accrued. With a median follow-up of 55 months, there were no differences in gastrointestinal, urinary, and quality-of-life patient reported outcomes between the two groups (52).
3. Ontario Clinical Oncology Group: testing 60.0 Gy at 3.0 Gy versus 78.0 Gy at 2.0 Gy. A total of 1200 patients were accrued to the trial. Results are still pending.
4. RTOG 04–15: testing 70.0 Gy at 2.5 Gy versus 73.8 Gy at 1.8 Gy. A total of 1067 patients were accrued to the trial. Results are still pending.

Specifically, for SBRT experiences, there are many recent reports. However, these patient series suffer from being relatively small with short follow-up. The relevant series are the following:

1. Virginia Mason: testing 6.70 Gy × 5 = 33.5 Gy

   A total of 40 favorable-risk prostate cancer patients were treated with a stereotactic technique. With a median follow-up of 5 years, the 5-year bRFS rate was 93%. The grade ≥3 rectal and urinary toxicity rates were 0% and 3%, respectively (53).
2. Stanford: testing 7.25 Gy × 5 = 36.25 Gy

   This is the most thoroughly analyzed and reported series of patients treated with SBRT. This Phase II trial was started in 2003 (47,54–56). A total of 67 favorable-risk patients were treated, with 57 evaluable at the last report. The eligibility criteria were stage T1-T2a, PSA ≤10, GS 3+3, or low volume 3+4, no TURP or other treatment, and a low IPSS score (<20). Treatment was delivered either daily or every other day. The planning target volume margins were 3 mm posteriorly and 5 mm elsewhere. Intraprostatic fiducials were used for guidance and no endorectal balloon was used. With a median follow-up of 2.7 years (maximum 5.9 years), the 5-year bRFS rate was 93%. The grade ≥3 rectal and urinary toxicity rates were 0% and 3%, respectively. An important observation was made that every other day treatment was associated with relatively less toxicity compared to daily treatments.

Pros: External beam radiotherapy is effective and well tolerated. The main advantage is the noninvasive nature. If proven effective, approaches such as SBRT will also provide significant convenience.

Cons: The schedules with established conventional fractionation are still inconvenient due to the daily treatment over as long as 9 weeks.

■ CONCLUSION

Finally, radiotherapeutic approaches to favorable-risk prostate cancer are effective and well tolerated. Brachytherapy approaches provide high probability of cure. Modifications in external beam radiotherapy regimens, while incorporating better shaping and aiming techniques, allow more convenient treatments with the use of hypofractionation. Results with extreme hypofractionation, that is, with SBRT, are encouraging.

■ REFERENCES

1. Klotz L. Active surveillance for prostate cancer: a review. *Curr Urol Rep*. 2010;11(3):165–171.
2. Krakowsky Y, Loblaw A, Klotz L. Prostate cancer death of men treated with initial active surveillance: clinical and biochemical characteristics. *J Urol*. 2010;184(1):131–135.
3. Lawrentschuk N, Klotz L. Active surveillance for favorable-risk prostate cancer: a short review. *Korean J Urol*. 2010;51(10):665–670.
4. Thompson IM, Klotz L. Active surveillance for prostate cancer. *JAMA*. 2010;304(21):2411–2412.
5. D'Amico AV, Whittington R, Malkowicz SB, et al. Biochemical outcome after radical prostatectomy, external beam radiation therapy, or interstitial radiation therapy for clinically localized prostate cancer. *JAMA*. 1998;280(11):969–974.
6. Kupelian PA, Potters L, Khuntia D, et al. Radical prostatectomy, external beam radiotherapy <72 Gy, external beam radiotherapy > or =72 Gy, permanent seed implantation, or combined seeds/external beam radiotherapy for stage T1-T2 prostate cancer. *Int J Radiat Oncol Biol Phys*. 2004;58(1):25–33.
7. Zelefsky MJ, Eastham JA, Cronin AM, et al. Metastasis after radical prostatectomy or external beam radiotherapy for patients with clinically localized prostate cancer: a comparison of clinical cohorts adjusted for case mix. *J Clin Oncol*. 2010;28(9):1508–1513.
8. D'Amico AV, Whittington R, Malkowicz SB, et al. A multivariate analysis of clinical and pathological factors that predict for prostate specific antigen failure after radical prostatectomy for prostate cancer. *J Urol*. 1995;154(1):131–138.
9. Loiselle CR, Waheed M, Sylvester J, et al. Analysis of the Pro-Qura Database: rectal dose, implant quality, and brachytherapist's experience. *Brachytherapy*. 2009;8(1):34–39.
10. Merrick GS, Butler WM, Wallner KE, et al. Variability of prostate brachytherapy pre-implant dosimetry: a multi-institutional analysis. *Brachytherapy*. 2005;4(4):241–251.
11. Zelefsky MJ, Worman M, Cohen GN, et al. Real-time intraoperative computed tomography assessment of quality of permanent interstitial seed implantation for prostate cancer. *Urology*. 2010;76(5):1138–1142.
12. Sharma NK, Cohen RJ, Eade TN, et al. An intraoperative real-time sleeved seed technique for permanent prostate brachytherapy. *Brachytherapy*. 2010;9(2):126–130.
13. Lee EK, Zaider M. Intraoperative dynamic dose optimization in permanent prostate implants. *Int J Radiat Oncol Biol Phys*. 2003;56(3):854–861.
14. Grimm P, Sylvester J. Advances in brachytherapy. *Rev Urol*. 2004;6(suppl 4):S37–S48.
15. Grimm PD, Blasko JC, Sylvester JE, et al. Technical improvement in permanent seed implantation: a two-stage brachytherapy system. Description and comparison with current technique. *Brachytherapy*. 2004;3(1):34–40.
16. Sylvester JE, Grimm PD, Wong J, Galbreath RW, Merrick G, Blasko JC. Fifteen-year biochemical relapse-free survival, cause-specific survival, and overall survival following I(125) prostate brachytherapy in clinically localized prostate cancer: Seattle experience. *Int J Radiat Oncol Biol Phys*. 2010.
17. Sylvester JE, Blasko JC, Grimm PD, Meier R, Malmgren JA. Ten-year biochemical relapse-free survival after external beam radiation and brachytherapy for localized prostate cancer: the Seattle experience. *Int J Radiat Oncol Biol Phys*. 2003;57(4):944–952.
18. Taira AV, Merrick GS, Butler WM, et al. Long-term outcome for clinically localized prostate cancer treated with permanent interstitial brachytherapy. *Int J Radiat Oncol Biol Phys*. 2010.
19. Taira AV, Merrick GS, Galbreath RW, Wallner KE, Butler WM. Natural history of clinically staged low- and intermediate-risk prostate cancer treated with monotherapeutic permanent interstitial brachytherapy. *Int J Radiat Oncol Biol Phys*. 2010;76(2):349–354.
20. Sanda MG, Dunn RL, Michalski J, et al. Quality of life and satisfaction with outcome among prostate-cancer survivors. *N Engl J Med*. 2008;358(12):1250–1261.
21. Taira AV, Merrick GS, Galbreath RW, et al. Erectile function durability following permanent prostate brachytherapy. *Int J Radiat Oncol Biol Phys*. 2009;75(3):639–648.
22. Martinez AA, Demanes J, Vargas C, Schour L, Ghilezan M, Gustafson GS. High-dose-rate prostate brachytherapy: an excellent accelerated-hypofractionated treatment for favorable prostate cancer. *Am J Clin Oncol*. 2010;33(5):481–488.
23. Noel C, Parikh PJ, Roy M, et al. Prediction of intrafraction prostate motion: accuracy of pre- and post-treatment imaging and intermittent imaging. *Int J Radiat Oncol Biol Phys*. 2009;73(3):692–698.

24. Langen KM, Lu W, Willoughby TR, et al. Dosimetric effect of prostate motion during helical tomotherapy. *Int J Radiat Oncol Biol Phys.* 2009;74(4):1134–1142.

25. Kupelian PA, Langen KM, Willoughby TR, Zeidan OA, Meeks SL. Image-guided radiotherapy for localized prostate cancer: treating a moving target. *Semin Radiat Oncol.* 2008;18(1):58–66.

26. de Crevoisier R, Melancon AD, Kuban DA, et al. Changes in the pelvic anatomy after an IMRT treatment fraction of prostate cancer. *Int J Radiat Oncol Biol Phys.* 2007;68(5):1529–1536.

27. Litzenberg DW, Balter JM, Hadley SW, et al. Influence of intrafraction motion on margins for prostate radiotherapy. *Int J Radiat Oncol Biol Phys.* 2006;65(2):548–553.

28. Kupelian PA, Langen KM, Willoughby TR, Wagner TH, Zeidan OA, Meeks SL. Daily variations in the position of the prostate bed in patients with prostate cancer receiving postoperative external beam radiation therapy. *Int J Radiat Oncol Biol Phys.* 2006;66(2):593–596.

29. Johnston H, Hilts M, Beckham W, Berthelet E. 3D ultrasound for prostate localization in radiation therapy: a comparison with implanted fiducial markers. *Med Phys.* 2008;35(6):2403–2413.

30. Langen KM, Pouliot J, Anezinos C, et al. Evaluation of ultrasound-based prostate localization for image-guided radiotherapy. *Int J Radiat Oncol Biol Phys.* 2003;57(3):635–644.

31. Nichol AM, Brock KK, Lockwood GA, et al. A magnetic resonance imaging study of prostate deformation relative to implanted gold fiducial markers. *Int J Radiat Oncol Biol Phys.* 2007;67(1):48–56.

32. Ullman KL, Ning H, Susil RC, et al. Intra- and inter-radiation therapist reproducibility of daily isocenter verification using prostatic fiducial markers. *Radiat Oncol.* 2006;1:2.

33. Langen KM, Zhang Y, Andrews RD, et al. Initial experience with megavoltage (MV) CT guidance for daily prostate alignments. *Int J Radiat Oncol Biol Phys.* 2005;62(5):1517–1524.

34. Gayou O, Miften M. Comparison of mega-voltage cone-beam computed tomography prostate localization with online ultrasound and fiducial markers methods. *Med Phys.* 2008;35(2):531–538.

35. Langen KM, Willoughby TR, Meeks SL, et al. Observations on real-time prostate gland motion using electromagnetic tracking. *Int J Radiat Oncol Biol Phys.* 2008;71(4):1084–1090.

36. Litzenberg DW, Willoughby TR, Balter JM, et al. Positional stability of electromagnetic transponders used for prostate localization and continuous, real-time tracking. *Int J Radiat Oncol Biol Phys.* 2007;68(4):1199–1206.

37. Willoughby TR, Kupelian PA, Pouliot J, et al. Target localization and real-time tracking using the Calypso 4D localization system in patients with localized prostate cancer. *Int J Radiat Oncol Biol Phys.* 2006;65(2):528–534.

38. Sandler HM, Liu PY, Dunn RL, et al. Reduction in patient-reported acute morbidity in prostate cancer patients treated with 81-Gy Intensity-modulated radiotherapy using reduced planning target volume margins and electromagnetic tracking: assessing the impact of margin reduction study. *Urology.* 2010;75(5):1004–1008.

39. Rosewall T, Chung P, Bayley A, et al. A randomized comparison of interfraction and intrafraction prostate motion with and without abdominal compression. *Radiother Oncol.* 2008;88(1):88–94.

40. Nichol AM, Warde PR, Lockwood GA, et al. A cinematic magnetic resonance imaging study of milk of magnesia laxative and an antiflatulent diet to reduce intrafraction prostate motion. *Int J Radiat Oncol Biol Phys.* 2010;77(4):1072–1078.

41. Smitsmans MH, Pos FJ, de Bois J, et al. The influence of a dietary protocol on cone beam CT-guided radiotherapy for prostate cancer patients. *Int J Radiat Oncol Biol Phys.* 2008;71(4):1279–1286.

42. Smeenk RJ, Teh BS, Butler EB, van Lin EN, Kaanders JH. Is there a role for endorectal balloons in prostate radiotherapy? A systematic review. *Radiother Oncol.* 2010;95(3):277–282.

43. Prada PJ, Gonzalez H, Menéndez C, et al. Transperineal injection of hyaluronic acid in the anterior perirectal fat to decrease rectal toxicity from radiation delivered with low-dose-rate brachytherapy for prostate cancer patients. *Brachytherapy.* 2009;8(2):210–217.

44. Diez P, Vogelius IS, Bentzen SM. A new method for synthesizing radiation dose-response data from multiple trials applied to prostate cancer. *Int J Radiat Oncol Biol Phys.* 2010;77(4):1066–1071.

45. Viani GA, Stefano EJ, Afonso SL. Higher-than-conventional radiation doses in localized prostate cancer treatment: a meta-analysis of randomized, controlled trials. *Int J Radiat Oncol Biol Phys.* 2009;74(5):1405–1418.

46. Michalski JM, Bae K, Roach M, et al. Long-term toxicity following 3D conformal radiation therapy for prostate cancer from the RTOG 9406 phase I/II dose escalation study. *Int J Radiat Oncol Biol Phys.* 2010;76(1):14–22.

47. Wiegner EA, King CR. Sexual function after stereotactic body radiotherapy for prostate cancer: results of a prospective clinical trial. *Int J Radiat Oncol Biol Phys.* 2010;78(2):442–448.

48. Kupelian PA, Willoughby TR, Reddy CA, Klein EA, Mahadevan A. Hypofractionated intensity-modulated radiotherapy (70 Gy at 2.5 Gy per fraction) for localized prostate cancer: Cleveland Clinic experience. *Int J Radiat Oncol Biol Phys.* 2007;68(5):1424–1430.

49. Ritter M, Forman J, Kupelian P, Lawton C, Petereit D. Hypofractionation for prostate cancer. *Cancer J.* 2009;15(1):1–6.

50. Ritter M. Rationale, conduct, and outcome using hypofractionated radiotherapy in prostate cancer. *Semin Radiat Oncol.* 2008;18(4):249–256.

51. Martin JM, Rosewall T, Bayley A, et al. Phase II trial of hypofractionated image-guided intensity-modulated

radiotherapy for localized prostate adenocarcinoma. *Int J Radiat Oncol Biol Phys.* 2007;69(4):1084–1089.

52. Pollack A, Hanlon AL, Horwitz EM, et al. Dosimetry and preliminary acute toxicity in the first 100 men treated for prostate cancer on a randomized hypofractionation dose escalation trial. *Int J Radiat Oncol Biol Phys.* 2006;64(2):518–526.

53. Madsen BL, Hsi RA, Pham HT, Fowler JF, Esagui L, Corman J. Stereotactic hypofractionated accurate radiotherapy of the prostate (SHARP), 33.5 Gy in five fractions for localized disease: first clinical trial results. *Int J Radiat Oncol Biol Phys.* 2007;67(4):1099–1105.

54. King CR, Brooks JD, Gill H, Pawlicki T, Cotrutz C, Presti JC Jr. Stereotactic body radiotherapy for localized prostate cancer: interim results of a prospective phase II clinical trial. *Int J Radiat Oncol Biol Phys.* 2009;73(4):1043–1048.

55. Pawlicki T, Cotrutz C, King C. Prostate cancer therapy with stereotactic body radiation therapy. *Front Radiat Ther Oncol.* 2007;40:395–406.

56. King CR, Lehmann J, Adler JR, Hai J. CyberKnife radiotherapy for localized prostate cancer: rationale and technical feasibility. *Technol Cancer Res Treat.* 2003;2(1):25–30.

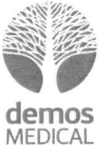

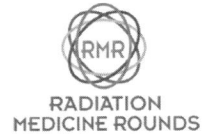

Intermediate-Risk Prostate Cancer: Role of Androgen Deprivation

Sravana K. Chennupati and Arthur Y. Hung*

Oregon Health & Science University, Portland, OR

■ ABSTRACT

Intermediate-risk prostate cancer is possibly the most significant category for radiation oncologists. Patients with intermediate-risk prostate cancer are most likely to have sufficiently aggressive disease that improvements in local control can be demonstrated. Treatment intensification with dose escalation and/or androgen deprivation has been demonstrated to improve outcomes mainly for patients with intermediate-risk features. This article covers the definition and uncertainty of the categorization of intermediate prostate cancer. The data for treatment intensification with dose escalation and/or androgen deprivation is reviewed and summarized in detail.

Keywords: dose escalation, androgen deprivation

Intermediate-risk prostate cancer can be a difficult category to define (1). In many ways, it is a category for radiation oncologists. For a surgeon, after patients undergo a radical prostatectomy, the patients have their disease completely confined to the prostate and resected with negative margins, or the patients have features more likely to be associated with a recurrence and would benefit from adjuvant radiation. Thus the category only exists for surgeons in discussing management in relation to radiation. For radiation oncologists, the decision tree is more complicated because treatment intensification is possible. The radiation oncologist must make decisions regarding the dose to use, the number of fractions, and whether or not to use hormone therapy.

Categorizing intermediate-risk prostate cancer is a relatively new development in the evolution of radiation treatment for prostate cancer. High-risk patients have traditionally been identified with high Gleason scores and high pretreatment prostate-specific antigens (PSAs) (2–5). As the experience with the treatment of prostate cancer in the PSA era evolved, separate categories could be created using patients' preoperative characteristics. One of the largest and earliest reports demonstrated that patients who underwent a prostatectomy could be categorized into three distinct groups based on pretreatment PSA, Gleason score, and clinical stage. Using these criteria, the 10-year PSA failure-free survival was 83% for the 1,020 patients with low-risk features, 46% for the

*Corresponding author, Department of Radiation Medicine—KPV4, Oregon Health & Science University, Portland, OR 97239

E-mail address: hunga@ohsu.edu

Radiation Medicine Rounds 2:1 (2011) 27–34.
DOI: 10.5003/2151–4208.2.1.27

693 patients with intermediate-risk features, and 29% for the 414 patients with high-risk features (6).

Presently, consensus categories are defined in the National Comprehensive Cancer Network Clinical Practice Guidelines: low (T1-T2a and Gleason score 2–6 and PSA < 10 ng/mL), intermediate (T2b-T2c or Gleason score of 7 or PSA 10–20 ng/mL), and high (T3a or Gleason score 8–10 or PSA > 20 ng/mL) (7).

One of the difficulties in defining risk categories is that the pretreatment factors do not always predict the actual pathology. Historically, interobserver variability was a much greater problem with early reports suggesting that only 2/3 of pathology specimens at the same institution would be identical between the biopsy and the prostatectomy specimen (8). The correlation was even less (<50%) for patients who had their biopsies read at a different institution.

Template sextant biopsies have reduced the incidence of under sampling higher grade disease, but the risk still persists.

The use of surgical data can help predict which patients may be harboring higher-risk features, and in some cases, these factors should be included in evaluating patients for treatment. Utilizing all available data from the biopsy, multiple studies have attempted to identify other factors that may contribute to identifying more aggressive disease. The risk of under-staging and/or under-grading is very significant. In a study from Johns Hopkins, examining the correlation between biopsy and prostatectomy specimens demonstrated that >1/3 of patients with a biopsy Gleason score of <7 ended up with a Gleason grade ≥7 after prostatectomy (8). First of all, the amount of disease identified during biopsy, and quantified by the number of cores and the percentage of the cores involved with disease, has been analyzed in the hope of identifying which patients are more likely to harbor more aggressive disease. In a study from the National Health Services analyzing the correlation between the radical prostatectomy specimen and the biopsy Gleason score, the correlation increased with the number of cores submitted from the biopsy. The agreement increased with the number of cores submitted: 37% agreement with ≤5 cores, 48% with six cores, 56% with ≥7 cores, $P = .006$ (9). In addition to the number of cores removed, the percentage of positive cores has been identified as a factor that can predict under staging and/or under grading. In a study from CaPSURE database (Cancer of the Prostate Strategic Urologic Research Endeavor), under grading (when a pattern of 1 to 3 was converted to a

pattern of 4 or 5) of primary and secondary Gleason patterns occurred for 13% and 29% of the patients from their biopsy to their prostatectomy. Unexpected extraprostatic disease (under staging) was identified 24% of the time. The percentage of positive biopsies appeared to be the most important for predicting the likelihood of extraprostatic disease extension in intermediate or high-risk disease categories (10). Other investigators have identified the percentage of positive biopsies to be independently prognostic, in addition to our standard features for biochemical recurrence, prostate cancer–specific mortality, and overall survival after radical prostatectomy or radiation (11–14,63). Still, the utility of incorporating the percentage of positive biopsies in contemporary practice has been questioned. The radiation doses used in the treatment of the patients that supply the majority of the dataset for analysis were treated with radiation doses considered to be low by current standards (16). And while the percentage of positive biopsies may be a significant factor, the largest study assessing the overall impact of the factor on predictive models demonstrated that it has limited ability to further improve our modeling efficiency above our conventional variables (17,18). Thus the percentage of positive biopsies has not routinely supplemented the current variables for discriminating risk.

Another factor to be potentially incorporated into pretreatment risk assessment is the pretreatment PSA velocity. Postoperative PSA doubling time may be used as a surrogate for prostate cancer–specific mortality in patients with biochemical recurrence after radical prostatectomy (19–31). Pretreatment PSA velocity has been reported in some series to be associated with prostate cancer–specific mortality following RP and external beam radiation therapy (32,33). In a large dataset from a screening study where all patients that were analyzed underwent a radical prostatectomy, the patients with a PSA velocity greater than 2.0 ng/mL per year had a statistically significant higher risk of biochemical recurrence and prostate cancer–specific mortality than patients with a PSA velocity <2.0 ng/mL per year. Men with low-risk disease and a PSA velocity >2.0 ng/mL per year had a 7-year estimated rate of prostate cancer–specific mortality of 19% (95%CI 2%–39%) compared with 0% for men whose PSA velocity was 2.0 ng/mL per year or less. The corresponding values for men with higher-risk disease were 24% (95%CI 12%–37%) and 4% (95%CI, 0%–11%), respectively (34,35). However, other investigators have not been able to confirm similarly strong associations in datasets of a similar size and treatment (36–38).

One of the reasons for identifying patients with intermediate-risk prostate cancer is that this is the category where treatment intensification with radiation dose has been shown to make a singular difference. Randomized trials have demonstrated that increasing dose confers longer term biochemical control. Pollack et al reported the long-term results of a randomized dose escalation trial, comparing 70 Gy versus 78 Gy in a total of 301 patients with stage T1b-T3 prostate cancer. The median follow up was 8.7 years and PSA failure was defined as nadir+2. Freedom from biochemical or clinical failure was significantly greater in the 78-Gy arm compared to the 70-Gy arm (78% versus 59%, $P = 0.001$). Interestingly, the benefit of a higher dose was greatest in patients with an initial PSA >10 ng/mL (78% versus 39%, $P = 0.001$). A GI toxicity of grade 2 or greater occurred more often in the 78-Gy arm (26% versus 13%, $P = 0.013$). The number of patients with a GU toxicity of grade 2 or more was not statistically significant when comparing the two groups. Since the M.D. Anderson Cancer Center trial was first reported, other trials have confirmed that higher dose are associated with higher rates of long-term biochemical control (39–41).

Other studies have confirmed the benefit of dose escalation in patients with intermediate-risk prostate cancer. The Proton Radiation Oncology Group conducted a randomized controlled trial of 393 men with T1b-T2b prostate cancer with PSA <15 ng/mL, treated to receive external beam radiation at a dose of 70.2 Gy or 79.2 Gy by using a combination of conformal photon and proton beams. For intermediate-risk patients, the 5-year freedom from biochemical failure was 62.7% for patients treated with 70.2 Gy and 81% for patients treated with 79.2 Gy ($P = 0.02$) using the ASTRO definition (42). Fox Chase Cancer reviewed their results with dose escalation. They evaluated a cohort of 1,530 men treated with 3DCRT and divided into four groups: <70 Gy, 70–74.9 Gy, 75–79.9 Gy, >80 Gy. Using a definition of nadir +2 to define biochemical failure, they found adjusted 5-year estimates of freedom from biochemical failure to be 70%, 81%, 83%, and 89%, respectively. Among the 367 patients that were treated with >80 Gy, the majority (2/3) were intermediate risk (43).

Other institutions have demonstrated equivalent control rates for patients with intermediate-risk cancers. Between 1996 and 2000, 561 patients with

clinically localized prostate cancer were treated with IMRT at Memorial Sloan Kettering Cancer Center. All patients were treated to a dose of 81 Gy prescribed to the planning target volume. For patients that were intermediate risk, the 8-year biochemical relapse-free survival rate was 78% when failure was defined using the nadir+2 definition (44,45). A phase III trial in the Netherlands compared 68 Gy versus 78 Gy in patients with T1b-4 prostate cancer. About 664 patients were included in the study, and the median follow up was 51 months. Freedom from failure was significantly improved in the 78 Gy arm compared to the 68 Gy arm (64% vs. 54%). There were 15% less failures for patients that were intermediate risk and treated with a higher dose, compared to 68Gy. In the subgroup analysis, this was statistically significant (46). The majority of the benefit from the dose escalation studies is most evident in the intermediate-risk patients. The patients with low-risk disease have excellent outcomes regardless, while the patients with high-risk disease are treated with concurrent androgen deprivation and have a much higher risk of metastatic disease development, which can obfuscate the improved local control. Table 1 lists several studies that demonstrate the expected outcomes and the improvement with dose escalation when treating patients with intermediate-risk prostate cancer.

TABLE 1 Dose escalation studies with intermediate-risk patients

Study	Dose	No. of Patients	bRFS (Years)
MDACC*	70 Gy		76% (8)
	78 Gy		86% (8)*
PROG	70.2 Gy	68	62.7% (5)
	79.2 Gy	61	81.0% (5)
FCCC	<70 Gy	13	70% (5)
	70–74.9 Gy	164	81% (5)
	75–79.9 Gy	174	83% (5)
	≥80 Gy	247	89% (5)**
MSKCC	81 Gy	255	78% (8)
Dutch	68 Gy	90	64% (5)
	78 Gy	92	79% (5)***

*Not statistically significant.
**30, 31, 31, and 67%, respectively, of patients in these group were intermediate risk.
***Actual percentage at 5 years.

Dose escalation has also been accomplished with brachytherapy, where some investigators argue that the permanent prostate implants or temporary HDR implants can provide a higher dose to the prostate than an external beam can (36,47,48,49,61).

An alternative is to supplement external beam radiation with brachytherapy implants. Some investigators have reported excellent results. Intermediate-risk patients treated with I-125 or Pd-103 implants, after 45 Gy of neoadjuvant external beam radiation, had a 15-year bRFS of 80.3% (17,50–55).

In addition to dose, the other means for treatment intensification is with androgen deprivation. We know from the landmark EORTC trial that 3 years of androgen deprivation improved biochemical control, disease-free survival, and overall survival for patients with high-risk (WHO grade 3 and/or cT3) disease. Prior to that study, we had results from both RTOG 85–31 and RTOG 86–10 that demonstrated statistically significant improvements in outcome for biochemical disease-free survival and distant metastases failure, with the addition of hormones. Patients on 85–31 received long-term hormones starting in the last week of RT and continuing indefinitely. Patients on 86–10 received goserelin and flutamide, 2 months prior to and during RT. Radiation doses for both these studies would be considered low by conventional criteria (56–58).

RTOG 92–02 investigated whether the addition of 2 years of androgen deprivation to a regimen that already included 4 months of neoadjuvant and concurrent hormonal therapy, with definitive radiation, improved outcomes. All endpoints except overall survival showed statistically significant improvements, including disease-free survival, disease-specific survival, local progression, distant metastasis, and biochemical failure (59). A difference in overall survival was significant when the subgroup of patients with Gleason 8–10 tumors was analyzed.

D'Amico reported on a small trial randomizing 206 patients with PSA of at least 10 ng/mL, a Gleason score of at least 7, or radiographic evidence of extra-prostatic disease (60). The patient characteristics showed a mix of both intermediate and high-risk patients. Over the entire group, about 15% had a Gleason score of 8–10 and/or a PSA of 20 to 40 ng/mL. At most, 1/3 of the group was high-risk, and thus the overwhelming majority had intermediate-risk disease by contemporary criteria. Patients received 70 Gy of radiation, alone or in combination with 6 months of androgen deprivation therapy. After a median

follow-up of only 4.5 years, patients randomized to radiation and androgen deprivation had a significantly higher survival and a lower prostate cancer–specific mortality rate. The differences in 5-year survival rates were 88% versus 78%. After a median follow-up of 7.6 years, the Kaplan-Meier 8-year survival estimates were 74% in the combined therapy arm and 61% in the only radiation arm ($P = 0.01$) (14,61).

RTOG 94–08 attempted to answer whether the addition of 4 months of androgen deprivation therapy improved on definitive radiation for what was considered "Good Prognosis" at that time. 2,000 patients with PSA < 20 ng/mL and < Stage T2c disease were enrolled. Patients were stratified by grade, but high grades were not excluded. Patients received only 66.6 to 68.4 Gy. With a median follow-up of 9 years, the 10-year overall survival rate is 62% versus 57% ($P = 0.03$). Disease-specific survival rate was improved from 93% to 96%. 10 year biochemical failure rate was 26% versus 41% ($P \leq 0.01$). They reported that the majority of the benefit was in patients classified as intermediate risk by today's measures (62).

To summarize our current knowledge of utilizing androgen deprivation for treatment intensification, the addition of a short-term (4–6 months) of androgen deprivation to standard doses of radiation can improve overall survival and biochemical, relapse-free survival. At this time, there are no published randomized controlled trials for the combination of dose escalation and androgen deprivation. RTOG 0815 is titled "A Phase III Prospective Randomized Trial of Dose-Escalated Radiotherapy With or Without Short-Term Androgen Deprivation Therapy for Patients with Intermediate-Risk Prostate Cancer." The protocol is designed to define the magnitude of the benefit from adding androgen deprivation to dose-escalated radiation specifically in the treatment of intermediate-risk prostate cancer. The protocol will allow the dose escalation to be delivered via external beam radiation alone, external beam and low dose rate permanent prostate implant, or external beam and high dose rate prostate implant (63).

In conclusion, intermediate-risk prostate cancer is a category where major advances in the treatment of prostate cancer have been made. The patients with intermediate-risk prostate cancer are most likely to have such sufficiently aggressive disease that recurrence is a likely possibility with inadequate treatment, and simultaneously, patients have disease that is unlikely to harbor occult metastatic disease.

Intermediate-risk prostate cancer is the category where researchers and oncologists will be most able to efficiently and accurately augment our understanding of how to attain complete local control of prostate cancer.

■ REFERENCES

1. Williams SG, Millar JL, Dally MJ, Sia S, Miles W, Duchesne GM. What defines intermediate-risk prostate cancer? Variability in published prognostic models. *Int J Radiat Oncol Biol Phys.* 2004;58(1):11–18.

2. Babaian RJ, Zagars GK, Ayala AG. Radiation therapy of stage C prostate cancer: significance of Gleason grade to survival. *Semin Urol.* 1990;8(4):225–231.

3. Zagars GK, Sherman NE, Babaian RJ. Prostate-specific antigen and external beam radiation therapy in prostate cancer. *Cancer.* 1991;67(2):412–420.

4. Zagars GK. Prostate-specific antigen as a prognostic factor for prostate cancer treated by external beam radiotherapy. *Int J Radiat Oncol Biol Phys.* 1992;23(1):47–53.

5. Zagars GK, von Eschenbach AC, Ayala AG. Prognostic factors in prostate cancer. Analysis of 874 patients treated with radiation therapy. *Cancer.* 1993;72(5):1709–1725.

6. D'Amico AV, Whittington R, Malkowicz SB, et al. Predicting prostate specific antigen outcome preoperatively in the prostate specific antigen era. *J Urol.* 2001;166(6):2185–2188.

7. Mohler J, Bahnson RR, Boston B, et al. NCCN clinical practice guidelines in oncology: prostate cancer. *J Natl Compr Canc Netw.* 2010;8(2):162–200.

8. Steinberg DM, Sauvageot J, Piantadosi S, Epstein JI. Correlation of prostate needle biopsy and radical prostatectomy Gleason grade in academic and community settings. *Am J Surg Pathol.* 1997;21(5):566–576.

9. Bott SR, Freeman AA, Stenning S, Cohen J, Parkinson MC. Radical prostatectomy: pathology findings in 1001 cases compared with other major series and over time. *BJU Int.* 2005;95(1):34–39.

10. Grossfeld GD, Chang JJ, Broering JM, et al. Under staging and under grading in a contemporary series of patients undergoing radical prostatectomy: results from the Cancer of the Prostate Strategic Urologic Research Endeavor database. *J Urol.* 2001;165(3):851–856.

11. D'Amico AV, Whittington R, Malkowicz SB, et al. Clinical utility of the percentage of positive prostate biopsies in defining biochemical outcome after radical prostatectomy for patients with clinically localized prostate cancer. *J Clin Oncol.* 2000;18(6):1164–1172.

12. D'Amico AV, Keshaviah A, Manola J, et al. Clinical utility of the percentage of positive prostate biopsies in predicting prostate cancer-specific and overall survival after radiotherapy for patients with localized prostate cancer. *Int J Radiat Oncol Biol Phys.* 2002;53(3):581–587.

13. Kestin LL, Goldstein NS, Vicini FA, Martinez AA. Percentage of positive biopsy cores as predictor of clinical outcome in prostate cancer treated with radiotherapy. *J Urol.* 2002;168(5):1994–1999.

14. D'Amico AV, Renshaw AA, Cote K, et al. Impact of the percentage of positive prostate cores on prostate cancer-specific mortality for patients with low or favorable intermediate-risk disease. *J Clin Oncol.* 2004;22(18):3726–3732.

15. Merrick GS, Butler WM, Wallner KE, Galbreath RW, Lief JH, Adamovich E. Prognostic significance of percent positive biopsies in clinically organ-confined prostate cancer treated with permanent prostate brachytherapy with or without supplemental external-beam radiation. *Cancer J.* 2004;10(1):54–60.

16. Nurani R, Wallner K, Merrick G, Virgin J, Orio P, True LD. (2007). Optimized prostate brachytherapy minimizes the prognostic impact of percent of biopsy cores involved with adenocarcinoma. *J Urol.* 178(5):1968–1973; discussion 1973.

17. Merrick GS, Butler WM, Wallner KE, et al. Impact of supplemental external beam radiotherapy and/or androgen deprivation therapy on biochemical outcome after permanent prostate brachytherapy. *Int J Radiat Oncol Biol Phys.* 2005;61(1):32–43.

18. Williams SG, Buyyounouski MK, Pickles T, et al. Percentage of biopsy cores positive for malignancy and biochemical failure following prostate cancer radiotherapy in 3,264 men: statistical significance without predictive performance. *Int J Radiat Oncol Biol Phys.* 2008;70(4):1169–1175.

19. Pound CR, Partin AW, Eisenberger MA, Chan DW, Pearson JD, Walsh PC. Natural history of progression after PSA elevation following radical prostatectomy. *JAMA.* 1999;281(17):1591–1597.

20. Egawa S, Arai Y, Tobisu K, et al. Use of pretreatment prostate specific antigen doubling time to predict outcome after radical prostatectomy. *Prostate Cancer Prostatic Dis.* 2000;3(S1):S11.

21. Cannon GM Jr, Walsh PC, Partin AW, Pound CR. Prostate-specific antigen doubling time in the identification of patients at risk for progression after treatment and biochemical recurrence for prostate cancer. *Urology.* 2003;62 Suppl 1:2–8.

22. Loberg RD, Fielhauer JR, Pienta BA, et al. Prostate-specific antigen doubling time and survival in patients with advanced metastatic prostate cancer. *Urology.* 2003;62(suppl 1):128–133.

23. D'Amico AV, Moul J, Carroll PR, Sun L, Lubeck D, Chen MH. Prostate specific antigen doubling time as a surrogate end point for prostate cancer specific mortality following radical prostatectomy or radiation therapy. *J Urol.* 2004;172(5 Pt 2):S42–6; discussion S46.

24. Shulman MJ, Karam JA, Benaim EA. Prostate-specific antigen doubling time predicts response to deferred antiandrogen therapy in men with androgen-independent prostate cancer. *Urology.* 2004;63(4):732–736.

25. Ward JF, Zincke H, Bergstralh EJ, Slezak JM, Blute ML. Prostate specific antigen doubling time subsequent to radical prostatectomy as a prognosticator of outcome

following salvage radiotherapy. *J Urol*. 2004;172(6 Pt 1):2244–2248.

26. Eastham JA. Prostate-specific antigen doubling time as a prognostic marker in prostate cancer. *Nat Clin Pract Urol*. 2005;2(10):482–491.

27. Lee AK, Levy LB, Cheung R, Kuban D. Prostate-specific antigen doubling time predicts clinical outcome and survival in prostate cancer patients treated with combined radiation and hormone therapy. *Int J Radiat Oncol Biol Phys*. 2005;63(2):456–462.

28. Semeniuk RC, Venner PM, North S. Prostate-specific antigen doubling time is associated with survival in men with hormone-refractory prostate cancer. *Urology*. 2006;68(3):565–569.

29. Sengupta S, Blute ML, Bagniewski SM, et al. Increasing prostate specific antigen following radical prostatectomy and adjuvant hormonal therapy: doubling time predicts survival. *J Urol*. 2006;175(5):1684–90; discussion 1690.

30. Valicenti RK, DeSilvio M, Hanks GE, et al. Posttreatment prostatic-specific antigen doubling time as a surrogate endpoint for prostate cancer-specific survival: an analysis of Radiation Therapy Oncology Group Protocol 92–02. *Int J Radiat Oncol Biol Phys*. 2006;66(4):1064–1071.

31. Maffezzini M, Bossi A, Collette L. Implications of prostate-specific antigen doubling time as indicator of failure after surgery or radiation therapy for prostate cancer. *Eur Urol*. 2007;51(3):605–13; discussion 613.

32. Sengupta S, Myers RP, Slezak JM, Bergstralh EJ, Zincke H, Blute ML. Preoperative prostate specific antigen doubling time and velocity are strong and independent predictors of outcomes following radical prostatectomy. *J Urol*. 2005;174(6):2191–2196.

33. Palma D, Tyldesley S, Pickles T. Pretreatment prostate-specific antigen velocity is associated with development of distant metastases and prostate cancer mortality in men treated with radiotherapy and androgen-deprivation therapy. *Cancer*. 2008;112(9):1941–1948.

34. D'Amico AV, Chen MH, Roehl KA, Catalona WJ. Preoperative PSA velocity and the risk of death from prostate cancer after radical prostatectomy. *N Engl J Med*. 2004;351(2):125–135.

35. D'Amico AV, Renshaw AA, Sussman B, Chen MH. Pretreatment PSA velocity and risk of death from prostate cancer following external beam radiation therapy. *JAMA*. 2005;294(4):440–447.

36. Bittner N, Merrick GS, Andreini H, et al. Prebiopsy PSA velocity not reliable predictor of prostate cancer diagnosis, Gleason score, tumor location, or cancer volume after TTMB. *Urology*. 2009;74(1):171–176.

37. O'Brien MF, Cronin AM, Fearn PA, et al. Pretreatment prostate-specific antigen (PSA) velocity and doubling time are associated with outcome but neither improves prediction of outcome beyond pretreatment PSA alone in patients treated with radical prostatectomy. *J Clin Oncol*. 2009;27(22):3591–3597.

38. Loeb S, Kan D, Yu X, Roehl KA, Catalona WJ. Preoperative prostate specific antigen doubling time is not a useful predictor of biochemical progression after radical prostatectomy. *J Urol*. 2010;183(5):1816–1821.

39. Pollack A, Zagars GK, Smith LG, et al. Preliminary results of a randomized radiotherapy dose-escalation study comparing 70 Gy with 78 Gy for prostate cancer. *J Clin Oncol*. 2000;18(23):3904–3911.

40. Pollack A, Zagars GK, Starkschall G, et al. Prostate cancer radiation dose response: results of the M. D. Anderson phase III randomized trial. *Int J Radiat Oncol Biol Phys*. 2002;53(5):1097–1105.

41. Kuban DA, Tucker SL, Dong L, et al. Long-term results of the M. D. Anderson randomized dose-escalation trial for prostate cancer. *Int J Radiat Oncol Biol Phys*. 2008;70(1):67–74.

42. Zietman AL, DeSilvio ML, Slater JD, et al. Comparison of conventional-dose vs high-dose conformal radiation therapy in clinically localized adenocarcinoma of the prostate: a randomized controlled trial. *JAMA*. 2005;294(10):1233–1239.

43. Eade TN, Hanlon AL, Horwitz EM, Buyyounouski MK, Hanks GE, Pollack A. What dose of external-beam radiation is high enough for prostate cancer? *Int J Radiat Oncol Biol Phys*. 2007;68(3):682–689.

44. Zelefsky MJ, Chan H, Hunt M, Yamada Y, Shippy AM, Amols H. Long-term outcome of high dose intensity modulated radiation therapy for patients with clinically localized prostate cancer. *J Urol*. 2006;176(4 Pt 1):1415–1419.

45. Zelefsky MJ, Yamada Y, Fuks Z, et al. Long-term results of conformal radiotherapy for prostate cancer: impact of dose escalation on biochemical tumor control and distant metastases-free survival outcomes. *Int J Radiat Oncol Biol Phys*. 2008;71(4):1028–1033.

46. Peeters ST, Heemsbergen WD, Koper PC, et al. Dose-response in radiotherapy for localized prostate cancer: results of the Dutch multicenter randomized phase III trial comparing 68 Gy of radiotherapy with 78 Gy. *J Clin Oncol*. 2006;24(13):1990–1996.

47. Martinez AA, Gustafson G, Gonzalez J, et al. Dose escalation using conformal high-dose-rate brachytherapy improves outcome in unfavorable prostate cancer. *Int J Radiat Oncol Biol Phys*. 2002;53(2):316–327.

48. Martinez AA, Gonzalez J, Ye H, et al. Dose escalation improves cancer-related events at 10 years for intermediate- and high-risk prostate cancer patients treated with hypofractionated high-dose-rate boost and external beam radiotherapy. *Int J Radiat Oncol Biol Phys*. 2011;79(2):363–370.

49. Bittner N, Merrick GS, Wallner KE, Butler WM. Interstitial brachytherapy should be standard of care for treatment of high-risk prostate cancer. *Oncology* (Williston Park). 2008;22(9):995–1004; discussion 1006, 1011–1017.

50. Sylvester J, Blasko JC, Grimm PD, Meier R, Cavanagh W. Short-course androgen ablation combined with external-beam radiation therapy and low-dose-rate permanent brachytherapy in early-stage prostate cancer: a matched subset analysis. *Mol Urol*. 2000;4(3):155–9; discussion 161.

51. Sylvester JE, Blasko JC, Grimm PD, Meier R, Malmgren JA. Ten-year biochemical relapse-free survival after external beam radiation and brachytherapy for localized prostate cancer: the Seattle experience. *Int J Radiat Oncol Biol Phys.* 2003;57(4):944–952.

52. Dattoli M, Wallner K, True L, Cash J, Sorace R. Long-term outcomes after treatment with brachytherapy and supplemental conformal radiation for prostate cancer patients having intermediate and high-risk features. *Cancer.* 2007;110(3):551–555.

53. Frank SJ, Grimm PD, Sylvester JE, et al. Interstitial implant alone or in combination with external beam radiation therapy for intermediate-risk prostate cancer: a survey of practice patterns in the United States. *Brachytherapy.* 2007;6(1):2–8.

54. Sylvester JE, Grimm PD, Blasko JC, et al. 15-Year biochemical relapse free survival in clinical Stage T1-T3 prostate cancer following combined external beam radiotherapy and brachytherapy; Seattle experience. *Int J Radiat Oncol Biol Phys.* 2007;67(1):57–64.

55. Sylvester JE, Grimm PD, Wong J, Galbreath RW, Merrick G, Blasko JC. Fifteen-year biochemical relapse-free survival, cause-specific survival, and overall survival following I(125) prostate brachytherapy in clinically localized prostate cancer: Seattle experience. *Int J Radiat Oncol Biol Phys.* 2010.

56. Horwitz EM, Winter K, Hanks GE, Lawton CA, Russell AH, Machtay M. Subset analysis of RTOG 85–31 and 86–10 indicates an advantage for long-term vs. short-term adjuvant hormones for patients with locally advanced nonmetastatic prostate cancer treated with radiation therapy. *Int J Radiat Oncol Biol Phys.* 2001;49(4):947–956.

57. Pilepich MV, Winter K, John MJ, et al. Phase III radiation therapy oncology group (RTOG) trial 86–10 of androgen deprivation adjuvant to definitive radiotherapy in locally advanced carcinoma of the prostate. *Int J Radiat Oncol Biol Phys.* 2001;50(5):1243–1252.

58. Roach M 3rd, Bae K, Speight J, et al. Short-term neoadjuvant androgen deprivation therapy and external-beam radiotherapy for locally advanced prostate cancer: long-term results of RTOG 8610. *J Clin Oncol.* 2008;26(4):585–591.

59. Horwitz EM, Bae K, Hanks GE, et al. Ten-year follow-up of radiation therapy oncology group protocol 92–02: a phase III trial of the duration of elective androgen deprivation in locally advanced prostate cancer. *J Clin Oncol.* 2008;26(15):2497–2504.

60. D'Amico AV, Chen MH, Renshaw AA, Loffredo M, Kantoff PW. Androgen suppression and radiation vs radiation alone for prostate cancer: a randomized trial. *JAMA.* 2008;299(3):289–295.

61. D'Amico AV, Manola J, Loffredo M, Renshaw AA, DellaCroce A, Kantoff PW. 6-month androgen suppression plus radiation therapy vs radiation therapy alone for patients with clinically localized prostate cancer: a randomized controlled trial. *JAMA.* 2004;292(7):821–827.

62. McGowan DG, Hunt D, Jones CU, et al. Short-term endocrine therapy prior to and during radiation therapy improves overall survival in patients with T1b-T2b adenocarcinoma of the prostate and PSA # 20: initial results of RTOG 94–08. *Int J Radiat Oncol Biol Phys.* 2009;72(1 (Late-Breaking Abstracts)):1.

63. RTOG. (2008). RTOG 0815 a phase III prospective randomized trial of dose-escalated radiotherapy with or without short-term androgen deprivation therapy for patients with intermediate-risk prostate cancer.

RADIATION
MEDICINE ROUNDS

High-Risk Prostate Cancer

Chirag Shah, Nasiruddin Mohammed, Michel Ghilezan, and Alvaro Martinez*
Rose Cancer Center, William Beaumont Hospital, Royal Oak, MI

■ ABSTRACT

High-risk prostate cancer is decreasing in incidence with the advent of PSA screening. However, management of this disease requires a multi-modality approach with a focus on radiation therapy and long-term androgen-deprivation therapy. Multiple series have demonstrated the efficacy of dose-escalated radiation therapy utilizing 3-D conformal radiation therapy, intensity-modulated radiation therapy, or brachytherapy. Further, multiple prospective randomized trials have demonstrated a benefit to the administration long-term hormonal therapy compared with no adjuvant hormonal therapy or short-term androgen deprivation. There is currently a limited role for surgical intervention in high-risk prostate cancer. While chemotherapy has been utilized in the setting of metastatic hormone-refractory prostate cancer for some time, more recent trials have looked at the role of adjuvant chemotherapy following definitive radiotherapy in high-risk patients. Results are pending at this time. With the advent of modern technologies, including image-guided radiation therapy, acute and chronic GI, and GU toxicities are relatively low compared to traditional techniques.

Keywords: prostate cancer, dose escalation, hormonal therapy, toxicity

■ INTRODUCTION

High-risk prostate cancer (PCA) represents a wide spectrum of disease which requires a multi-disciplinary approach involving radiation oncology, urology, and medical oncology. The definition of high-risk disease varies by organization and institution. The National Comprehensive Cancer Network (NCCN) definition for high-risk PCA includes patients with Gleason 8–10 disease, prostate-specific antigen (PSA)

> 20 ng/mL, or T3a or higher disease (1). The Radiation Therapy Oncology Group (RTOG) risk classification stratifies high-risk patients as patients with T1–2 disease with a Gleason score 8–10 or T3 disease/N1 disease with Gleason 7 histology (2). The D'Amico classification system defines high-risk disease as T2c or greater, PSA > 20 ng/mL, or a Gleason score of greater than 8 (3). Workup for patients with high-risk PCA includes preparing a history, a physical examination with digital rectal examination, PSA, bone scan, CT or MRI scan of the pelvis, and biopsy. While bone scan and imaging of the pelvis has a low yield in low and intermediate risk PCA, the risk of finding more advanced disease on bone scan or CT scan is 10% and 20%, respectively, in high-risk patients (4). The NCCN currently gives radiation therapy with

*Corresponding author, Rose Cancer Center, Oakland University William Beaumont School of Medicine, William Beaumont Hospital, 3601 W. 13 Mile Rd, Royal Oak, MI 48073

E-mail address: amartinez@beaumont.edu

Radiation Medicine Rounds 2:1 (2011) 35–42.
DOI: 10.5003/2151–4208.2.1.35

long-term (2–3 years) androgen-deprivation therapy (ADT) a Category 1 recommendation. Radical prostatectomy with pelvic lymph node (LN) dissection is an alternative, but is a Category 2A recommendation for high-risk patients, at this time (1). The purpose of this chapter is to review the data on treatment modalities available for high-risk patients and potential toxicities following radiation therapy.

■ TREATMENT

Radiation Therapy

It is well established with the publication of multiple randomized Phase III trials that dose escalation improves biochemical control for patients with high-risk PCA (5–8). The MDACC trial randomized patients to receive 70 Gy versus 78 Gy to the isocenter, utilizing a 3D conformal boost technique.

At 8 years, there was a significant improvement in freedom from biochemical failure in the high-risk group (63% vs. 26%) (8). Similar studies with dose escalation were performed by the MRC and Dutch groups and found improvements in biochemical progression-free survival (PFS) with dose escalation in high-risk PCA (6,7). Various modalities may be utilized to provide dose escalation, including 3D conformal radiation therapy, intensity-modulated radiation therapy with or without image guidance, and low-dose rate or high-dose rate (HDR) boosts to traditional external beam radiation therapy (EBRT). The results from multiple trials evaluating various forms of dose escalation with long-term outcomes in high-risk PCA patients are presented in Table 1 (7–11). Recently, Martinez et al. examined outcomes in patients with GS 8–10 disease receiving a hypofractionated regimen with 5 weeks of pelvic EBRT combined with a dose escalated HDR interstitial

TABLE 1 Summary of radiation therapy outcomes for high-risk prostate cancer

Author (year)	Dearnaley 2007 (7)	Kuban 2008 (8)	Zelefsky 2008 (9)	Stock 2009 (10)	Martinez 2010 (11)	
Dose escalation technique	EBRT 74 Gy	EBRT 78 Gy	EBRT 70.2–86.4 Gy	EBRT + LDR	EBRT + HDR	
No. of patients	184 (high-risk); 50 (GS 8–10)	53 (high-risk); 27 (GS 8–10)	752 (high-risk); 350 (GS 8–10)	181 (GS 8–10)	488	
Pretreatment PSA	12.8 ng/mL (median)	NR	NR	9 (mean); 14 (median)	11.0 ng/mL (median); 19.3 ng/mL (mean)	
PSA failure	nadir + 2 ng/mL	nadir + 2 ng/mL	nadir + 2 ng/mL	nadir + 2 ng/mL	PSA nadir + 2 ng/mL	
Median FU	5.25 years	8.7 years	6.6 years	5.42	4.7 years (median); 5.5 years (mean)	
BC	57% @ 5 years	63% @ 8 years	44% @ 7 years	73% @ 8 years	74.8% @ 5 years	57.4% @ 10 years
DMFS	NR	96% @ 8 years	76% @ 7 years	80% @ 8 years	88.0% @ 5 years	77.9% @ 10 years
Clinical PFS	NR	NR	NR	NR	84.0% @ 5 years	72.0% @ 10 years
CSS	NR	NR	NR	87% @ 8 years	93.9% @ 5 years	83.8% @ 10 years
OS	NR	NR	NR	79% @ 8 years	86.5% @ 5 years	65.1% @ 10 years
Adjuvant Tx	NR	NR	NR	NR	13% ADT for salvage	

NR, not reported; GS, Gleason Score; BC, biochemical control; DMFS, distant metastasis-free survival; PFS, progression-free survival; CSS, cause-specific survival; OS, overall survival.

boost. The 5- and 10-year rates of biochemical control were 74.8% and 57.4%, respectively, with a 10-year cause-specific survival (CSS) of 83.8% (11). Currently, the NCCN recommends a dosage of 78 to 80 Gy to the prostate, with our without the utilization of pelvic LN irradiation (1). While hypofractionation could potentially reduce treatment duration, data at this time is limited to single institution studies or studies with limited follow up; for example, a study from the Cleveland Clinic has found a 5-year biochemical PFS rate of 72%, utilizing 2.5 Gy per fraction to a total dosage of 70 Gy (12). Future studies will examine the potential role of hypofractionation and gastrointestinal (GI) and genitourinary (GU) toxicities that may develop due to following this form of treatment.

Pelvic radiation therapy has been a traditional part of treatment of high-risk PCA patients with the hypothesis being that the use of the pelvic field could eradicate potential un-diagnosed micro-metastatic disease within the pelvis. While still utilized frequently in high-risk patients, controversy exists at this time regarding the role of pelvic radiation therapy in high-risk cancer patients. RTOG 94–13 utilized a 2 × 2 factorial design that examined the role of pelvic radiation therapy and the sequencing of hormonal therapy. A total of 1,323 patients with PSA < 100 ng/mL and an LN risk of greater than 15% (by Roach formula) were randomized to whole pelvis treatment or prostate only treatment. While the trial was not powered to show a difference in any one arm, no benefit in clinical outcomes was noted with pelvis therapy (13). The GETUG-01 trial randomized 444 patients with T1–3bN0 disease in a treatment with 66 to 70 Gy, with or without the incorporation of 46 Gy of pelvic treatment. While limited by a large number of patients that were not high-risk, no benefit to pelvic treatment was noted (14).

LN-positive patients represent a challenging subset of high-risk PCA patients. Review of RTOG 75–06 demonstrated that a small subset of node-positive patients were cured at 10 years with radiation therapy (15). A review of 255 LN positive patients found that patients receiving RT in addition to ADT improved 10-year overall survival (OS) by 21% and freedom from relapse by 55% (16). A subset analysis of 173 patients enrolled on RTOG 85–31, that were LN positive, found that hormonal therapy, in addition to radiation therapy, improved biochemical control, distant metastases, and OS, suggesting that the management of patients with LN disease should include radiation therapy and ADT (17).

Surgery

At this time, surgery is not the recommended treatment for patients with high-risk PCA (1). Multiple surgical series have examined outcomes following radical prostatectomy in high-risk patients. One of the largest series was reported by Lau et al, which examined 407 patients with GS 8–10 disease. Within the cohort, 45% received adjuvant treatment and 38% received hormonal therapy. 27% of the patients were found to be node positive and 48% were with pathological T3. At 10 years, the PFS rate and OS rate were only 36% and 67%, respectively; however, the CSS rate was 85% (18). Table 2 summarizes multiple surgical series evaluating outcomes following RP for GS 8–10 disease (11,19–22). On the far right of the table, for comparison, are the outcomes of a recent radiation therapy trial of high-risk patients. In comparison, the surgical outcomes had much worse biochemical control outcomes, with 5-year rates of 20% to 62%, compared to 75% from the radiation trial (11).

Androgen-Deprivation Therapy

ADT is considered standard of care for high-risk PCA patients at this time (1). Multiple trials have evaluated the efficacy, sequencing, and duration of hormonal therapy.

Short-Term

Short-term ADT was evaluated in RTOG 86–10 which randomized 456 patients with palpable, bulky (5 × 5) T2–4 tumors, with or without LN involvement, to radiation therapy (66–70 Gy, with 44–46 Gy of the whole pelvis) with or without 4 months of ADT (2 months neoadjuvant, 2 months concurrent). After 10 years, there was a significant improvement in CSS, biochemical failure, and distant metastases (23). This benefit was confirmed in a trial from MGH which examined 206 intermediate and high-risk patients, randomized to receive 6 months (2 months neoadjuvant, 2 months concurrent, and 2 months adjuvant) of ADT or not with radiation therapy. This trial found an 8-year OS benefit (74% vs. 61%) which held for high-risk patients (24).

Long-Term

Long-term ADT is defined as more than 6 months of treatment. However, the typical duration of ADT

TABLE 2   Summary of radical prostatectomy outcomes for Gleason 8–10 prostate cancer

Author (year)	Do (19) 2001	Manoharan (20) 2003	Boorjian (21) 2007	Audenet (22) 2009	Martinez (11)	
Publication year	2001	2003	2007	2009	2010	
No. of patients GS 8–10	87	54	584	62	488	
Pretreatment PSA	16.2 ng/mL (median)	13 ng/mL (mean)	NR	11.9 ng/mL (mean)	11.0 ng/mL (median); 19.3 ng/mL (mean)	
PSA failure	ASTRO	PSA ≥ 0.4 ng/mL	PSA ≥ 0.4 ng/mL	PSA ≥ 0.2 ng/mL	PSA nadir + 2 ng/mL	
Median FU	6.22 years	4.1 years	8.3 years	7.0 years	4.7 years (median); 5.5 years (mean)	
BC	20% @ 5 years	62%	42% @ 7 years	44 % @ 5 years	74.8% @ 5 years	57.4%@ 10 years
DMFS	NR	NR	82% @ 7 years	NR	88.0% @ 5years	77.9% @ 10 years
Clinical PFS	35% @ 5 years	NR	NR	NR	84.0% @ 5 years	72.0% @ 10 years
CSS	NR	NR	89% @ 7 years	NR	93.9% @ 5 years	83.8% @ 10 years
OS	NR	NR	NR	NR	86.5% @ 5 years	65.1% @ 10 years
Adjuvant Tx	NR	NR	38% adj. ADT; 28% salvage ADT	5% adj. ADT; 31% adj. RT; 8% adj. ADT+RT	13% ADT for salvage	

NR, not reported; GS, Gleason Score; BC, biochemical control; DMFS, distant metastasis-free survival; PFS, progression-free survival; CSS, cause-specific survival; OS, overall survival; Adj, adjuvant.

in high-risk patients is 2 to 3 years, based on published studies. RTOG 85–31 initially evaluated the role of long-term ADT on a heterogeneous population of patients. 945 patients with clinical T3 disease or node positive disease, or postprostatectomy patients with pathological T3 disease, were randomized to receive radiation therapy (65–70 Gy, 44–46 Gy to the pelvis) with or without indefinite goserelin, which began during the last week of radiation therapy. At 10 years, the OS was improved (49% vs. 39%), as was local failure (23% vs. 38%), DM (24% vs. 39%), and disease-specific mortality (16% vs. 22%). A subset analysis of this trial found that the OS and CSS benefit was limited only to GS 7–10 patients, who were primarily high risk (25). RTOG 92–02 randomized 1,554 patients with T2-T4 disease and a PSA < 150 ng/mL, to radiation therapy (65–70 Gy, 44–46 Gy to the pelvis), with or without ADT for 2 years. At 10 years, there was no difference in OS, but an improvement in CSS, DFS, BF, and

DM. A subset analysis of this trial found that there was an OS benefit for patients with GS 8–10 (45% vs. 32%) (26). EORTC 22863 randomized 415 patients with T1–2 disease and GS of 7 or greater, or T3–4 disease, to radiation therapy (70 Gy, 50 Gy to the pelvis), with or without ADT for 3 years (goserelin + cyproterone for 1 month), beginning on the first day of RT. At 10 years, there was a significant benefit in OS and CSS, with the addition of ADT. Further, DM were decreased by 20% and DFS increased by 24% (27). To compare short-term with long-term ADT, EORTC 22961 randomized 970 patients displaying T2c-T4 disease with PSA < 160 ng/mL, or node-positive patients to radiation therapy (70 Gy, 50 Gy to the pelvis) and 6 months versus 3 years of ADT. At 5 years, there was an improvement in BF (22% vs. 41%), PCA mortality (3% vs. 5%), and OS (85% vs. 81%) with 3 years of ADT (28). Despite the evidence for long-term ADT, the role of ADT with dose escalated RT remains to be answered as the majority of studies performed were done with substandard dosing based on current recommendations. However, recent data suggests that the benefit of ADT might not be as significant with dose-escalated RT (29).

Chemotherapy

There is limited prospective Phase III data regarding the use of chemotherapy in nonmetastatic PCA. A trial performed at Nihon University in Japan randomized 39 patients with intermediate or high-risk PCA by NCCN guidelines to radiation therapy accompanied by ADT, with or without neoadjuvant and concurrent estramustine for 6 months. With a 2-year follow-up period, there was a statistically significant improvement in biochemical control with good toxicity profiles, for both arms (30). RTOG 9902 was a Phase III trial with 397 patients with high-risk PCA (PSA 20–100 and GS ≥ 7 or T2+ with GS 8, PSA < 100) who received radiation therapy with ADT (2/2/2 scheme), with or without four cycles of TEE (paclitaxel, estramustine, and etoposide) chemotherapy. The trial closed early, secondary to increased thromboembolic events in the chemotherapy arm, but no clinical outcomes have been published at this time (31). In metastatic PCA, the combination of docetaxel and prednisone was found to lead to improved survival compared to mitoxantrone and prednisone (32). Based on this data, RTOG 05–21 opened, enrolling high-risk patients (GS ≤ 9 with a PSA ≤ 150 ng/mL or T2 or higher with a GS 8, PSA < 20 ng/mL or GS 7–8 with a PSA 20–150 ng/mL) with clinically negative LNs. Patients received RT of 72 to 75.6 Gy with 24 months of ADT (2/2/2 scheme) with or without the addition of six cycles of docetaxel and prednisone following RT. This trial recently closed to accrual, with no outcomes available at this time.

■ TOXICITY

Toxicity from treatment can be broken down into toxicity secondary to radiation therapy and secondary to ADT. Adverse effects with ADT can include osteoporosis and subsequent fractures, obesity, insulin resistance, changes in lipid profiles, and cardiovascular disease (1). The greatest controversy regarding ADT is the risk of cardiovascular disease, and conflicting reports exist. A review of

RTOG 85–31, 86–10, and 92–02 has not found any increase in fatal cardiac events, which was confirmed by analysis of the EORTC 22863 and EORTC 22961 (27,28,33).

With regard to radiation therapy, toxicity is primarily limited to GI and GU toxicity and can be broken down into acute and chronic toxicities. A recent review of approximately 2,000 patients treated with definitive radiation at William Beaumont Hospital outlines the acute and long-term toxicities experienced by patients, according to the NCI-CTC (v 3.0). This study found that the rate of any acute toxicity that is Grade 2 or greater was 49% for dose-escalated EBRT utilizing image guidance (IGRT) and 55% for EBRT + HDR boost (Table 3). IGRT had a 43% rate of any GU Grade 2+ toxicity and a 16% rate of any GI Grade 2+ toxicity, while EBRT + HDR Boost had a 50% rate of any GU Grade 2+ toxicity and a 26% rate of any GI Grade 2+ toxicity (34). Table 4 lists rates of chronic GU and GI toxicities, utilizing IGRT and EBRT with HDR boost. The rate of any late GU toxicity Grade 2+ is 21% for IGRT and 28% for EBRT + HDR Boost, while the rate of any late GI toxicity Grade 2+ is 20% for IGRT

TABLE 3 Acute genitourinary (GU) and gastrointestinal (GI) toxicity ≥ grade 2

	EB-IGRT (%)	EBRT + HDR (%)
Percent of patients receiving hormones	24	53
Acute GU		
Dysuria	8	25
Frequency	39	38
Retention	6	6
Hematuria	3	0.6
Incontinence	2	1
Any acute GU	43	50
Acute GI		
Diarrhea	9	21
Tenesmus	16	21
Bleeding	3	1
Any acute GI	16	26
Any acute toxicity	49	55

EB-IGRT, image-guided external beam radiotherapy; EBRT + HDR, external beam radiotherapy with HDR BT boost; GU, genitourinary; GI, gastrointestinal.

TABLE 4 Late genitourinary (GU) and gastrointestinal (GI) toxicity ≥ grade 2

	EB-IGRT (%)	EBRT + HDR (%)
Percent of patients receiving hormones	24	53
Late GU		
Dysuria	0.5	3
Frequency/urgency	14	17
Retention	3	12
Hematuria	7	4
Incontinence	3	5
Urethral stricture	2	11
Any late GU	21	28
Late GI		
Diarrhea	2	2
Rectal bleeding	16	7
Proctitis	5	3
Rectal incontinence	3	0.8
Nausea	0	0
Any late GI	20	9

EB-IGRT, image-guided external beam radiotherapy; EBRT+HDR, external beam radiotherapy with HDR BT boost; GU, genitourinary.

and 9% for EBRT + HDR Boost. The rates of Grade 3, and higher, toxicity are relatively rare with modern IGRT and EBRT + HDR boost treatments.

■ REFERENCES

1. NCCN Clinical Practice Guidelines in Oncology: Prostate Cancer, V.1.2011. http://www.nccn.org/professionals/physician_gls/PDF/prostate.pdf. Accessed December 13, 2010.
2. Roach M, Lu J, Pilepich MV, et al. Predicting long-term survival, and the need for hormonal therapy: a meta-analysis of RTOG prostate cancer trials. *Int J Radiat Oncol Biol Phys.* 2000;47(3):617–627.
3. D'Amico AV, Whittington R, Malkowicz SB, et al. Biochemical outcome after radical prostatectomy, external beam radiation therapy, or interstitial radiation therapy for clinically localized prostate Cancer. *JAMA.* 1998;280(11):969–974.
4. Albertsen PC, Hanley JA, Harlan LC, et al. The positive yield of imaging studies in the evaluation of men with newly diagnosed prostate cancer: a population based analysis. *J Urol.* 2000;163(4):1138–1143.
5. Zietman AL, Bae K, Slater JD, et al. Randomized trial comparing conventional-dose with high-dose conformal radiation therapy in early-stage adenocarcinoma of the prostate: long-term results from Proton Radiation Oncology Group/American College of Radiology 95–09. *J Clin Oncol.* 2010;28(7):1106–1111.
6. Peeters ST, Heemsbergen WD, Koper PC, et al. Dose-response in radiotherapy for localized prostate cancer: results of the Dutch multicenter randomized phase II trial comparing 68 Gy of radiotherapy with 78 Gy. *J Clin Oncol.* 2006;24(13):1990–1996.
7. Dearnaley DP, Sydes MR, Graham JD, et al. Escalated-dose versus standard-dose conformal radiotherapy in prostate cancer: first results from the MRC RT01 randomised controlled trial. *Lancet Oncol.* 2007;8(6):475–487.
8. Kuban DA, Tucker SL, Dong L, et al. Long-term results of the M.D. Anderson randomized dose-escalation trial for prostate cancer. *Int J Radiat Oncol Biol Phys.* 2008;70(1):67–74.
9. Zelefsky MJ, Yamada Y, Fuks Z, et al. Long-term results of conformal radiotherapy for prostate cancer: impact of dose escalation on biochemical tumor control and distant metastases-free survival outcomes. *Int J Radiat Oncol Biol Phys.* 2008;71(4):1028–1033.
10. Stock RG, Cesaretti JA, Hall SJ, et al. Outcomes for patients with high-grade prostate cancer treated with a combination of brachytherapy, external beam radiotherapy and hormonal therapy. *BJU Int.* 2009;104(11):1631–1636.
11. Martinez AA, Mohammed N, Demanes DJ, et al. Improved 10-year outcomes for prostate cancer patients with Gleason 8–10 treated with external beam radiation and high dose rate brachytherapy boost in the PSA era. *J Urol.* Publication pending.
12. Kupelian PA, Willoughby TR, Reddy CA, et al. Hypofractionated intensity-modulated radiotherapy (70 Gy at 2.5 Gy per fraction) for localized prostate cancer: Cleveland Clinic experience. *Int J Radiat Oncol Biol Phys.* 2007;68(5):1424–1430.
13. Lawton CA, DeSilvio M, Roach M, et al. An update of the phase III trial comparing whole pelvic to prostate only radiotherapy and neoadjuvant to adjuvant total androgen suppression: updated analysis of RTOG 94–13, with emphasis on unexpected hormone/radiation interactions. *Int J Radiat Oncol Biol Phys.* 2007;69(3);646–655.
14. Pommier P, Chabaud S, Lagrange JL, et al. Is there a role for pelvic irradiation in localized prostate adenocarcinoma? Preliminary results of GETUG-01. *J Clin Oncol.* 2007;25(34):5366–5373.
15. Hanks GE, Buzydlowski J, Sause WT, et al. Ten-year outcomes for pathologic node-positive patients treated in RTOG 75–06. *Int J Radiat Oncol Biol Phys.* 1998;40(4), 765–768.
16. Zagars GK, Pollack A, von Eschenbach AC. Addition of radiation therapy to androgen ablation improves outcomes for subclinically node-positive prostate cancer. *Urology.* 2001;58(2):233–239.

17. Lawton CA, Winter K, Grignon D, et al. Androgen suppression plus radiation versus radiation alone for patients with stage D1/pathologic node-positive adenocarcinoma of the prostate. Updated results based on national prospective randomized trial Radiation Therapy Oncology Group 85–31. *J Clin Oncol*. 3005;23(4): 800–807.

18. Lau WK, Bergstralh EJ, Blute ML, et al. Radical prostatectomy for pathological Gleason 8 or greater prostate cancer: influence of concomitant pathological variables. *J Urol*. 2002;167(1):117–122.

19. Do TM, Parker RG, Smith RB, et al. High-grade carcinoma of the prostate: a comparison of current local therapies. *Urology*. 2001;57(6):1121–1126.

20. Manoharan M, Bird VG, Kim SS, et al. Outcome after radical prostatectomy with a pretreatment prostate biopsy Gleason score of ≥8. *BJU Int*. 2003;92(6): 539–544.

21. Boorjian SA, Karnes RJ, Rangel LJ, et al. Impact of prostate-specific antigen testing on the clinical and pathological outcomes after radical prostatectomy for Gleason 8–10 cancers. *BJU Int*. 2008;101(3):299–304.

22. Audenet F, Comperat E, Seringe E, et al. Oncologic control obtained after radical prostatectomy in men with a pathological Gleason score ≥8: a single-center experience. *Urol Oncol*. 2009 Nov 17. [Epub ahead of print].

23. Roach M, Bae K, Speight J. Short-term neoadjuvant androgen deprivation therapy and external beam radiotherapy for locally advanced prostate cancer: long-term results of RTOG 8610. *J Clin Oncol*. 2008;26(4):585–591.

24. Nguyen PL, Chen MH, Beard CJ, et al. Radiation with or without 6 months of androgen suppression therapy in intermediate- and high-risk clinically localized prostate cancer: a postrandomization analysis by risk group. *Int J Radiat Oncol Biol Phys*. 2010;77(4):1046–1052.

25. Pilepich MV, Winter K, Lawton CA, et al. Androgen suppression adjuvant to definitive radiotherapy in prostate carcinoma—long-term results of phase III RTOG 85–31. *Int J Radiat Oncol Biol Phys*. 2005;61(5): 1285–1290

26. Horwitz EM, Bae K, Hanks GE, et al. Ten-year follow-up of Radiation Therapy Oncology Group protocol 92–02: a phase III trial of the duration of elective androgen deprivation in locally advanced prostate cancer. *J Clin Oncol*. 2008;26(15):2497–2504.

27. Bolla M, Collette L, Blank L, et al. Long-term results with immediate androgen suppression and external irradiation in patients with locally advanced prostate cancer (an EORTC study): a phase III randomised trial. *Lancet*. 2002;360:103–106.

28. Bolla M, de Reijke TM, Van Tienhoven G, et al. Duration of androgen suppression in the treatment of prostate cancer. *NEJM*. 2009;360(24):2516–2527.

29. Krauss D, Kestin L, Ye H, et al. Lack of benefit for the addition of androgen deprivation therapy to dose-escalated radiotherapy in the treatment of intermediate and high-risk prostate cancer. *Int J Radiat Oncol Biol Phys*. 2010 June 26. [Epub ahead of print].

30. Hirano D, Nagane Y, Satoh K, et al. Neoadjuvant LHRH analog plus estramustine phosphate combined with three-dimensional conformal radiotherapy for intermediate-to high-risk prostate cancer: a randomized study. *Int Urol Nephrol*. 2010;42(1):81–88.

31. Rosenthal SA, Bae K, Pienta KJ, et al. Phase III multi-institutional trial of adjuvant chemotherapy with paclitaxel, estramustine, and oral etoposide combined with long-term androgen suppression therapy and radiotherapy versus long-term androgen suppression plus radiotherapy alone for high-risk prostate cancer: preliminary toxicity analysis of RTOG 99–02. *Int J Radiat Oncol Biol Phys*. 2009;73(3):672–678.

32. Berthold DR, Pond GR, Soban F, et al. Docetaxel plus prednisone or mitxantrone plus prednisone for advanced prostate cancer: updated survival in the TAX 327 study. *J Clin Oncol*. 2008;26(2):242–245.

33. Lawton CA, Bae K, Pilepich M, et al. Long-term treatment sequelae after external beam irradiation with or without hormonal manipulation for adenocarcinoma of the prostate: analysis of Radiation Therapy Oncology Group studies 85–31, 86–10, and 92–02. *Int J Radiat Oncol Biol Phys*. 2008;70(2):437–441.

34. Mohammed N, Kestin L, Ghilezan M, et al. Comparison of acute and late toxicities for three modern high-dose radiation treatment techniques for localized prostate cancer. *Int J Radiat Oncol Biol Phys*. 2010 Dec 16. [Epub ahead of print].

Duration and Timing of Neoadjuvant/Adjuvant Androgen Deprivation in Nonmetastatic Prostate Cancer

Ronald C. Chen[1]*, Jordan A. Holmes[1], and Anthony V. D'Amico[2]

[1]*University of North Carolina, Chapel Hill, NC*

[2]*Dana-Farber Cancer Institute/Brigham and Women's Hospital, Boston, MA*

■ ABSTRACT

External beam radiation therapy (EBRT) plus androgen-deprivation therapy (ADT) is a well-established treatment regimen for patients with high-risk localized and locally advanced prostate cancer. Two trials randomizing patients on ADT, with versus without EBRT, have established a survival benefit from EBRT in these patients. In addition, multiple randomized trials have consistently demonstrated a benefit from adding short-term or long-term ADT to EBRT. Recently, the toxicity of ADT has been better elucidated, including a potential association between ADT and cardiovascular disease. Data on the benefit of adding ADT to EBRT, optimal timing and duration of ADT, choice and extent of ADT agents, toxicity of treatment, and appropriate patient selection will be reviewed. Potential treatments for ADT-associated hot flashes, sexual dysfunction, and fatigue are also described.

Keywords: prostate cancer, radiation therapy, androgen deprivation therapy

External beam radiation therapy (EBRT) plus androgen-deprivation therapy (ADT) is the most well-established treatment regimen for patients with high-risk localized and locally advanced prostate cancer. Two trials randomizing patients on ADT, with versus without EBRT, have established a survival benefit from EBRT in these patients (1,2). In addition, multiple randomized trials, many conducted by the Radiation Therapy Oncology Group (RTOG) and European Organisation for Research and Treatment of Cancer (EORTC), have consistently demonstrated a benefit from adding ADT to EBRT. Recently, the toxicity of ADT has been better elucidated, including a potential association between ADT treatment and cardiovascular disease. In this chapter, data on the benefit of adding ADT to EBRT, optimal timing and duration of ADT, choice and extent of ADT agents, toxicity of treatment, and appropriate patient selection will be reviewed.

*Corresponding author, Department of Radiation Oncology, University of North Carolina, CB #7512, Chapel Hill, NC 27599

E-mail address: ronald_chen@med.unc.edu

Radiation Medicine Rounds 2:1 (2011) 43–58.
DOI: 10.5003/2151–4208.2.1.43

■ COMMONLY USED AGENTS FOR ANDROGEN DEPRIVATION AND MECHANISMS OF ACTION

Two classes of ADT agents are commonly used with radiation therapy (Table 1). Luteinizing hormone-releasing hormone (LHRH) agonists—also called gonadotropin-releasing hormone (GnRH) agonists—are synthetic peptides which bind to the GnRH receptors on pituitary gonadotropin-producing cells, causing the release of leuteinizing hormone (LH) and follicle stimulating hormone (FSH). This, in turn, leads to an initial increase in testosterone production from testicular Leydig cells. In a recent prospective study, 80% of the patients experienced a testosterone surge after receiving an LHRH agonist (3). Over time, LHRH agonists induce downregulation of the GnRH receptors in the pituitary, leading to a decline in LH and FSH production, and testosterone down to castrate levels (4,5). The time from start of treatment to maximal testosterone suppression is approximately 4 weeks (3). Available LHRH agonists include leuprolide, goserelin, and triptorelin.

Antiandrogens are compounds which bind to androgen receptors and competitively inhibit their interaction with testosterone and dihydrotestosterone. Antiandrogens are commonly used either before the start of LHRH agonist therapy, to prevent a disease flare due to the acute testosterone surge, or in conjunction with an LHRH agonist to provide maximal androgen blockade. In the treatment of prostate cancer, antiandrogens are not commonly used alone without an LHRH agonist. Available formulations include flutamide, bicalutamide, and nilutamide.

TABLE 1 Commonly used androgen deprivation therapy agents

Luteinizing Hormone-Releasing Hormone Agonists

    Leuprolide

    Goserelin

    Triptorelin

    Buserelin (not available in US)

Antiandrogens

    Flutamide

    Bicalutamide

    Nilutamide

    Cyproterone acetate (Europe)

■ TRIALS DEMONSTRATING A BENEFIT FROM ADDING ADT TO EBRT

At least eight randomized trials have compared EBRT alone versus EBRT plus ADT in the treatment of nonmetastatic prostate cancer. It is instructive to examine these trials based on the disease characteristics of the enrolled patients: five trials included mainly patients with localized prostate cancer (T1-T2, intermediate or high-risk), and three included mainly patients with locally advanced disease (T3-T4 or node positive).

Benefit of Adding ADT to EBRT in Localized Prostate Cancer

The Dana-Farber trial randomized 206 patients with EBRT versus EBRT plus 6 months of ADT (6,7) (Table 2). All patients had localized disease: 74% were intermediate-risk using the D'Amico criteria (8), and 26% were high-risk. EBRT plus ADT demonstrated an improved prostate cancer–specific survival and overall survival compared to EBRT alone. The 8-year overall survival rates were 74% (EBRT plus ADT) versus 61% (EBRT alone, $P = .01$) (6). In subgroup analysis, the survival benefit from the addition of ADT was similar for both intermediate and high-risk patients (9). In a Cox multivariable regression model for patients with intermediate-risk prostate cancer, after adjusting for age, Gleason score, prostate-specific antigen (PSA), and comorbidity, treatment with EBRT alone was associated with a three-fold higher risk of death compared with EBRT plus ADT. Similarly, in a separate model for men with high-risk disease, the risk of death for EBRT alone was 3.3-fold higher, compared to EBRT plus ADT.

RTOG 94–08 also demonstrated an overall survival benefit from the addition of short-term ADT to EBRT (10). This trial included patients with low (35%), intermediate (54%) and high-risk prostate cancer (11%), and randomized patients to EBRT alone versus EBRT plus 4 months of ADT. Ten-year overall survival rates were 57% (EBRT) versus 62% (EBRT plus ADT, $P = .03$), and a subgroup analysis demonstrated the most benefit for intermediate- and high-risk patients.

The Trans-Tasman Radiation Oncology Group (TROG) 96.01 trial included a mixture of patients with intermediate-risk localized prostate cancer (16%), high-risk localized (44%), and locally advanced

TABLE 2 Randomized trials comparing EBRT vs. EBRT plus different durations of ADT in patients with localized prostate cancer

	Median FU (Years)	Patient Inclusion	Treatment Arms	OS (%)	CSS (%)	DF (%)	bFFS (%)	LF (%)
Dana-Farber (6) (N = 206)	7.6	T1-T2 (74% intermediate risk, 26% high-risk)	EBRT EBRT + 6 months ADT	(8 year) 74 61 (P = .01)	(8 year) HR 4.1 (P = .01)	NA	NA	NA
RTOG 94-08 (10) (N = 1,979)	9.1	T1b-T2b (35% low-risk, 54% intermediate-risk, 11% high-risk)	EBRT EBRT + 4 months ADT	(10 year) 57 62 (P = .03)	(10 year) 93 96 (P < .01)	NA	NA	(2 year)++ 39 21 (P < .01)
TROG 96.01 (11) (N = 802)	5.9	60% T2 (16% intermediate-risk, 44% high-risk), 40% T3-T4	EBRT EBRT + 3 months ADT EBRT + 6 months ADT	NA	(5 year) 91 92 94 (P = .04)	(5 year) 19 22 13 (P = .05)	(5 year)* 38 52 (P < .01) 56 (P < .01)	(5 year) 28 17 (P < .01) 12 (P < .01)
Quebec 1 (12) (N = 161)	5	~70% T2, ~30% T3	EBRT EBRT + 3 months ADT EBRT + 10 months ADT	NA	NA	NA	(7 year)** 42 66 (P < .01) 69 (P < .01)	NA
Quebec 2 (12) (N = 296)	3.7	86% T2, 14% T3	EBRT + 5 months ADT EBRT + 10 months ADT	NA	NA	NA	(4 year)** 70 70 (P = .55)	NA
Canadian (15) (N = 361)	6.6	87% T2 (25% low-risk, 43% intermediate-risk, 18% high-risk), 13% T3	EBRT + 3 months ADT EBRT + 8 months ADT	(7 year) 81 79 (P = .7)	(7 year) 94 93 (P = .24)	NA	(7 year)*** 58 65 (P = .18)	NA
Quebec (16) (N = 120)	NA	74% T2, 26% T3	EBRT EBRT + 3 months ADT EBRT + 9 months ADT	NA	NA	NA	NA	(1 year)*+ 62 30 4 (P < .01)
RTOG 92-02 (19) (N = 1,521)	11.3*++	T2c (45%), T3 (52%), T4 (3%)	EBRT + 4 months ADT EBRT + 28 months ADT	(10 year) 52 54 (P = .36)	(10 year) 84 89 (P < .01)	(10 year) 23 15 (P < .01)	(10 year)++ 13 23 (P < .01)	(10 year) 22 12 (P < .01)

FU, follow-up; OS, overall survival; CSS, cancer-specific survival; DF, distant failure; bFFS, biochemical failure-free survival; LF, local failure; EBRT, external beam radiation therapy; ADT, androgen deprivation therapy; HR, hazard ratio; NA, not available.

*Biochemical failure defined as nadir+2

**Biochemical failure defined as two consecutive rises in PSA with PSA value at least 1.5 ng/mL.

***Freedom from any failure. Biochemical failure defined as nadir+2.

*+Positive biopsy rate at 12 months.

*++Disease-free survival. Biochemical failure defined as three consecutive rises in PSA, PSA > 4 ng/mL, or receiving additional ADT.

++Positive biopsy rate at 2 years.

**+Median follow-up for survivors.

disease (T3-T4, 40%) (11). Patients were randomized to receive EBRT alone, EBRT plus 3 months of ADT, or EBRT plus 6 months of ADT. Compared to EBRT alone, EBRT plus 3 months of ADT reduced local failure, improved biochemical failure-free survival, and disease-free survival. EBRT plus 6 months of ADT (compared to EBRT alone) improved upon these endpoints, as well as distant failures and prostate cancer–specific survival. In the subgroup of patients with high-risk or locally advanced disease, the addition of 6 months of ADT improved disease-free survival (hazard ratio [HR] = .52, 95% confidence interval [CI] .42–.66) and prostate cancer–specific survival (HR = .56, 95% CI .32–.96). There also appeared to be a benefit for intermediate-risk patients (HR = .80 for disease-free survival) but the sample size was too small to be of statistical significance.

Laverdière et al. reported results of two randomized trials from Quebec that included, mostly, patients with localized prostate cancer (12). The first trial included approximately 70% patients with T2 disease, randomized to receive EBRT alone versus EBRT plus 3 months of ADT versus EBRT plus 10 months of ADT. After 5 years of follow-up, the two arms with ADT (either for 3 months or 10 months) achieved similar biochemical relapse-free survival, and both were better, compared to EBRT alone. The second Quebec trial included 86% patients with T2 disease, and randomized patients to EBRT plus 5 versus 10 months of ADT. After 3.7 years of follow-up, no difference was found between the two groups in biochemical relapse-free survival rates (70% in both groups).

These trials demonstrate that for patients with localized, intermediate- or high-risk prostate cancer, the addition of short-term ADT to EBRT improves disease control and overall survival. It is important to note that only one of the trials described above included patients with low-risk prostate cancer (RTOG 94–08), and a survival benefit was not seen in the low-risk subgroup (10). For patients with low-risk disease, dose escalated radiation therapy alone has demonstrated excellent outcomes (13,14) and the addition of ADT is of unproven benefit.

Optimal Timing and Duration of ADT When Added to EBRT for Patients with Localized Prostate Cancer

Several randomized trials have examined the outcomes of different durations of ADT, when combined with EBRT, for patient with localized prostate cancer. In addition to TROG 96.01 (11) and the Quebec trials (12), a Canadian multi-center study randomized patients with EBRT plus 3 versus 8 months of ADT (15). In the Canadian trial, 87% of patients had localized prostate cancer (25% low-risk, 43% intermediate risk, 18% high risk), and 13% had T3 disease. Overall, the trial showed no difference in overall survival, cause-specific survival or freedom from any failure between the two arms. In a subgroup analysis, 8 versus 3 months of ADT resulted in improved freedom from any failure for patients with high-risk and locally-advanced disease (59% vs. 33%, P = .01).

For patients with intermediate-risk prostate cancer, EBRT plus 4 (RTOG 94–08) to 6 months (Dana-Farber) of ADT is appropriate. When used in the neoadjuvant and concurrent setting, ADT appears to potentiate the local effects of EBRT via cytoreduction (neoadjuvant) and radiosensitization (concurrent). In TROG 96.01, the use of neoadjuvant and concurrent ADT decreased local failures when compared to EBRT alone (11). In RTOG 94–08, patients underwent prostate biopsies 2 years after treatment (10). The addition of ADT significantly reduced the rate of positive biopsies (39% for EBRT alone vs. 21% for EBRT plus ADT, P < .01). Another trial compared EBRT alone versus EBRT plus 3 month of ADT versus EBRT plus 9 months of ADT (16). Patients underwent prostate biopsies 12 and 24 months after completion of radiation treatment. The rate of positive biopsies at 12 months were 62% (EBRT alone), 30% (EBRT plus 3 months ADT) and 4% (EBRT plus 9 months ADT, P < .01). Results for the 24-month biopsies were almost identical, confirming a local effect in neoadjuvant and concurrent ADT with EBRT. This trial, which showed an additional local control benefit when ADT lasted longer than 3 months, along with the two trials demonstrating an overall survival advantage of adding ADT to EBRT for intermediate-risk patients (Dana-Farber and RTOG 94–08), lends support to the use of 4 months (neoadjuvant and concurrent) or 6 months (neoadjuvant, concurrent, and adjuvant) of ADT in this patient group.

Attempts to better define the optimal timing and duration of ADT in relation to EBRT are being studied. In a Phase II trial from Columbia University, neoadjuvant ADT was used to maximally cytoreduce the prostate in each individual patient before the start of radiation treatment (17). This study used a combination of PSA nadir and digital rectal examinations to individualize the start of EBRT. This regimen was found to be feasible and safe, but disease control and survival results have not been reported. RTOG 99–10, which randomized patients with intermediate-risk prostate cancer to 2 versus 7 months of neoadjuvant ADT prior to EBRT, has finished accrual and the results are pending.

The addition of ADT may also be beneficial because of an effect on distant micrometastatic disease, which may be important for patients with intermediate-risk prostate cancer, and even more so for high-risk disease. In patients with high-risk prostate cancer, the trials suggest that long-term ADT may be necessary. In TROG 96.01, although both 3 and 6 months of ADT improved local control compared to EBRT alone, only 6 months of ADT reduced distant failures and improved cancer-specific survival (11). In accord with these findings, the Canadian trial demonstrated a benefit in 8 versus 3 months of ADT for the subgroup of patients with high-risk disease (15). Taken together, these trials demonstrate that 3 months of ADT may not be sufficient for patients with high-risk prostate cancer, despite localized disease.

RTOG 92–02 included a mixture of patients with high-risk localized (T2, 45%) and locally advanced disease (T3–4, 55%), and compared short-term versus long-term ADT (18,19). In this trial, patients received 4 months of neoadjuvant and concurrent ADT with EBRT and were randomized to no further treatment versus 24 months of additional ADT (total ADT duration: 4 months vs. 28 months). Long-term ADT improved local control, disease-free survival, and cancer-specific survival (19). Overall survival was improved in the subgroup of patients with Gleason 8–10 disease (10-year rates 31% for short-term ADT vs. 45% for long-term, $P < .01$). Analysis based on patients with high-risk localized versus locally advanced prostate cancer was not performed. RTOG 92–02 provides support for the use of EBRT with long-term neoadjuvant, concurrent, and adjuvant ADT, for patients with high-risk localized prostate cancer.

Benefit of Adding ADT to EBRT in Locally Advanced Prostate Cancer

RTOG 85–31 randomized patients with locally advanced prostate cancer (T3 or node positive) to EBRT versus EBRT plus indefinite ADT; 28% of

patients in this study were node positive (20–22) (Table 3). The addition of ADT improved all endpoints, including overall survival (22). In subgroup analysis, a survival benefit was seen in patients with Gleason 2–6, 7, and 8–10 disease; however, the benefit for the Gleason 2–6 subgroup (6% absolute difference) was not of sufficient magnitude to be statistically significant, potentially reflecting a lack of power for this subgroup comparison.

EORTC 22863 randomized patients with T3 (82%) or T4 (9%) disease to EBRT versus EBRT plus 3 years of ADT (23,24). Similar to RTOG 85–31, long-term ADT improved all endpoints, including overall survival, compared to EBRT alone.

RTOG 86–10 tested the potential benefit of adding short-term ADT to EBRT in this patient population (25,26). This trial included patients with bulky primary tumors (5 × 5 cm²), the majority of whom had locally advanced prostate cancer (70% with stage C disease). Patients were randomized to receive EBRT alone versus EBRT plus 4 months of ADT. The addition of short-term ADT improved local control, disease-free survival, cancer-specific survival but not overall survival, although the P-value (.12) approached statistical significance (26).

Overall, these studies demonstrated a consistent benefit in adding ADT to EBRT for patients with locally advanced prostate cancer. However, because both long-term and short-term ADT improved outcomes over EBRT alone, the optimal timing and duration of ADT for patients with locally advanced prostate cancer became the subject of further study.

Optimal Timing and Duration of ADT When Added to EBRT for Patients with Locally Advanced Prostate Cancer

Two randomized trials compared short-term versus long-term ADT, when combined with EBRT, for the treatment of locally advanced prostate cancer. RTOG 92–02, described above, included patients with localized and locally advanced (55%) disease, and demonstrated improved local control, disease-free survival, and cancer-specific survival from long-term (28 months) versus short-term (4 months) of ADT (18,19). EORTC 22961 had a similar randomization: patients received EBRT with 6 months of ADT, then were randomized to no further treatment versus 30 months of additional ADT (total ADT duration 6 months versus 36 months) (27). The

TABLE 3 Randomized trials comparing EBRT vs. EBRT plus different durations of ADT in patients with locally advanced prostate cancer

	Median FU (Years)	Patient Inclusion	Treatment Arms	OS (%)	CSS (%)	DF (%)	bFFS (%)	LF (%)
RTOG 85-31 (22) (N = 945)	7.6	T3 or N+ (28%)		(10 year)	(10 year)	(10 year)	(10 year)*	(10 year)
			EBRT	39	78	39	9	38
			EBRT + indef ADT	49 ($P < .01$)	84 ($P < .01$)	24 ($P < .01$)	31 ($P < .01$)	23 ($P < .01$)
EORTC 22863 (23) (N = 412)	5.5	T1–2 (7%), T3 (82%), T4 (9%)		(5 year)	(5 year)	(5 year)	(5 year)	(5 year)**
			EBRT	62	79	29	45	16
			EBRT + 3 year ADT	79 ($P < .01$)	94 ($P < .01$)	10 ($P < .01$)	76 ($P < .01$)	2 ($P < .01$)
RTOG 86-10 (26) (N = 456)	13*+	Bulky tumors (5 × 5 cm). 70% with Stage C (locally advanced)		(10 year)	(10 year DSM)	(10 year)	(10 year)***	
			EBRT	34	36	47	3	NA
			EBRT + 4 months ADT	43 ($P = .12$)	23 ($P = .01$)	35 ($P < .01$)	11 ($P <. 01$)	
RTOG 92-02 (19) (N = 1,521)	11.3*+	T2c (45%), T3 (52%), T4 (3%)		(10 year)	(10 year)	(10 year)	(10 year)*++	(10 year)
			EBRT + 4 months ADT	52	84	23	13	22
			EBRT + 28 months ADT	54 ($P = .36$)	89 ($P < .01$)	15 ($P < .01$)	23 ($P < .01$)	12 ($P < .01$)
EORTC 22961 (27) (N = 970)	6.4	T2c-T4N0 (92%), N+ (8%)		(5-year OM)	(5-year CSM)	(5 year)++	(5-year BP)	
			EBRT + 6 months ADT	19	4.7	14	38	NA
			EBRT + 36 months ADT	15 ($P < .05$)	3.2 ($P < .01$)	6 ($P < .01$)	15	

FU, follow-up; OS, overall survival; CSS, cancer-specific survival; DF, distant failure; bFFS, biochemical failure-free survival; LF, local failure; EBRT, external beam radiation therapy; Indef, indefinite; DSM, disease-specific mortality; ADT, androgen deprivation therapy; OM, overall mortality; CSM, cancer-specific mortality; BP, biochemical progression; NA, not available.

*Disease-free survival. Biochemical failure defined as PSA > 1.5 ng/mL.

**Locoregional failure.

*+Median follow-up for survivors.

***Disease-free survival. Biochemical failure defined as PSA > 2 ng/mL at ≥ 1 year from randomization.

*++Disease-free survival. Biochemical failure defined as three consecutive rises in PSA, PSA > 4 ng/mL, or receiving additional ADT.

++Distant metastasis or death due to disease.

EORTC trial included patients with more advanced disease than RTOG 92–02, with almost all patients having locally advanced or node-positive (8%) disease. It was designed as a noninferiority trial. At 5 years, the primary null-hypothesis of noninferiority in overall mortality for 6 months of ADT could not be rejected. Post hoc, two-sided statistical analysis demonstrated that short-term ADT was inferior to long-term ADT for overall survival.

One potential reason for the lack of an observed overall survival benefit in RTOG 92–02 may be its relatively lower-risk patient population (45% patients with T1-T2 disease) compared to that from the EORTC trial (26). Longer follow-up may be needed in RTOG 92–02 for the benefits of local and distant disease control to translate into a statistically significant overall survival benefit. Another possibility is a potential interaction of ADT with underlying coronary artery disease in the treated patients (discussed further in the ADT Associated Toxicity section). It may be that since coronary artery disease is more prevalent in the United States as compared to Europe, this interaction was more apparent in the US study.

Taken together, results from RTOG 92–02 and EORTC 22961 support the use of long-term ADT (28 or 36 months) with EBRT for the treatment of patients with locally advanced prostate cancer. A secondary analysis of RTOG 85–31, examining the disease control and survival outcomes of patients who completed >5 years of ADT versus those who stopped ADT before 5 years, similarly showed an improvement in all endpoints, including overall survival, for long-term ADT (28). The additional benefit from long-term versus short-term ADT in these patients may be due to its ability to better treat micrometastatic disease; an important risk for patients with locally advanced prostate cancer. This is evidenced by the reduction in the rates of distant metastasis by long-term versus short-term ADT in both RTOG 92-02 and EORTC 22961 trials.

The timing of ADT in relation to EBRT in patients with high-risk and locally advanced prostate cancer has been specifically studied by RTOG 94–13 (29,30). This trial had a 2 × 2 design, randomizing patients to neoadjuvant and concurrent ADT versus adjuvant ADT (4 months total duration in both arms), and whole pelvis versus prostate-only radiation therapy. No difference in progression-free survival was found between the two ADT schedules, but an unexpected interaction was found between the timing of ADT and extent of radiation treatment. Given the inconclusive findings from this trial, it would be reasonable to give patients with locally advanced prostate cancer neoadjuvant/concurrent/adjuvant ADT (RTOG 92–02) or concurrent/adjuvant ADT (EORTC) with EBRT.

■ **TESTOSTERONE RECOVERY AFTER CESSATION OF ADT**

One potentially important consideration regarding the duration of ADT use is the length of time that the testosterone level is suppressed in a patient. Several studies have shown that recovery of testosterone is dependent upon the duration of ADT, patient age, and baseline testosterone level (31–35). Not all patients experience testosterone recovery after cessation of ADT.

In a prospective study of 129 patients treated with 6 months of LHRH agonist, Gulley et al. reported a median time of 15.4 weeks to testosterone normalization (defined as >211 ng/dL) (31,32). The time of recovery differed for patients with normal baseline testosterone levels (median 14.4 weeks) versus those with low baseline testosterone levels (31.3 weeks, $P < .001$), and also for patients younger than 67 years (14.7 weeks) versus older (17.1 weeks, $P = .02$). These results are consistent with findings from the Canadian randomized trial of EBRT plus 3 versus 8 months of ADT (15). The Canadian trial documented testosterone recovery in 95.5% of patients in the 3-month ADT arm and 88.7% in the 8-month arm; median time to recovery was 6 months.

Patients who receive EBRT with short-term ADT but have delayed testosterone recovery may derive benefits from prolonged androgen suppression. In a retrospective study of 220 men who received EBRT with 6 months of ADT, an increasing duration of androgen suppression was associated with a decreased risk of prostate cancer specific mortality (adjusted HR = .89, $P = .003$) and all-cause mortality (adjusted HR = .94, $P = .007$), after adjusting for other prognostic factors (36). Similarly, in a postrandomization analysis of the Dana-Farber trial, an increased time to testosterone recovery was significantly associated with a decreased risk of prostate cancer specific mortality and improved overall survival in men with little or no comorbidity (37). For these patients with time to testosterone recovery of 0, ≤ 2 years, and > 2 years, 8-year prostate cancer specific mortality rates were 14%, 6%, and 0% ($P = .006$), respectively; overall survival rates were 65%, 81%, and 93% ($P < .001$). Because testosterone recovery time increases with age, these results suggest that older men may need less ADT when used in conjunction with EBRT to attain the same survival benefit as younger men.

For patients who receive long-term ADT, recovery is slower. In a prospective study of prostatic bed EBRT plus 2 years of ADT, Yoon et al. found that testosterone recovery to baseline levels occurred at a median of 22 months (35). Overall, 93% of patients were able to achieve noncastrate testosterone levels within 36 months after the cessation of ADT, but only 72% recovered to baseline testosterone levels. Older age was associated with a lower likelihood of testosterone recovery and a longer recovery time. Patients older than 60 had a cumulative incidence of testosterone recovery of 66% (vs. 86% for those younger than 60) and median recovery time of 28 months (vs. 16 months). Two other studies of patients receiving long-term ADT also showed a significant relationship between age (33,34) and baseline testosterone level (34) with speed of testosterone recovery.

■ **EXTENT OF ANDROGEN SUPPRESSION**

There is a relative paucity of published data examining the relationship between the extent of ADT and the outcome in men who receive radiation-based primary therapy for nonmetastatic prostate cancer. In all the randomized trials that demonstrated a benefit from adding short-term ADT to EBRT, ADT consisted of maximum androgen blockade (MAB, LHRH agonist plus antiandrogen) (7,10–12,15,16) (Table 4). In contrast, trials that evaluated the addition of long-term ADT to EBRT used LHRH agonist alone (19,22,23,27). When combined with

TABLE 4   Treatment details of randomized trials comparing EBRT vs. EBRT plus different durations of ADT

	Duration of ADT	Timing of ADT*	Choice of ADT	Radiation Dose (Gy)
Trials utilizing EBRT with short-term ADT				
Dana-Farber (6)	6 months	N + C + A	LHRH agonist (leuprolide or goserelin) + antiandrogen (flutamide)	70.35
RTOG 9408 (10)	4 months	N + C	LHRH agonist (leuprolide or goserelin) + antiandrogen (flutamide)	66.6
TROG 96.01 (11)	3 vs. 6 months	3 months: N + C 6 months: N + C	LHRH agonist (goserelin) + antiandrogen (flutamide)	66
Quebec 1 (12)	3 vs. 10 months	3 months: N 10 months: N + C + A	LHRH agonist + antiandrogen	64
Quebec 2 (12)	5 vs. 10 months	5 months: N + C 10 months: N + C + A	LHRH agonist + antiandrogen	64
Canadian (15)	3 vs. 8 months	3 months: N 8 months: N	LHRH agonist (goserelin) + antiandrogen (flutamide)	66,67
Quebec (16)	3 vs. 9 months	3 months: N 9 months: N + C + A	LHRH agonist + antiandrogen	64
RTOG 8610 (26)	4 months	N + C	LHRH agonist (goserelin) + antiandrogen (flutamide)	65–70
Trials utilizing EBRT with long-term ADT				
RTOG 8531 (22)	Indefinite	A	LHRH agonist (goserelin)	65–70**
EORTC 22863 (23)	3 years	C + A	LHRH agonist (goserelin)	70
RTOG 9202 (19)	4 vs. 28 months	4 months: N + C 28 months: N + C + A	LHRH agonist (goserelin) + antiandrogen (flutamide) for 4 months, then LHRH agonist alone for 24 months	65–70 (T2c) 67.5–70 (T3-T4)
EORTC 22961 (27)	6 vs. 36 months	6 months: C + A 36 months: C + A	LHRH agonist (triptorelin) + antiandrogen (flutamide or bicalutamide) for 6 months, then LHRH agonist alone for 30 months	70

EBRT, external beam radiation therapy; ADT, androgen-deprivation therapy.
*N, neoadjuvant; C, concurrent; A, adjuvant.
**Postprostatectomy patients received 60–65 Gy.

radiation-based primary therapy, whether MAB is associated with improved outcomes compared to LHRH agonist alone is unclear. As a result, current practice patterns vary.

In a secondary analysis of the Dana-Farber randomized trial, comparing EBRT alone to EBRT plus 6 months of MAB for localized prostate cancer, D'Amico et al. found that men who completed 6 months of MAB had a lower risk of PSA recurrence compared to those who discontinued flutamide early (38,39). In these patients, all of whom received an LHRH agonist for the full 6-month duration, the recurrence risk decreased for each additional month of flutamide completed (HR = 0.81, P = .001). Thus, the risk of PSA recurrence was the lowest in patients who completed the prescribed 6 months of MAB, higher for those who completed partial-course ADT (discontinued flutamide early), and highest for the no-ADT group. A second study that has examined this question was a multi-institutional retrospective review of 628 patients with high-risk prostate cancer treated by high-dose radiation therapy (EBRT plus brachytherapy boost) plus short-term ADT (40). In a multivariable analysis that adjusted for known prognostic factors, men who received MAB had a significantly lower risk of prostate cancer–specific mortality, compared to those treated with an LHRH agonist alone (HR = .18, P = .04).

These results suggest a potential benefit of MAB, compared to an LHRH agonist alone, when used in conjunction with EBRT for the treatment of patients with localized prostate cancer. However, further investigation is needed to confirm the findings of these studies.

■ RADIATION DOSE ESCALATION AND ADT, ARE BOTH NECESSARY?

The randomized trials which have demonstrated a benefit from adding short-term ADT to EBRT in the treatment of prostate cancer, all used radiation doses between 64 and 70 Gy (7,10–12,15,16) (Table 4). An important benefit from short-term ADT in these trials may be to compensate for inadequate radiation dosage, as evidenced by the improvement in local control with the addition of ADT in several of the trials (10,11,16). In the modern era of 3D conformal and intensity-modulated radiation therapy, higher doses can be safely delivered. Therefore, whether short-term ADT is needed in the setting of dose escalated EBRT is a subject of debate. This issue is most relevant for patients with intermediate-risk disease; for those with high-risk and locally advanced prostate cancer, the risk of distant micrometastatic disease is higher and long-term ADT is indicated. Conversely, whether dose escalated EBRT provides an incremental benefit in patients receiving concurrent ADT also needs to be defined. In short, are both dose escalation and short-term ADT necessary for prostate cancer treatment?

Several randomized trials have compared dose escalated versus lower-dose EBRT for localized prostate cancer. The Proton Radiation Oncology Group (PROG) 95–09 trial randomized patients with low-risk and intermediate-risk prostate cancer to 70.2 versus 79.2 Gy without ADT (13,41) Patients received photon radiation at an initial course of 50.4 Gy, followed by proton radiation boosts for an additional 19.8 versus 28.8 Gy. The 10-year biochemical failure rates were 32.0% (low dose) versus 17.4% (high dose, P < .001) (13). In the subgroup analysis, there appeared to be a benefit from dose escalation for low-risk and intermediate-risk patients. No overall survival benefit was seen (78.4% vs. 83.4%, P = .41). An MD Anderson Cancer Center (MDACC) trial included patients with more advanced disease (32% of patients had high-risk or T3 disease), randomized to receive 70 versus 78 Gy prescribed to the isocenter, without ADT (14,42). The 10-year freedom from failure rates were 50% (low dose) versus 73% (high dose, P = .004) (14). In subgroup and multivariable analyses for freedom from failure, patients with PSA >10 ng/mL derived the most benefit from dose escalation. In addition, this trial demonstrated that dose escalation may reduce distant metastasis (P = .059), but no overall survival difference was seen. A Dutch trial included 56% of patients with high-risk or locally advanced prostate cancer, randomized to receive 68 versus 78 Gy (43,44). Approximately 22% of patients in each arm received 3 to 6 months of ADT, as per institutional practice. With 70 months median follow-up, dose escalated EBRT improved the 7-year freedom from failure rates (45% vs. 56%, P = .03) compared to lower-dose EBRT (43). In contrast to PROG 95–09, this study found the benefit of dose escalation to be apparent in patients with intermediate- and high-risk prostate cancer, but not low-risk disease. However, only 18% of patients in the Dutch trial had low-risk prostate cancer so the study may not be adequately powered for this examination. No distant metastasis or overall survival difference was seen.

Taken together, these three trials clearly show that dose escalated radiation therapy has a local control benefit over lower-dose treatment which may, over time, translate into decreased distant metastasis (14). Compared to lower-dose EBRT, the magnitude of the local control benefit from short-term ADT versus that from dose escalation appear similar (45). However, none of the dose escalation trials have yet demonstrated an overall survival benefit with up to 9 years of median follow-up (13,14). It is possible that 10 to 15 years of follow-up may be required for a potential survival benefit to become apparent from dose escalation (46). In contrast, both RTOG 94–08 (8 years) and the Dana-Farber trials (4.5 years) have demonstrated an overall survival benefit from the addition of short-term ADT to lower-dose EBRT for patients with intermediate-risk prostate cancer (7,10).

This earlier demonstration of a survival benefit suggests that short-term ADT not only compensated for lower-dose radiation therapy in terms of improving local control, but likely had an effect on distant micrometastatic disease as well. Because dose escalated radiation therapy does not directly treat distant disease, these results suggest a possible incremental benefit in adding ADT to dose escalated EBRT. Results from RTOG 08–15 and EORTC 22991 (47) will further provide information on this question.

There also appears to be a benefit from dose escalation in patients receiving concurrent ADT (48,49). In a Phase II study by the Grupo de Investigacion Clinica en Oncologia Radioterapica, patients with intermediate-risk prostate cancer received EBRT plus 4 to 6 months of neoadjuvant and concurrent ADT, and high-risk patients received EBRT plus 2 years of ADT (49). Radiation dose was not prescribed by the protocol and varied according to the treating institutions. Comparing patients who received <70 Gy versus ≥ 72 Gy, the higher dose resulted in an improved biochemical disease-free survival for both intermediate-risk (56% vs. 94%) and high-risk patients (64% vs. 84%). However, the difference in intermediate-risk patients was not statistically significant, likely due to the small sample size. These results were confirmed by the Medical Research Council RT01 trial, which randomized patients to 64 versus 74 Gy of EBRT; all patients received an LHRH agonist that started 3 to 6 months prior to EBRT and throughout radiation treatment (48). This study included a mixture of patients with low-risk (24%), intermediate-risk (32%) and high-risk and locally advanced prostate cancer (43%). At 63-month median follow-up, patients who received high-dose EBRT had improved biochemical progression-free survival (60% vs. 71% at 5 years, $P < .001$). In subgroup analysis, the benefit of dose escalation was seen in all prostate cancer risk groups. There was no statistically significant difference in metastasis-free survival; overall survival was not reported.

Thus, the available evidence supports the use of both dose escalated EBRT and ADT in the treatment of patients with prostate cancer, assuming that the patient's life expectancy is long enough (>10 years) to achieve a survival benefit from dose escalation.

■ **ADT-ASSOCIATED TOXICITY**

While ADT has consistently demonstrated a disease control and survival benefit when added to EBRT, it

also causes well-described adverse effects, including hot flashes, sexual dysfunction, fatigue and a possible increased risk of cardiovascular disease. The symptoms caused by ADT can impact a patient's quality of life (50), leading to treatment intolerability. In RTOG 85–31, which randomized patients with EBRT alone versus EBRT plus indefinite ADT, 44% of patients in the ADT arm stopped treatment before 2 years (21). In EORTC 22961, which randomized patients to EBRT plus 6 versus 36 months of ADT, approximately 5% of patients discontinued ADT before 6 months, and 22% in the long-term ADT arm stopped treatment early. Therefore, the treatment decision-making process should include proper selection of patients who are likely to benefit from the addition of ADT to EBRT. When ADT is indicated, supportive therapies may improve treatment tolerability.

Risk of Cardiovascular Disease and Patient Selection Considerations

Recently, several studies have examined the potential association between ADT and risk of cardiovascular disease (Table 5). While ADT has been shown to cause increased obesity and fat mass (51–53), dyslipidemia (52,54), insulin resistance (55,56), and diabetes (57–59), studies show mixed results on a potential association with frank cardiovascular disease and cardiovascular mortality. Several population-based or large cohort studies using the SEER/Medicare (58,60), Veteran's Administration (57) and Cancer of the Prostate Strategic Urologic Research Endeavor (CaPSURE) (61) databases, reported a statistically significant association between ADT and time to cardiovascular disease and mortality. LHRH agonist, but not antiandrogen, appears to be the associated agent (57,58), and the absolute increase in cardiovascular mortality due to ADT is approximately 4 to 10 deaths per 1,000 person-years (57,58). Of note, changes in fat mass, lipids, and insulin resistance often become apparent within a few months of ADT; in the studies that demonstrated a statistically significant association, the increased risk of cardiovascular morbidity and mortality were observed even for patients receiving short-term ADT (58,60,62,63). In a post-randomization pooled analysis of the Dana-Farber, Canadian, and TROG 96.01 trials, 6 months of ADT was associated with a shorter time to fatal myocardial infarction in men 65 years or older,

TABLE 5 Studies Examining the Potential Relationship Between ADT in Prostate Cancer and Risk of Cardiovascular Morbidity and Mortality

	Median FU (Years)	Comparison Arms	Time to Cardiovascular Morbidity (ADT vs. no ADT): AHR (95% CI)	Time to Cardiovascular Death (ADT vs. no ADT): AHR or Point Estimates (95%CI)
Studies Demonstrating a Significant Relationship				
Observational Studies				
SEER/Medicare (58) (N = 73,196)	4.6	ADT vs. No ADT	CAD: AHR:1.16 (1.10–1.21) MI: AHR:1.11 (1.01–1.21)	Sudden Cardiac Death AHR: 1.16 (1.05–1.27)
SEER/Medicare (60) (N = 22,816)	NA	ADT vs. No ADT	AHR 1.20 (1.15–1.26)	NA
Veterans Healthcare Administration (57) (N = 37,443)	2.6	ADT vs. No ADT	CAD: AHR:1.19 (1.10–1.28) MI: AHR:1.28 (1.08–1.52)	Sudden Cardiac Death AHR: 1.35 (1.18–1.54)
CaPSURE (61) (N = 4,892)	3.8	Local tx + ADT vs. Local tx	NA	Surgery: AHR:2.6 (1.4–4.7) RT or cryo: AHR:1.2 (0.8–1.9)
Post-randomization Analysis				
Pooled analysis of Dana-Farber, Canadian, and TROG 96.01 trials (63) (N = 1,372)	~6	EBRT + ADT vs. EBRT	NA	Shorter time to fatal MI in patients ≥ 65 receiving ADT compared to those not treated with ADT (*P* = .017)
	Median FU (Years)	Treatment Arms	Time to Cardiovascular Morbidity (ADT vs. no ADT): AHR (95% CI)	Time to Cardiovascular Death (ADT vs. no ADT): AHR or Point Estimates (95%CI)
Studies Demonstrating No Significant Relationship				
Observational Studies				
Ontario (59) (N = 19,079)	6.5	ADT ≥ 6 months vs. No ADT	MI: AHR: 0.91 (0.84–1.00)	Sudden cardiac death: AHR: 0.96 (0.83–1.10)
Post-randomization Analysis				
RTOG 85–31 (65) (N = 945)	8.1	EBRT + indef ADT vs. EBRT	NA	AHR: 0.99 (0.58–1.69)*
RTOG 86–10 (26) (N = 456)	13*+	EBRT + 4 months ADT vs. EBRT	NA	10-year fatal cardiac events: 9.1% (EBRT) vs. 12.5% (EBRT + ADT), *P* = .32

ADT, androgen deprivation therapy; FU, follow-up; AHR, adjusted hazard ratio; CI, confidence interval; CAD, coronary artery disease; MI, myocardial infarction; Tx, treatment; RT, radiation therapy; Cryo, cryotherapy; EBRT, external beam radiation therapy; NA, not available; Indef, indefinite.
*Analysis based on censoring at time of salvage LHRH agonist therapy. Without censoring, AHR 0.73 (95% CI: 0.47–1.15)
*+Median follow-up for survivors.

compared to patients who received EBRT alone (63). Long-term versus short-term ADT does not appear to further increase the risk of cardiovascular disease. In EORTC 22961, the rates of fatal cardiac events were similar among patients receiving short-term (4.0%) versus long-term (3.0%) ADT (27). In a post-randomization analysis of RTOG 92–02, the risk of cardiovascular mortality on multivariable analysis was also found to be similar in the two arms (adjusted HR = 1.02, P = .90) (64).

In contrast, several studies showed no significant association between ADT and the development of cardiovascular disease or mortality. These include a study using the Ontario Cancer Registry linked with administrative data (59), as well as post-randomization analyses of RTOG 85–31 (65) and RTOG 86–10 (26). It is important to note that none of the population-based, cohort or post-randomization studies described above were designed to assess cardiovascular disease, so the inconsistent findings may reflect differences in study design, patient selection, and other inherent biases of retrospective studies. Also, these prior studies did not specifically examine outcomes in subsets of men with baseline coronary artery disease, in whom an interaction with ADT treatment is most plausible. The risk of cardiovascular morbidity and mortality from ADT may be increased only in certain patient subgroups, in which the prostate cancer-specific benefit of ADT may be negated by its harm. In a retrospective study of 5,077 prostate cancer patients treated with brachytherapy, 30% received neoadjuvant ADT for a mean duration of 4 months (66). The use of ADT was associated with an increased risk of all-cause mortality only for the subgroup of patients with preexisting coronary artery disease-induced congestive heart failure or myocardial infarction (comprising 5% of the overall patient cohort). These results are consistent with results from a post-randomization analysis of the Dana-Farber trial, which showed that the survival benefit from the addition of 6 months of ADT to EBRT was seen only in patients with no or minimal, comorbidity at baseline, but not in those with moderate or severe comorbidity (6). Future trials which stratify patients by baseline comorbid conditions would be able to address this question more directly.

A recent joint consensus panel report published by the American Heart Association, the American Cancer Society, and the American Urological Association states that there "may be a relationship between ADT and cardiovascular events and death (67)."

The group recommends that the treating physician weigh the potential risks and benefits of ADT in each patient's specific clinical scenario. For patients with aggressive prostate cancer to whom the addition of ADT is necessary, no further evaluation by an internist, cardiologist or endocrinologist is recommended. Patients with cardiac disease should receive appropriate secondary preventive measures (such as statins, aspirin, and antihypertensive medications) and be monitored by their primary care physicians.

Management of ADT-Associated Symptoms

When ADT is indicated, supportive therapies may help some patients complete the prescribed treatment. Potential management of ADT-associated hot flashes, sexual dysfunction, and fatigue are described below.

Approximately 80% of men undergoing ADT experience hot flashes (68), an intense feeling of warmth, usually in the face and upper body, which may be accompanied by sweating and nausea. Hot flashes can occur at any time and are particularly distressing to patients when they occur at night and cause sleep disturbance. Selective serotonin uptake inhibitors have demonstrated efficacy in reducing hot flashes for men receiving ADT. In a pilot study by Quella et al., patients with moderate to severe hot flashes were treated with venlafaxine 12.5 mg twice a day. Treatment reduced the incidence of severe and very severe hot flashes from 2.3 to 0.6 events per day (P = .003) (69). Ten of 16 patients experienced a greater than 50% decrease in hot flash score (frequency x severity) by week 4 of treatment. Similar efficacy has also been shown for paroxetine (70). Recently, two randomized trials also demonstrated the ability of gabapentin (300 mg three times a day) (71) and pregabalin (75 mg or 150 mg, twice daily) (72) to reduce the frequency and intensity of hot flashes in men receiving ADT. Gabapentin reduced hot flash frequency by 46% (vs. 22% for placebo) and hot flash score by 44% (vs. 27% for placebo) (71). Pregabalin reduced hot flash frequency by approximately 60% (vs. 36% for placebo) and hot flash score by approximately two-thirds (vs. 50% for placebo) (72).

Sexual dysfunction is a common side effect of ADT (50,73). The Prostate Cancer Outcomes Study found that ADT increased the proportion of men reporting no sexual interest (32% at baseline compared to 58% with ADT), no sufficient erections for intercourse (52% vs. 84%) and having no sexual activity (45% vs. 80%) (50). While there are no available treatments to increase sex drive in men treated with ADT, phosphodiesterase type 5 (PDE5) inhibitors have been used for erectile dysfunction in these patients. Teloken et al. studied 152 men with functional erections prior to EBRT or brachytherapy with or without ADT, who experienced erectile dysfunction following treatment completion (74). The mean age of this patient cohort was 62 years, and the duration of ADT was 3.8 months. Sildenafil achieved a response rate (defined as erections sufficient for intercourse) in 61% of patients who received radiation therapy alone, and 47% of patients who received radiation therapy with ADT.

Fatigue is another potentially modifiable side effect of ADT. In a cross-sectional study of prostate cancer survivors who have completed EBRT, 39% of those who continue to receive ADT reported chronic fatigue, significantly higher than those who never received ADT (26%) (75). In randomized trials, physical activity has been shown to reduce fatigue in men receiving ADT for prostate cancer (76,77). Segal et al. randomly assigned 155 patients receiving ADT to 12 weeks of a resistance exercise program versus a waiting list (77). Using a questionnaire at 12 weeks, the authors documented reduced fatigue and improved quality of life for patients in the exercise arm. In a subsequent and complementary trial, resistance exercise was also found to have similar benefits for men receiving radiation therapy for prostate cancer (78).

SUMMARY

In multiple randomized trials, the addition of ADT to EBRT improved disease control and overall survival in men with intermediate-risk, high-risk, and locally advanced prostate cancer. Patients with intermediate-risk prostate cancer should receive short-term (4–6 months) neoadjuvant and concurrent ADT with EBRT. Those with high-risk and locally advanced disease should receive long-term (28–36 months) neoadjuvant, concurrent, and adjuvant ADT with EBRT. However, short-term ADT may be adequate in older men with high-risk localized prostate cancer, because testosterone recovery time in these men is prolonged. There appears to be an incremental benefit in adding ADT to dose escalated EBRT and vice versa.

ADT causes well-described adverse effects including hot flashes, sexual dysfunction, fatigue, and a possible increase in the risk of cardiovascular morbidity and mortality. Whether patients with significant baseline comorbidity or cardiovascular disease benefit from the addition of ADT to EBRT needs to be further studied.

■ REFERENCES

1. Widmark A, Klepp O, Solberg A, et al. Endocrine treatment, with or without radiotherapy, in locally advanced prostate cancer (SPCG-7/SFUO-3): an open randomised phase III trial. *Lancet.* 2009;373(9660):301–308.
2. Warde PR, Mason MD, Sydes MR, et al. Intergroup randomized phase III study of androgen deprivation therapy (ADT) plus radiation therapy (RT) in locally advanced prostate cancer (CaP). *J Clin Oncol.* 2010;28(18 suppl): CRA4504.
3. Klotz L, Boccon-Gibod L, Shore ND, et al. The efficacy and safety of degarelix: a 12-month, comparative, randomized, open-label, parallel-group phase III study in patients with prostate cancer. *BJU Int.* 2008;102(11):1531–1538.
4. Conn PM, Crowley WF Jr. Gonadotropin-releasing hormone and its analogues. *N Engl J Med.* 1991;324(2):93–103.
5. Limonta P, Montagnani Marelli M, Moretti RM. LHRH analogues as anticancer agents: pituitary and extrapituitary sites of action. *Expert Opin Investig Drugs.* 2001;10(4):709–720.
6. D'Amico AV, Chen MH, Renshaw AA, Loffredo M, Kantoff PW. Androgen suppression and radiation vs radiation alone for prostate cancer: a randomized trial. *JAMA.* 2008;299(3):289–295.
7. D'Amico AV, Manola J, Loffredo M, Renshaw AA, DellaCroce A, Kantoff PW. 6-month androgen suppression plus radiation therapy vs radiation therapy alone for patients with clinically localized prostate cancer: a randomized controlled trial. *JAMA.* 2004;292(7):821–827.
8. D'Amico AV, Whittington R, Malkowicz SB, et al. Biochemical outcome after radical prostatectomy, external beam radiation therapy, or interstitial radiation therapy for clinically localized prostate cancer. *JAMA.* 1998;280(11):969–974.
9. Nguyen PL, Chen MH, Beard CJ, et al. Radiation with or without 6 months of androgen suppression therapy in intermediate- and high-risk clinically localized prostate cancer: a postrandomization analysis by risk group. *Int J Radiat Oncol Biol Phys.* 2010;77(4):1046–1052.
10. McGowan D, Hunt D, Jones C, et al. Effect of short-term endocrine therapy prior to and during radiation therapy on overall survival in patients with T1b-T2b adenocarcinoma of the prostate and PSA equal to or less than 20: initial results of RTOG 94–08. *Genitourinary Cancers Symposium.* Abstract No. 6., 2010.
11. Denham JW, Steigler A, Lamb DS, et al. Short-term androgen deprivation and radiotherapy for locally

advanced prostate cancer: results from the Trans-Tasman Radiation Oncology Group 96.01 randomised controlled trial. *Lancet Oncol.* 2005;6(11):841–850.

12. Laverdière J, Nabid A, De Bedoya LD, et al. The efficacy and sequencing of a short course of androgen suppression on freedom from biochemical failure when administered with radiation therapy for T2-T3 prostate cancer. *J Urol.* 2004;171(3):1137–1140.

13. Zietman AL, Bae K, Slater JD, et al. Randomized trial comparing conventional-dose with high-dose conformal radiation therapy in early-stage adenocarcinoma of the prostate: long-term results from proton radiation oncology group/American College Of Radiology 95–09. *J Clin Oncol.* 2010;28(7):1106–1111.

14. Kuban DA, Tucker SL, Dong L, et al. Long-term results of the M. D. Anderson randomized dose-escalation trial for prostate cancer. *Int J Radiat Oncol Biol Phys.* 2008;70(1):67–74.

15. Crook J, Ludgate C, Malone S, et al. Final report of multicenter Canadian Phase III randomized trial of 3 versus 8 months of neoadjuvant androgen deprivation therapy before conventional-dose radiotherapy for clinically localized prostate cancer. *Int J Radiat Oncol Biol Phys.* 2009;73(2):327–333.

16. Laverdière J, Gomez JL, Cusan L, et al. Beneficial effect of combination hormonal therapy administered prior and following external beam radiation therapy in localized prostate cancer. *Int J Radiat Oncol Biol Phys.* 1997;37(2):247–252.

17. Heymann JJ, Benson MC, O'Toole KM, et al. Phase II study of neoadjuvant androgen deprivation followed by external-beam radiotherapy with 9 months of androgen deprivation for intermediate- to high-risk localized prostate cancer. *J Clin Oncol.* 2007;25(1):77–84.

18. Hanks GE, Pajak TF, Porter A, et al. Phase III trial of long-term adjuvant androgen deprivation after neoadjuvant hormonal cytoreduction and radiotherapy in locally advanced carcinoma of the prostate: the Radiation Therapy Oncology Group Protocol 92–02. *J Clin Oncol.* 2003;21(21):3972–3978.

19. Horwitz EM, Bae K, Hanks GE, et al. Ten-year follow-up of radiation therapy oncology group protocol 92–02: a phase III trial of the duration of elective androgen deprivation in locally advanced prostate cancer. *J Clin Oncol.* 2008;26(15):2497–2504.

20. Lawton CA, Winter K, Murray K, et al. Updated results of the phase III Radiation Therapy Oncology Group (RTOG) trial 85–31 evaluating the potential benefit of androgen suppression following standard radiation therapy for unfavorable prognosis carcinoma of the prostate. *Int J Radiat Oncol Biol Phys.* 2001;49(4):937–946.

21. Pilepich MV, Caplan R, Byhardt RW, et al. Phase III trial of androgen suppression using goserelin in unfavorable-prognosis carcinoma of the prostate treated with definitive radiotherapy: report of Radiation Therapy Oncology Group Protocol 85–31. *J Clin Oncol.* 1997;15(3):1013–1021.

22. Pilepich MV, Winter K, Lawton CA, et al. Androgen suppression adjuvant to definitive radiotherapy in prostate

carcinoma–long-term results of phase III RTOG 85–31. *Int J Radiat Oncol Biol Phys.* 2005;61(5):1285–1290.

23. Bolla M, Collette L, Blank L, et al. Long-term results with immediate androgen suppression and external irradiation in patients with locally advanced prostate cancer (an EORTC study): a phase III randomised trial. *Lancet.* 2002;360(9327):103–106.

24. Bolla M, Gonzalez D, Warde P, et al. Improved survival in patients with locally advanced prostate cancer treated with radiotherapy and goserelin. *N Engl J Med.* 1997;337(5):295–300.

25. Pilepich MV, Winter K, John MJ, et al. Phase III radiation therapy oncology group (RTOG) trial 86–10 of androgen deprivation adjuvant to definitive radiotherapy in locally advanced carcinoma of the prostate. *Int J Radiat Oncol Biol Phys.* 2001;50(5):1243–1252.

26. Roach M 3rd, Bae K, Speight J, et al. Short-term neoadjuvant androgen deprivation therapy and external-beam radiotherapy for locally advanced prostate cancer: long-term results of RTOG 8610. *J Clin Oncol.* 2008;26(4):585–591.

27. Bolla M, de Reijke TM, Van Tienhoven G, et al. Duration of androgen suppression in the treatment of prostate cancer. *N Engl J Med.* 2009;360(24):2516–2527.

28. Souhami L, Bae K, Pilepich M, Sandler H. Impact of the duration of adjuvant hormonal therapy in patients with locally advanced prostate cancer treated with radiotherapy: a secondary analysis of RTOG 85–31. *J Clin Oncol.* 2009;27(13):2137–2143.

29. Lawton CA, DeSilvio M, Roach M 3rd, et al. An update of the phase III trial comparing whole pelvic to prostate only radiotherapy and neoadjuvant to adjuvant total androgen suppression: updated analysis of RTOG 94–13, with emphasis on unexpected hormone/radiation interactions. *Int J Radiat Oncol Biol Phys.* 2007;69(3):646–655.

30. Roach M 3rd, DeSilvio M, Lawton C, et al. Phase III trial comparing whole-pelvic versus prostate-only radiotherapy and neoadjuvant versus adjuvant combined androgen suppression: Radiation Therapy Oncology Group 9413. *J Clin Oncol.* 2003;21(10):1904–1911.

31. Gulley JL, Aragon-Ching JB, Steinberg SM, et al. Kinetics of serum androgen normalization and factors associated with testosterone reserve after limited androgen deprivation therapy for nonmetastatic prostate cancer. *J Urol.* 2008;180(4):1432–1437; discussion 1437.

32. Gulley JL, Figg WD, Steinberg SM, et al. A prospective analysis of the time to normalization of serum androgens following 6 months of androgen deprivation therapy in patients on a randomized phase III clinical trial using limited hormonal therapy. *J Urol.* 2005;173(5):1567–1571.

33. Kaku H, Saika T, Tsushima T, et al. Time course of serum testosterone and luteinizing hormone levels after cessation of long-term luteinizing hormone-releasing hormone agonist treatment in patients with prostate cancer. *Prostate.* 2006;66(4):439–444.

34. Pickles T, Agranovich A, Berthelet E, et al. Testosterone recovery following prolonged adjuvant androgen ablation for prostate carcinoma. *Cancer.* 2002;94(2):362–367.

35. Yoon FH, Gardner SL, Danjoux C, et al. Testosterone recovery after prolonged androgen suppression in patients with prostate cancer. *J Urol*. 2008;180(4):1438–1443; discussion 1443–1444.

36. D'Amico AV, Renshaw AA, Loffredo B, Chen MH. Duration of testosterone suppression and the risk of death from prostate cancer in men treated using radiation and 6 months of hormone therapy. *Cancer*. 2007;110(8):1723–1728.

37. D'Amico AV, Chen MH, Renshaw AA, Loffredo M, Kantoff PW. Interval to testosterone recovery after hormonal therapy for prostate cancer and risk of death. *Int J Radiat Oncol Biol Phys*. 2009;75(1):10–15.

38. D'Amico AV, Chen MH, Renshaw AA, Loffredo B, Kantoff PW. Risk of prostate cancer recurrence in men treated with radiation alone or in conjunction with combined or less than combined androgen suppression therapy. *J Clin Oncol*. 2008;26(18):2979–2983.

39. D'Amico AV, Kantoff PW, Chen MH. Aspirin and hormone therapy for prostate cancer. *N Engl J Med*. 2007;357(26):2737–2738.

40. Nanda A, Chen MH, Moran BJ, et al. Total androgen blockade versus a luteinizing hormone-releasing hormone agonist alone in men with high-risk prostate cancer treated with radiotherapy. *Int J Radiat Oncol Biol Phys*. 2010;76(5):1439–1444.

41. Zietman AL, DeSilvio ML, Slater JD, et al. Comparison of conventional-dose vs high-dose conformal radiation therapy in clinically localized adenocarcinoma of the prostate: a randomized controlled trial. *JAMA*. 2005;294(10):1233–1239.

42. Pollack A, Zagars GK, Smith LG, et al. Preliminary results of a randomized radiotherapy dose-escalation study comparing 70 Gy with 78 Gy for prostate cancer. *J Clin Oncol*. 2000;18(23):3904–3911.

43. Al-Mamgani A, van Putten WL, Heemsbergen WD, et al. Update of Dutch multicenter dose-escalation trial of radiotherapy for localized prostate cancer. *Int J Radiat Oncol Biol Phys*. 2008;72(4):980–988.

44. Peeters ST, Heemsbergen WD, Koper PC, et al. Dose-response in radiotherapy for localized prostate cancer: results of the Dutch multicenter randomized phase III trial comparing 68 Gy of radiotherapy with 78 Gy. *J Clin Oncol*. 2006;24(13):1990–1996.

45. Zelefsky MJ, Leibel SA, Gaudin PB, et al. Dose escalation with three-dimensional conformal radiation therapy affects the outcome in prostate cancer. *Int J Radiat Oncol Biol Phys*. 1998;41(3):491–500.

46. Nanda A, D'Amico AV. Combined radiation and hormonal therapy or dose escalation for men with unfavourable-risk prostate cancer: an evidence-based approach using a synthesis of randomized clinical trials. *BJU Int*. 2008;102(10):1366–1368.

47. Matzinger O, Duclos F, van den Bergh A, et al. Acute toxicity of curative radiotherapy for intermediate- and high-risk localised prostate cancer in the EORTC trial 22991. *Eur J Cancer*. 2009;45(16):2825–2834.

48. Dearnaley DP, Sydes MR, Graham JD, et al. Escalated-dose versus standard-dose conformal radiotherapy in prostate cancer: first results from the MRC RT01 randomised controlled trial. *Lancet Oncol*. 2007;8(6):475–487.

49. Zapatero A, Valcárcel F, Calvo FA, et al. Risk-adapted androgen deprivation and escalated three-dimensional conformal radiotherapy for prostate cancer: Does radiation dose influence outcome of patients treated with adjuvant androgen deprivation? A GICOR study. *J Clin Oncol*. 2005;23(27):6561–6568.

50. Potosky AL, Knopf K, Clegg LX, et al. Quality-of-life outcomes after primary androgen deprivation therapy: results from the Prostate Cancer Outcomes Study. *J Clin Oncol*. 2001;19(17):3750–3757.

51. Smith MR. Changes in fat and lean body mass during androgen-deprivation therapy for prostate cancer. *Urology*. 2004;63(4):742–745.

52. Smith MR, Finkelstein JS, McGovern FJ, et al. Changes in body composition during androgen deprivation therapy for prostate cancer. *J Clin Endocrinol Metab*. 2002;87(2):599–603.

53. Smith MR, Lee H, McGovern F, et al. Metabolic changes during gonadotropin-releasing hormone agonist therapy for prostate cancer: differences from the classic metabolic syndrome. *Cancer*. 2008;112(10):2188–2194.

54. Eri LM, Urdal P, Bechensteen AG. Effects of the luteinizing hormone-releasing hormone agonist leuprolide on lipoproteins, fibrinogen and plasminogen activator inhibitor in patients with benign prostatic hyperplasia. *J Urol*. 1995;154(1):100–104.

55. Dockery F, Bulpitt CJ, Agarwal S, Donaldson M, Rajkumar C. Testosterone suppression in men with prostate cancer leads to an increase in arterial stiffness and hyperinsulinaemia. *Clin Sci*. 2003;104(2):195–201.

56. Smith MR, Lee H, Nathan DM. Insulin sensitivity during combined androgen blockade for prostate cancer. *J Clin Endocrinol Metab*. 2006;91(4):1305–1308.

57. Keating NL, O'Malley AJ, Freedland SJ, Smith MR. Diabetes and cardiovascular disease during androgen deprivation therapy: observational study of veterans with prostate cancer. *J Natl Cancer Inst*. 2010;102(1):39–46.

58. Keating NL, O'Malley AJ, Smith MR. Diabetes and cardiovascular disease during androgen deprivation therapy for prostate cancer. *J Clin Oncol*. 2006;24(27):4448–4456.

59. Alibhai SM, Duong-Hua M, Sutradhar R, et al. Impact of androgen deprivation therapy on cardiovascular disease and diabetes. *J Clin Oncol*. 2009;27(21):3452–3458.

60. Saigal CS, Gore JL, Krupski TL, Hanley J, Schonlau M, Litwin MS. Androgen deprivation therapy increases cardiovascular morbidity in men with prostate cancer. *Cancer*. 2007;110(7):1493–1500.

61. Tsai HK, D'Amico AV, Sadetsky N, Chen MH, Carroll PR. Androgen deprivation therapy for localized prostate cancer and the risk of cardiovascular mortality. *J Natl Cancer Inst*. 2007;99(20):1516–1524.

62. Tsai EC, Boyko EJ, Leonetti DL, Fujimoto WY. Low serum testosterone level as a predictor of increased visceral fat in Japanese-American men. *Int J Obes Relat Metab Disord*. 2000;24(4):485–491.

63. D'Amico AV, Denham JW, Crook J, et al. Influence of androgen suppression therapy for prostate cancer on the

frequency and timing of fatal myocardial infarctions. *J Clin Oncol.* 2007;25(17):2420–2425.

64. Efstathiou JA, Bae K, Shipley WU, et al. Cardiovascular mortality and duration of androgen deprivation for locally advanced prostate cancer: analysis of RTOG 92–02. *Eur Urol.* 2008;54(4):816–823.

65. Efstathiou JA, Bae K, Shipley WU, et al. Cardiovascular mortality after androgen deprivation therapy for locally advanced prostate cancer: RTOG 85–31. *J Clin Oncol.* 2009;27(1):92–99.

66. Nanda A, Chen MH, Braccioforte MH, Moran BJ, D'Amico AV. Hormonal therapy use for prostate cancer and mortality in men with coronary artery disease-induced congestive heart failure or myocardial infarction. *JAMA.* 2009;302(8):866–873.

67. Levine GN, D'Amico AV, Berger P, et al. Androgen-deprivation therapy in prostate cancer and cardiovascular risk: a science advisory from the American Heart Association, American Cancer Society, and American Urological Association: endorsed by the American Society for Radiation Oncology. *Circulation.* 2010;121(6):833–840.

68. Schow DA, Renfer LG, Rozanski TA, Thompson IM. Prevalence of hot flushes during and after neoadjuvant hormonal therapy for localized prostate cancer. *South Med J.* 1998;91(9):855–857.

69. Quella SK, Loprinzi CL, Sloan J, et al. Pilot evaluation of venlafaxine for the treatment of hot flashes in men undergoing androgen ablation therapy for prostate cancer. *J Urol.* 1999;162(1):98–102.

70. Loprinzi CL, Barton DL, Carpenter LA, et al. Pilot evaluation of paroxetine for treating hot flashes in men. *Mayo Clin Proc.* 2004;79(10):1247–1251.

71. Loprinzi CL, Dueck AC, Khoyratty BS, et al. A phase III randomized, double-blind, placebo-controlled trial of gabapentin in the management of hot flashes in men (N00CB). *Ann Oncol.* 2009;20(3):542–549.

72. Loprinzi CL, Qin R, Balcueva EP, et al. Phase III, randomized, double-blind, placebo-controlled evaluation of pregabalin for alleviating hot flashes, N07C1. *J Clin Oncol.* 2010;28(4):641–647.

73. Lubeck DP, Grossfeld GD, Carroll PR. The effect of androgen deprivation therapy on health-related quality of life in men with prostate cancer. *Urology.* 2001;58 (2 Suppl 1):94–100.

74. Teloken PE, Ohebshalom M, Mohideen N, Mulhall JP. Analysis of the impact of androgen deprivation therapy on sildenafil citrate response following radiation therapy for prostate cancer. *J Urol.* 2007;178(6):2521–2525.

75. Kyrdalen AE, Dahl AA, Hernes E, Hem E, Fosså SD. Fatigue in prostate cancer survivors treated with definitive radiotherapy and LHRH analogs. *Prostate.* 2010;70(13):1480–1489.

76. Culos-Reed SN, Robinson JW, Lau H, et al. Physical activity for men receiving androgen deprivation therapy for prostate cancer: benefits from a 16-week intervention. *Support Care Cancer.* 2010;18(5):591–599.

77. Segal RJ, Reid RD, Courneya KS, et al. Resistance exercise in men receiving androgen deprivation therapy for prostate cancer. *J Clin Oncol.* 2003;21(9):1653–1659.

78. Segal RJ, Reid RD, Courneya KS, et al. Randomized controlled trial of resistance or aerobic exercise in men receiving radiation therapy for prostate cancer. *J Clin Oncol.* 2009;27(3):344–351.

Current Role of Salvage and Adjuvant Radiotherapy for Prostate Cancer

Peter J. Rossi[1], Mariam Korah[1], Brandon Mancini[2], Anees H. Dhabaan[1], and Ashesh B. Jani[1]*

[1]The Winship Cancer Institute of Emory University, Atlanta, GA
[2]Wayne State University School of Medicine, Detroit, MI

■ ABSTRACT

Prostatectomy is commonly used for the treatment of adenocarcinoma of the prostate. Radiotherapy following prostatectomy has been offered as adjuvant or as salvage therapy. The results of this intervention demonstrate high prostate cancer–specific survival in either setting. The best results have been demonstrated when patients have been treated adjuvantly, in event of pathologic T3 disease or in the presence of positive margins. The toxicity of radiotherapy is modest and mostly related to urinary function. In this article we review post-prostatectomy radiotherapy—rationale, treatment techniques/doses, toxicity and cancer control outcomes (including single- and multi-institutional data), and current clinical trials.

Keywords: prostate cancer, adjuvant radiotherapy, salvage radiotherapy, postprostatectomy, outcome

■ INTRODUCTION

Prostatectomy is a standard of care for treatment of adenocarcinoma of the prostate. In a large multi center randomized controlled trial, prostatectomy has shown to provide a survival advantage over observation in patients with newly diagnosed prostate cancer. After prostatectomy, patients may fail. Studies demonstrate that a prostate-specific antigen (PSA) rise following prostatectomy, is associated with a decreased prostate cancer–specific survival (PCSS) in men. The predominant pattern of failure following prostatectomy is locoregional. Many factors have been identified to predict the likelihood of local or distant failure. Radiotherapy following prostatectomy has been offered as adjuvant or as salvage therapy. The results of this intervention demonstrate long-term PCSS in each setting. The best results following prostatectomy have been demonstrated when patients have been treated adjuvantly, in the event of pathologic T3 disease or in the presence of positive margins. Three randomized control trials support the use of radiotherapy in the adjuvant setting, and

*Corresponding author, Department of Radiation Oncology, Emory University, Atlanta, GA

E-mail address: abjani@emory.edu or jani_1969@yahoo.com

Radiation Medicine Rounds 2:1 (2011) 59–80.

DOI: 10.5003/2151–4208.2.1.59

long-term follow-up supports a metastatic disease-free survival and overall survival benefit of a magnitude similar to with prostatectomy. The toxicity is modestly increased and is mostly related to urinary function. The current techniques, dosing and field sizes, are reviewed, as well as the current data and current clinical trials. For a similar benefit and intent as prostatectomy, the authors maintain that postoperative radiotherapy is of significant benefit to select patients, and the appropriate counseling is required. Radiotherapy, offered to patients in the event of PSA failure or when high-risk pathologic features are found at the time of prostatectomy, is essential in preventing death due to prostate cancer.

■ THE TRENDS, SUCCESSES, AND FAILURES OF RADICAL PROSTATECTOMY

Prostatectomy is a mainstay in the treatment for adenocarcinoma of the prostate. Often referred to as the "gold standard," all other modalities must compare to the successes and failures of prostatectomy in terms of prostate cancer control and toxicity. In the modern era, there are several practiced techniques to remove the prostate and prostate cancer; much ado is made today of the robotic assisted technique, for example. The outcome data for prostatectomy control of prostate cancer is largely based on the "open" radical retro pubic approach, and less data exist for other procedures.

That being said, the majority of patients diagnosed with prostate cancer in the United States receive early surgical intervention (1). A recent SEER analysis of over 800,000 men documents that prostatectomy is attempted in 3 of 4 patients treated for prostate cancer de novo in the United States, and this data is further supported by other modern databases of prostate cancer trends (2). This has declined in recent years, as radiotherapy and brachytherapy have become more popular, but the role of prostatectomy is prominent and understanding its success and failures is paramount.

Investigators have understood for years about risk factors leading to failure after prostatectomy. Partin tables and popularized nomograms are commonly used to predict the likelihood of a successful procedure based on preoperative variables such as age, PSA level, Gleason score, percentage of cores with cancer, and T stage on clinical examination (3–5). Predicting such events as biochemical free survival

and prostate death is also attempted. These tools should be used with caution; they are retrospective, sometimes unvalidated and represent a select patient population. Important prognostic endpoints can be poorly estimated, for instance, in the use of Partin tables, older men and higher PSA scores are uncommon and many publications question the validity of the tool in predicting important clinical endpoints in other populations (6–9).

Many disease characteristics have been looked at historically for predicting failure from prostatectomy and the need for additional treatment. Researchers have looked to predict pathologic findings most significant for local recurrence to assist clinicians. Many variables have been evaluated and are predictive of recurrence following prostatectomy, such as pretreatment PSA, margin status and tumor stage at the time of prostatectomy, seminal vesicle invasion, lymph node invasion, PSA immediately after prostatectomy, disease-free interval if PSA levels become undetectable, and rate of PSA change or velocity after failure. It is likely that the initial pathologic tumor stage and margin status remain most important predictors of PSA failure (10–12).

Table 1 summarizes commonly referenced surgical outcome series. Table 2 is a summary of robotic-assisted radical prostatectomy (RP) series, limited currently by shorter follow-up to make comparisons. Of the nearly 20 select studies listed, three are controlled studies (13,14,28). The Scandinavian Prostate Cancer Group randomized study is familiar to all in our field. This study established the rationale of early intervention for treatment of adenocarcinoma of the prostate with definitive therapy. This landmark study randomized nearly 700 men with clinically discovered prostate cancer to immediate RP or watchful waiting. This was a study done is the pre-PSA era and the surgical approach was "open," (so arguably limited in application today), yet the results support an aggressive approach based on a significant reduction in risk of death at 10 years (15). In this study, absolute risk of death decreased by 5% and relative risk decreased by 40%. Other more significant reductions were seen with reduced risk of local progression, metastasis, and prostate cancer–specific mortality. The follow-up on this study was long, over 10 years, and of interest; most patients had intact disease and negative margins at the time of prostatectomy, yet a significant number were found to have adverse pathologic findings that, in the modern era, we would counsel for additional therapy (28). Of the men undergoing prostatectomy,

TABLE 1   Radical retropubic prostatectomy series

Investigators	Number of Cases (Patients)	Median Follow-Up in Years	pT2 (%)	GL < 8 (%)	Positive Surgical Margins (%)	Local Progression (%)	Biochemical Progression-Free Survival (%)	Prostate Cancer–Specific Survival (%)
Bill-Axelson et al. (15)	695	10.8	53%	86%	35%	22%	NR	12 years: 12.5% versus 18%
Giberti et al. (14)	100	5	84	97	<8	NR	5 years:91%	NR
Yee et al. (13)	148	8	51/61	67/79	19/38	1	7 years:80	99
Freedland et al. (18)	1,654	3.6	71%	92%	30%	NR	25%	NR
Han et al. (19)	2,091	5.9	50%	94%	NR	2%	17% overall 5 years:84 10 years:72 15 years:61	5 years:99 10 years:96 15%:89
Roehl et al. (20)	3,478	5.5	68	93	NR	NR	5 years:80 10 years:68	10 years:97
Bianco et al. (21) (Urology 2005)	1,746	6	66	96	12	NR	5 years:82 10 years:77 15 years:75	5 years:99 10 years:95 15 years:89
Porter et al. (22)	752	11	55	92	38	8	68	93
Berglund (23)	281	2.9	88	77	19	1	70	99
Kupelian (11)	423	3.3	35	90	46	8	5 years:59 (37% with positive margin)	5 years:79
Mian (17)	188	5	31	100	8	NR	68	71
Carver (16)	176	6.4	30	85	27	NR	5 years:48 10 years:44	5 years:94 10 years:85

NR, not reported.

47% were found to have disease outside the prostate and 35% had positive surgical margins, yet only 14% had a Gleason score at prostatectomy greater than 7. In the cohort who received upfront prostatectomy, 22% were ultimately found to have a loco-regional progression. Another way of interpreting the results of the study is using number needed to treat (NNT), and to prevent one death on this study, 20 needed

TABLE 2   Robotic assisted radical prostatectomy outcome series

Investigators	Number of Cases	Median Follow-Up in Years	pT2	Gl < 8	Positive Surgical Margins (%)	Biochemical Progression-Free Survival (%)
Zorn et al. (24)	300	1.5	84	98	21	NR
White et al. (25)	50		88	99	22	NR
Menon et al. (26)	2,652	1	78	89	13	5ry:91
Badani (27)	2,766	1.8	78	89	T3:35% T2:4%	5 years: 84

NR, not reported.

treatment, a number we will return to later in discussion of adjuvant therapy.

Yee and Giberti have reported other controlled series of open prostatectomy (13,14). Yee et al. studied the use of 3 months of neoadjuvant hormone therapy prior to RP in a phase III study completed at Memorial Sloan Kettering Cancer Center. For the entire cohort, pathologic T3 disease was discovered at prostatectomy in 45% of patients, and presence of positive margins was seen in 38% of patients on the control arm. Brachytherapy was compared to prostatectomy in a select low-risk patient population. In the prostatectomy arm, in this low-risk population, 16% had disease outside the prostate and about 8% of patients were found to have a positive margin. At 5 years, 1 in 10 men experienced PSA failure. Many other retrospective series are also presented in Table 1. Many of the studies have large numbers of patients, but are limited by short median follow-up time. Also note that patient populations range from very select, low-risk populations to men with higher risk disease. It's clear from these studies that adverse findings at prostatectomy predict poor disease outcome (11,16,17).

The robotic assisted RP experience is more limited due to low number of published series, and mostly because the experience is 7 to 8 years, at best, in any one institution. Zorn et al. has published a prospective quality of life study with surgical outcome data in men operated on at the University of Chicago. In their series of 300 cases, with 98% of men having low or intermediate-risk disease, preoperatively, the incidence of pathologic T3 (pT3) or greater disease was 16% and the incidence of positive margins was 21% (24). In comparing Tables 1 and 2, the incidence of pT3 disease

and positive surgical margin trends continue to be an issue, regardless of technique. Further, investigators in Virginia recently reported on nearly 800 patients enrolled in a quality of life study, prior to definitive therapy (29). The treatment was either open RP, robot assisted laparoscopic prostatectomy, brachytherapy or cryotherapy. Biochemical disease-free survival outcomes are not reported, but robot assisted prostatectomy surgical outcomes did not demonstrate superiority to an open approach. So, as treatment techniques change, changes in many significant endpoints have not been demonstrated, and adverse pathologic findings will continue to be a challenge to the surgical patient.

■ THE SIGNIFICANCE OF PSA FAILURE FOLLOWING PROSTATECTOMY

Tables 1 and 2 list multiple series where cancer outcomes have not been optimized by prostatectomy. The most immediate findings suggesting a good or poor cancer outcome is found in the pathology report of a surgical procedure. Further information is obtained from postoperative PSA values. Although the significance of a positive margin or disease outside the prostate or a PSA rise following prostatectomy have been topics of many publications and there has been historical debate as to their predictive value, data is presented within this article that refutes these findings as insignificant. These variables are, more often than not, associated with prostate cancer outcomes; most importantly, they have been helpful in predicting PCSS.

In a landmark publication, Pound et al. reported on the significance of a PSA rise following prostatectomy (30). In this retrospective study, 1,997 patients were treated with prostatectomy by a single physician, and salvage therapy was not given until the time of detection of clinical metastasis. The overall metastasis free survival for this cohort of men was 82% at 15 years, or roughly more than 1% per year. In total, they report that 315 men or 15% of patients had a PSA rise following prostatectomy. In these men with a PSA rise, the median time for biochemical recurrence to progression to metastases was 8 years, or approximately 40% at 5 years. After development of metastatic disease, the median time to death was less than 5 years. In this study, no man with metastatic disease died of any cause other than prostate cancer (30).

Of note, Pound reported on a fairly homogenous population of men with lower risk prostate cancer. The preoperative characteristics of these men included only 8% of men with Gleason scores greater than 7 and only 6% of men with a PSA values greater than 20 ng/mL (30,31). Pretreatment variables of Gleason score, time interval to recurrence, PSA doubling time (PSADT), and serum PSA at metastasis were not significant predictors of prostate cancer–specific mortality. Time to metastatic disease was important—the earlier metastatic disease appeared, the more likely a patient died of prostate cancer. Similar to other solid tumor disease sites, Pound et al. found that preventing metastatic disease reduced risk of prostate cancer–specific death.

Similar to the Pound study, and in a similar case series, Trock et al. validate the risk associated with a PSA rise following prostatectomy (31). Trock reported on 635 men with a PSA rise following RP with a median 6-year follow-up. The primary endpoint of this study was prostate cancer–specific mortality and the intent was to compare salvage therapies. Most men—397 or 63%—did not receive therapy for their PSA rise. The outcome of this cohort was 12% prostate cancer death at 5 years and 38% death at 10 years. In the author's analysis of variables associated with outcome; time from prostatectomy to recurrence, year of prostatectomy, and postoperative Gleason score, all demonstrated a statistically significant association with prostate cancer–specific mortality after prostatectomy (31).

The relationship of a PSA failure with prostate cancer–specific mortality can be learned from these series. With long-term follow-up, and likewise in a man with a 10 year or better life expectancy, the risk of prostate cancer-specific mortality is substantial,

nearly 40%, as seen in the Trock study (31), and intervention needs to be considered to improve outcomes.

■ INDICATIONS FOR POSTOPERATIVE THERAPY

Ultimately, PSA failure is important in any man with reasonable life expectancy. PSA failure is predictive of metastases and prostate cancer death (30,31). Beneficial intervention must be considered in these patients. Fortunately, PSA failure can be predicted. Surgical series early in the PSA era found an association between preoperative characteristics and pathologic findings and eventual biochemical failure (12,32–36).

It is evident that the higher the risk factors such as pretreatment PSA level, clinical T stage, and Gleason score, the more likely a patient is to experience a PSA failure. Pathologic T3 disease and the presence of a positive margin in controlled series predict PSA failure in a matter of months (37,38). T3 disease or greater is known to be associated with greater risk of local recurrence (39). Other risk factors important to predicting PSA failure include margin status, pathologic T stage and Gleason score, seminal vesicle or lymph node disease, and any combination of these variables. Analysis of these factors has led to many nomograms and tables that clinicians can use in counseling their patients (39–44).

Treatment options can be separated into two categories: local and distant. The intent and timing of intervention is distinct to both. For further categorization, local therapy can be separated further into salvage or adjuvant interventions. Salvage therapy commonly refers to treatment at the time of detection of disease, that is, PSA rise, whereas adjuvant therapy is treatment without detectable disease after surgery.

■ SALVAGE RADIOTHERAPY

Early in the PSA era, it became apparent that prostatectomy did not always eradicate all PSA producing tissue (45). Radiotherapy has been used in the event of PSA failure without clinical failure. Schild et al. reported in the early 1990s that nearly all patients with PSA failure following radiotherapy responded with a PSA decline (46). The durability of PSA control in early series was not good, but judiciously using radiotherapy when PSA levels are low was identified early as a predictor of future biochemical control (46,47). Other limitations existed from the early experiences; in additional to durable PSA response, it was unclear whether or not there was an impact on more meaningful endpoints such as metastases and death. Also, we had identifying occult local and distant disease. All these factors contribute to the controversy that surrounds the use of salvage radiotherapy.

Schild et al. reported on one of the earliest experiences of salvage therapy when their group treated eleven men upon repeated PSA rises after prostatectomy (46,48). At short follow-up, all had an initial PSA response. The response was sustained in 64% and there was no clinical progression or side effects to report in their treated cohort. This suggested to these investigators that local therapy could improve upon prostatectomy, but further study and follow-up was needed.

Hudson and Catalona at Washington University reported similar findings in an initial 21 patients treated for PSA failure after prostatectomy (48). This group identified variables associated with biochemical failure. In particular, they noted that patients with lower PSA levels at the start of radiation and patients who initially had undetectable PSA prior to failure benefited the most. They reported a biochemical progression-free survival rate of 53% to 67% for their entire cohort with 28 months of follow-up and concluded these were very promising results.

Not all studies shared these promising conclusions. The use of salvage radiotherapy was controversial as other series showed less benefit (49,50). Whereas most found the PSA to decline after radiotherapy, the durability of the change and therapeutic value was unknown and challenged. Radiotherapy was concluded to have limited impact and was not accepted as standard therapy.

Selecting patients more carefully was needed. In 1998, Cadeddu et al. reported on a cohort of patients whose selection for salvage radiotherapy was based on prior experience (47,51,52). Eighty-two men were treated with salvage radiotherapy and only 10% showed progression of disease. They were able to identify patients most likely to benefit from salvage local therapy. They suggested risk factors that are more likely to be associated with occult distant disease. Characteristics of the these men included Gleason scores 8 or higher, positive seminal vesicles or lymph nodes, and a PSA recurrence within the first year of prostatectomy (53).

Longer follow-up was needed and eventually reported. Schild et al. reported in their growing single institution experience with salvage radiotherapy that after 5 years of follow-up, biochemical progression-free survival was achieved in 50% of patients (54). Other investigators found similar results (55–57). Rogers et al. reported biochemical progression-free survival of 48% at 3 years and also that pretreatment PSA and Gleason predicted the best outcomes (58). The Stanford group published their long-term experience. They noted that in 110 patients treated in the early PSA era, 38% percent had sustained PSA control at greater than 12 years median follow-up. And notably, findings like advanced T stage and Gleason score, as well as a fast PSA velocity predicted distant disease (45).

Stephenson et al. recently update their retrospective multi institutional series of 1,540 men who received salvage radiotherapy (59,60). The patient population all had PSA failure following prostatectomy. Gleason 8–10 disease was present in 22%, seminal vesicle and lymph node disease was present in 24% and 3%, respectively. Approximately 30% of the men never had an undetectable PSA following prostatectomy. 65% had pT3a disease and 51% had positive margins after prostatectomy—known predictors of PSA. Their patient population had a median PSA prior to radiotherapy of approximately 1.0 ng/mL with a median disease free interval of 15 months from surgery. The median follow-up after prostatectomy was 90 months, and after radiotherapy was 53 months, for purposes of this report. For the entire cohort, the 6-year progression-free probability was 32% (95%CI 28–35). A nomogram was formed from statistically significant pretreatment variables including: PSA level before salvage radiotherapy, prostatectomy Gleason grade, PSADT, surgical margins status, use of hormonal therapy, and lymph node metastasis. Progression-free probability in this study was best predicted by PSA prior to salvage radiotherapy. If the PSA was equal or less than 2 ng/mL, 58% (54–62%) had sustained PSA survival at 6 years, but only 19% were disease free. The cohort most likely to be progression free in their analysis was a patient with pretreatment PSA less than 2, Gleason of 7 or less, positive surgical margins, and a slow PSADT (>10 months). This group had a predicted 4-year progression-free probability of 69% (95%CI 59–79) (59). Importantly, patients with high-risk disease by Gleason score (8–10) could beat the median as well if they had a presalvage radiotherapy PSA of 2 ng/mL or less, positive margins, and a slow PSADT. This cohort was found to have a 4-year progression-free probability of 50% (95%CI 16–86)—note the wide confidence interval due to small number of patients with these characteristics. This study has many limitations (low predictive accuracy, retrospective, many variations in data and treatment, shorter follow-up) but also a number of strengths (large patient population and it was multi-institutional). Hugen et al. found the predictive nomogram from Stephenson to be valid when tested on a separate independent cohort of patients (61). Despite fairly adverse pathologic features at prostatectomy and initial recurrence of disease, a large number of men in these studies remain free of PSA recurrence and clinical disease and cured by salvage radiotherapy.

Trock et al. report the most important study of salvage radiotherapy from their John Hopkins's experience (31). The intent was to compare observed to treated populations after prostatectomy and PSA failure. Trock et al. analyzed 635 men with long-term follow-up following PSA failure after prostatectomy (31). In total, 397 of these men were observed, 160 received radiotherapy, and 78 received combined radiotherapy and androgen-deprivation therapy. PCSS at 10 years was the primary endpoint and they had a 6-year median follow-up of patients. For the entire cohort, 18% died from prostate cancer and 8% died from other causes. Of note, men were less likely to receive salvage therapy in the event of positive lymph nodes, and men receiving salvage therapy that included hormonal therapy were more likely to have a shorter time to recurrence, shorter PSADT, and higher PSA level. Salvage therapy in this analysis improves survival from 88% to 96% at 5 years, and 62% to 86% at 10 years for the entire cohort. Most significant predictors of prostate cancer–specific mortality on multivariate analysis included time from prostatectomy to recurrence, year of prostatectomy, postoperative Gleason score, and PSADT at failure. The use of hormonal therapy did not show independent significance. The effect of hormonal therapy may be underpowered to detect a difference and represents sampling bias. The median time to prostate death in the observation group is approximately 12 years, consistent with previous reports (30), and a median prostate cancer–specific mortality was not found at last follow-up in the treated groups (31).

An important finding in the Trock study is the value of PSA velocity or PSADT and its use as a prognostic or predictive factor. As previously noted

(62), PSADT is a poor prognostic factor following PSA failure from prostatectomy; and in this study, it again proves to be associated with poorer outcome. Trock et al. confirm that a fast PSADT places men at an increased risk of death following PSA failure from prostatectomy. But what is important to note is that it may also be predictive of outcome when salvage radiotherapy is given. It turns out that the cohort who benefited the most from salvage radiotherapy were the patients with fast PSADT. The absolute 10-year PCSS improved 52%—from 30% to 82%—in patients with a fast PSADT (<6 months doubling time) when comparing observation to salvage radiotherapy. Similarly, patients with a slow PSADT still benefited from radiotherapy, just not with the same magnitude. The absolute benefit seen with salvage radiotherapy in this cohort was 11%, improving the 10-year PCSS to 85%. The cohort who fared best following salvage radiotherapy had a slow PSADT (>6 months) and positive margins at prostatectomy (10-year PCSS is approximately 90% with salvage radiotherapy), whereas the group that fared worse had a fast PSADT, positive margins, and a higher Gleason score (10-year PCSS of 5%).

Though retrospective, the value of their data is strengthened by the comparison with an observation group from the same surgeons and having 10-year PCSS data. Trock et al. solidify the role of salvage radiotherapy in practice today. Also, Trock et al. provide evidence for use of salvage radiotherapy in men with even the most adverse prognostic factors such as a fast PSADT and high Gleason score.

Time to initiating salvage therapy is raised as an important variable in this study as well as others (31,59). PSA at the time of salvage therapy and the time from PSA failure to the start of salvage therapy is associated with PCSS in these studies. The dilemma that presents itself is that we may still overtreat a population of men. But, waiting for failure may be detrimental to the population of men that are at high risk from PSA progression following prostatectomy. This finding begs the question whether adjuvant therapy would improve outcome in these men.

■ ADJUVANT RADIOTHERAPY

Adjuvant therapy—a means of supplemental treatment following cancer surgery—is a mainstay of therapy in many solid cancer sites. Clearly different from initiating therapy at the point of progression, adjuvant therapy in high-risk patients ideally eradicates microscopic residual disease that threatens to progress over time. Three randomized controlled studies have addressed the role of adjuvant therapy following RP in a population of men at high risk of failure (37,38,40,41). The objective of these randomized studies was to evaluate if early radiotherapy can improve outcomes. Table 3 is a summary of these three studies, which vary somewhat in size, patient population, follow-up and endpoints but all come to a similar conclusion: immediate radiotherapy following prostatectomy improves outcomes.

Bolla et al. reported on the EORTC study, which enrolled the most patients, in 2005 (40). Patients with pathologic T2 or T3 disease were eligible if they had one of the following: positive margin, extra capsular penetration or seminal vesicle invasion. 1,005 men were then randomized between immediate radiotherapy and observation. The radiotherapy was 60 Gray (Gy) prescribed to the prostate and surgical bed. The study was designed as an intention to treat analysis. The primary endpoint was biochemical progression-free survival. At first report, in the median follow-up of 5 years, adjuvant radiotherapy reduced that risk of a biochemical recurrence by nearly 50%, an absolute improvement of 21%, from 53% to 74%. The benefit was seen in all cohorts.

Additional details of the EORTC study are as follows: 11% had persistently elevated PSA prior to randomization, and poorly differentiated disease was present in 24%. Approximately 50% meet one criteria (16% positive margin, 27% extracapsular extension, 4% seminal vesicle invasion), and 12% had all risk factors. In the observation cohort, the median time to PSA failure was approximately 5 years. Of the patients who failed, 113 of 207 (55%) patients received radiotherapy. In addition to improved biochemical progression-free survival, clinical progression and locoregional control were improved (40). The absolute benefit for local control and clinical disease control were approximately 10% and 8%, respectively. The majority of failure was thought to be local. Hormonal therapy was more commonly used due to progression in the observation arm. At 5 years, no difference was seen in distant metastatic rate (6%) and overall survival. Of note however, is the fact that twice as many men died on the observation arm. We are eagerly anticipating an update of this trial with longer follow-up.

German investigators found a similar benefit to radiotherapy (41). Their study is different from the EORTC and Southwest Oncology Group (SWOG) study. It is a true adjuvant evaluation of the role of radiotherapy; eligible patients were required to have an undetectable PSA. The study enrolled 388 patients and randomized between radiotherapy, 60 Gy to the prostate bed, and observation. The primary endpoint was biochemical recurrence determined by two PSA rises during follow-up. By requiring an undetectable PSA for enrollment, the study likely excluded the higher risk patients seen on the other two controlled studies. For example, 10% of the population had Gleason 8 disease or worse upon central review, roughly half of the number seen in the other studies (38,40). Nonetheless, adjuvant radiotherapy significantly improved outcome. At the 54-month median follow-up, biochemical progression-free survival was 72% in the treatment arm and 52% in the wait and see arm, for a relative reduction of biochemical failure of approximately 50%, similar to the reduction

TABLE 3 Randomized trials of adjuvant radiotherapy, outcome by primary endpoints

Investigators	Number	Primary Endpoint	Follow-Up	PSA > 0.2	Seminal Vesicle Invasion	Local Control	bDFS 5 years/ Hazard Ratio	Metastatic-Free Survival/ Hazard Ratio	Overall Survival/ Hazard Ratio
EORTC (40)	1005	bDFS	5y	11	4	RT: 95 Obs:85	RT:85 Obs: 77/0.48	5 years 94 (NS)	93 (NS)
SWOG (37,38)	425	MFS	12y	33	10	NR	RT:65 OBS:35	10 years RT:57 OBS:46/0.71	RT:59 OBS:48/0.72
German researchers (41)	307	bDFS	4.4y	0	17	NR	RT:72 OBS:72/0.53	5 years 97–98%	NR

NR, not reported.

in failure seen in the EORTC study. Endpoints of disease-free survival, prostate cancer survival and overall survival, as well as toxicity, were not significantly different between arms, and due to the small number of patients enrolled, the study is underpowered to detect a difference if it exists. Local control was not assessed either. The authors note how a moderate dose of radiotherapy reduced the incidence of failure so substantially.

The third randomized study was completed by the SWOG and recently updated by Thompson et al. (37,38). This randomized controlled trial had similar eligibility to the EORTC study reported by Bolla et al.; namely, patients had positive margins, extra capsular extension of disease, or seminal vesicle invasion at the time of prostatectomy. Four hundred twenty-five men were randomized to receive immediate adjuvant radiotherapy or be observed. Adjuvant therapy consisted of radiotherapy to the prostate and surgical bed at 60 to 64 Gy. The primary endpoint was metastatic disease-free survival. With a median follow-up of 10.6 years, neither metastatic disease-free survival nor overall survival was significantly different between the two cohorts. However, the median time to relapse, which occurred at 3 years in the observation group but more than 10 years later in the treated population, was significantly improved. Adjuvant radiotherapy in the initial analysis improved biochemical free survival, relapse free survival and risk of salvage therapy (initiation of hormonal therapy). In similar magnitude to the EORTC and German studies, PSA relapse was reduced by 57% and salvage therapy was reduced by 45%.

Upon second report, at a median of 12.7 years of follow-up, radiotherapy improved endpoints of metastatic free survival and overall survival. Ultimately, this study showed that adjuvant radiotherapy reduced the risk of metastasis by 29%. Overall survival improved from 66% to 74% with therapy—this is an 8% absolute improvement. Therefore, to prevent one death from prostate cancer, 12 patients needed to be treated with adjuvant radiotherapy. Further subset analysis demonstrates that all subgroups benefitted. Evaluation of the men with seminal vesicle disease has shown that even with adjuvant radiotherapy, the PSA control at 10 years is merely 36%. Metastases-free survival and overall survival improved by approximately 20% in this cohort with the addition of radiotherapy, to 66% and 71%, respectively (64). Best results were observed in men with undetectable PSA levels prior to radiotherapy (39). Failure

was predominately local, and like other disease sites, when persistent local disease is eradicated, the result is less metastatic disease occurrence and improved survival (37).

Adjuvant radiotherapy in patients with pT3 disease or positive surgical margins improves biochemical free survival, hormonal therapy free survival, metastatic disease-free survival, disease-free survival, PCSS, and overall survival (37,40,41). Level 1 evidence supports that the magnitude of survival benefit in the SWOG study is similar to the benefit in the randomized study of RP versus watchful waiting (15). The NNT for survival benefit from prostatectomy is 12 and the NNT for adjuvant therapy is 12. If the intent of prostatectomy is curative, then when high-risk features are found at prostatectomy, there is strong data to support continuing treatment with adjuvant radiotherapy. Adjuvant radiotherapy confers the same benefit, with an equal level of evidence to surgical intervention. Although the suggested timing of radiotherapy after prostatectomy may be controversial, patients should be offered this discussion, preferably by a radiation oncologist.

■ THE ROLE OF HORMONAL THERAPY

There is currently no Level I evidence to support the routine use of hormone therapy with adjuvant or salvage radiotherapy. The RTOG is currently conducting a study to test the role in comparison to salvage prostate bed radiotherapy alone. Three controlled studies have established a PCSS benefit to the addition of hormonal therapy in patients with high-risk features in the intact, definitive setting, when compared to radiotherapy alone (65,66). Another RTOG study has demonstrated a progression-free survival benefit when hormonal therapy is added to pelvic radiation in the intact setting (67). In support of hormonal therapy in the adjuvant and salvage radiotherapy settings, at least one comprehensive report exists that finds a benefit in the patient inflicted with high-risk disease prior to prostatectomy (68).

The three prospective studies in adjuvant radiotherapy did not use hormonal therapy (38,40,41). The 5-year biochemical control of these studies is between 65% and 85% with radiotherapy alone. Perhaps adding concurrent hormonal therapy to the poorest performing cohorts found in these studies may improve outcome, but a phase III comparison is needed. RTOG 0534 is currently enrolling patients to address these questions in the setting of salvage radiotherapy.

Several retrospective series have looked at hormonal therapy with salvage radiotherapy. Trock et al. did not find a prostate cancer–specific survival benefit. The Johns Hopkins group compared patients who received hormonal therapy with radiotherapy and radiotherapy alone, and found no difference at 10 years (31). The median follow-up on this study was approximately 6 years and selection bias is a major limitation in interpreting this study. It is possible that hormonal therapy was used in the worst clinical scenarios and ameliorated the effects of worse disease.

Other studies have found benefit to the addition of androgen suppression. Spiotto et al. reported on a cohort of 160 men who received salvage radiotherapy following prostatectomy. Benefit was seen in men with high-risk disease who also had pelvic lymph node radiotherapy in addition to prostate bed treatment, analogous to the randomized study in the intact setting reported by Roach et al. (67,69). This is supported in a literature based review by Jani et al. (70). Significant benefit seems to be conferred by combined hormonal therapy and radiotherapy when patients have high-risk features de novo, prior to initiating treatment.

Our practice at Emory University is to use hormonal therapy in the setting of a clinical trial. RTOG 0534 is a three-arm randomized controlled trial designed to assess the benefit of adding hormonal therapy to radiotherapy in the setting of salvage radiotherapy. Patients may be randomized with 1) prostate bed radiotherapy alone or 2) neoadjuvant, concurrent, and adjuvant hormonal therapy (4–6 months total) plus prostate bed radiotherapy or 3) neoadjuvant, concurrent, and hormonal therapy plus pelvic lymph node radiotherapy with a prostate bed boost. Patients must have a negative metastatic work up and pathologic T2 or T3 disease, a PSA between 0.1 and 2.0 ng/mL and Gleason score of 9 or less. Off study, adding 4 months to 2 to 3 years of hormonal therapy in patients with high-risk disease de novo or with multiple high-risk features during adjuvant or salvage therapy is at the discretion of the treating physician.

RTOG 0622 is a single-arm phase II study evaluating the role of samarium-153 in conjunction with androgen deprivation and radiotherapy for high-risk postprostatectomy patients (PSA > 2.0 postoperatively and/or Gleason 9–10 disease and/or short PSADT). The goal, in addition to toxicity evaluation of this novel approach, is to see whether samarium-153 can aid in eradication of bone micrometastases and thereby improve distant failure rates.

■ TOXICITY

Over the past three decades, the toxicity of radiotherapy following RP has received considerable attention. Late complications associated with prostatectomy alone and with radiotherapy following prostatectomy are urinary incontinence, urinary stricture, and erectile dysfunction. Additionally, radiotherapy has a relationship with secondary malignancies, a conversation important to anyone with a long life expectancy.

Three randomized controlled studies exist to prospectively detail the side effect profile of adjuvant radiotherapy. The results of late toxicity seen on the EORTC, SWOG, and German studies are summarized in Table 4. Incontinence is probably the most clinically challenging. Symptoms of incontinence may be present in one out of four patients after prostatectomy (71). In the three randomized studies, radiotherapy was initiated within 4 months of prostatectomy, generally, by 3 months (38,40,41). In a quality of life study published by Sanda et al. (71), 12% of patients used at least one pad at 2 months following prostatectomy. This statistically decreased over a 2-year period to 4% at 2 years. Therefore, when offering radiotherapy in the adjuvant setting, we potentially irradiate healing tissue.

The SWOG study was the only study of the three that prospectively evaluated incontinence (38), although the EORTC study in an interim analysis found no difference between treatment arms (40). In contrast to the EORTC study, on the SWOG study, frank incontinence increased significantly from 3% to approximately 7% (38). Thus, in the adjuvant setting we may increase the risk of incontinence by 3% to 5%. The number of patients needed to treat to cause incontinence is approximately 25. We recommend initiating radiotherapy when symptoms have stabilized, if disease status allows, even if more than 4 months has passed since prostatectomy.

After prostatectomy and radiotherapy, urethral strictures and sexual dysfunction are common in this patient population. The incidence of urethral stricture increased from 10% to 18% with long-term follow-up on the SWOG study, but was uncommon on the German study (38,41). Finally, the incidence of sexual dysfunction has been addressed in the SWOG study as well. Swanson et al. reported on prospective health-related quality of life (HRQOL) data collected on 217 men enrolled in study. Important endpoints for analysis included bowel tenderness, frequent urination, and erectile dysfunction. At

TABLE 4 Late toxicity associated with adjuvant and salvage radiotherapy

Investigators	Grade ≥ 1	Grade 2	Grade 3	Grade 4
EORTC (40)*	NR	NR	4v3% p = NS	0
SWOG (37,38,63)	24v12% p = s	3v0% p = s GU stricture 18%v10% p = s GU incontinence 7v3%	0	0
German researchers (41)*	22v4% p = S	5 events (3GU/2GI) versus 0	1 patient (0.3%) (bladder)	0

*Did not assess incontinence.

5 years of follow-up, bowel and urinary function was significantly affected by radiotherapy but improved over time. The bowel symptoms were short lived and were not different between the two groups at last follow-up, but urinary bother persisted. Erectile dysfunction was not different between the two groups at follow-up (63). It is important to note that longer term assessment is confounded by increased use of hormonal therapy in the observed patients, due to treatment failure affecting HRQOL.

■ FIELD SIZE, DOSE, AND TECHNIQUE

The best results in controlled trials, to date, for the treatment of a higher risk patient with an intact prostate, have incorporated hormonal therapy and pelvic lymph node radiotherapy with the overall treatment plan (65,67,72–74). As discussed previously, less is known about the benefit of larger treatment fields to treat lymph nodes or of dose escalation in the postoperative radiotherapy treatment of men. The Stanford group has published a benefit for a larger field to include the pelvic lymph nodes, prior to a prostate bed boost in higher risk patients (69), and dose escalation to 70 Gy (75,76). Randomized studies have used a dose between 60 and 64 Gy (38,40,41). A consensus opinion from 2002 considers a dosage greater or equal to 64.8 Gy to be within standard practice guidelines (77). The current RTOG study specifies the dosage to be between 64.8 and 70.2 Gy in 1.8 Gy daily fractions. This study is designed to test field size to determine if treating the pelvic lymph nodes is of benefit. At Emory University, we treat the prostate bed with 66 to 70Gy in 2 Gy fractions or 68.4 to 70.2 Gy in 1.8 Gy daily fractions. Additionally, we will always consider treating the pelvic lymph nodes and adding hormonal therapy in high-risk patients.

Figures 1A and B show examples of treatment plans for patient treatment, postoperatively, with treatment to the prostate bed using intensity-modulated radiotherapy (IMRT) and volumetric modulated arc therapy (VMAT) (RapidArc) techniques. Figure 1C is an example of a treatment plan for a patient treated in the pelvic lymph nodes and prostate bed at 46 Gy followed by a prostate bed boost to a total of 70 Gy.

The technical aspects of treatment planning are as follows:

The treatments are planned using either IMRT or VMAT techniques on an Eclipse treatment planning system for treatment on a Trilogy linear accelerator (Varian Medical Systems) equipped with a 5-mm multileaf collimator (MLC120) system. A maximum dose rate of 600 monitor unit (MU)/minute was used for planning and treatment delivery. Other planning parameters were MLC motion speed 0 to 2.5 cm/second, dose rate 0 to 600 MU/minute, and gantry rotation speed of 0.5 to 5.54 degrees/second.

IMRT Beam Configuration

Five to seven beams are used, with beam angles selected based on the anatomical relationships of the planning target volumes (PTV) and the organ at risk (OAR). Most of the IMRT beams are directed from the anterior position to minimize the passage of radiation through the rectum. Using the prescribed dosage constraints, the inverse planning algorithm attempts to find the optimal solution, consisting of a set of intensity maps. Each individual beam has one intensity map. For each beam, a sliding window technique sequences the intensity map into multiple MLC segments. The total number of MLC segments per plan can be a few hundred to more than a thousand.

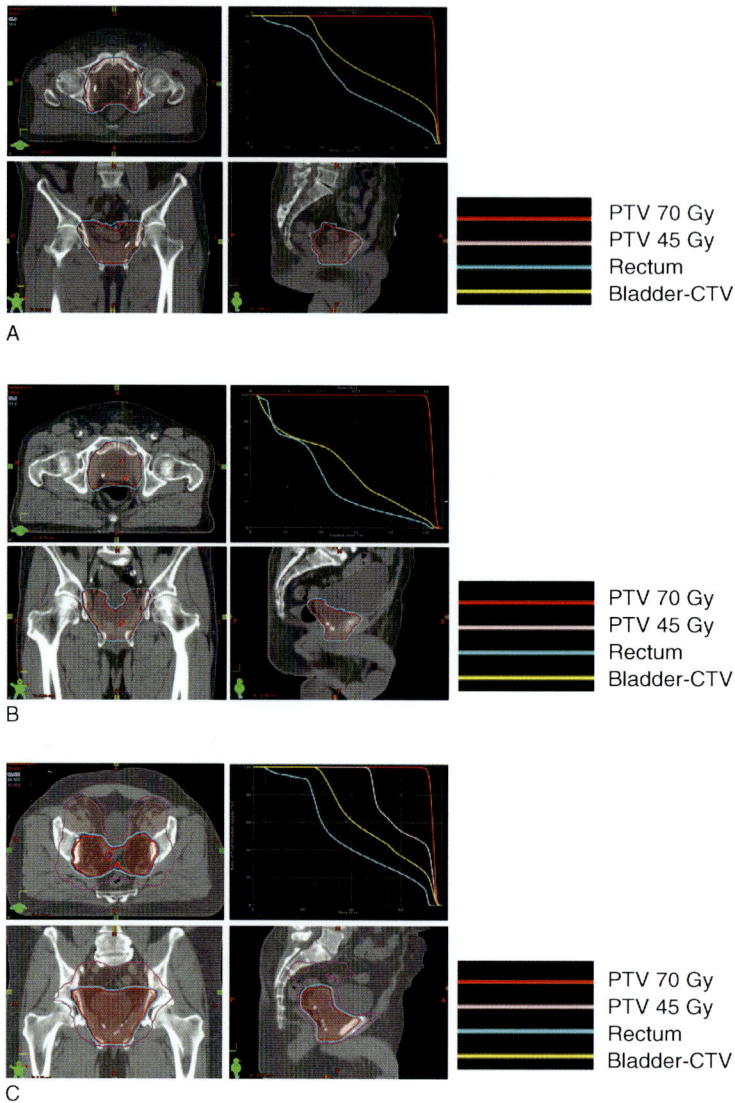

FIGURE 1 Demonstration of a treatment plan using (A) an IMRT technique for treatment of prostate bed, (B) a VMAT (RapidArc) technique for treatment of the prostate bed, and (C) VMAT technique for treatment of the pelvic lymph nodes and prostate bed.

VMAT Beam Configuration

The total arc length and the start/stop gantry positions are user defined, based on surrounding OAR and PTV location and shape. The arc is divided into 177 points or beamlets; each control point has only one MLC defined shape. In this study, two arcs were typically used; the first ARC is CW 340° with the collimator at 45° and the second is CCW 340° long with the collimator at 315°. The start and stop of the

arcs were arranged to avoid the rectum. The inverse planning algorithm optimizes the MLC shape and dose for each control point. Optimization constraints include the traditional IMRT constraints, in addition to the adjacent control points MLC shapes, gantry speed, and dose rate.

The clinical target volume may include the prostate bed or prostate bed and pelvic lymph nodes. It is decided upon after considering all clinical, pathologic, and radiographic information on an individual

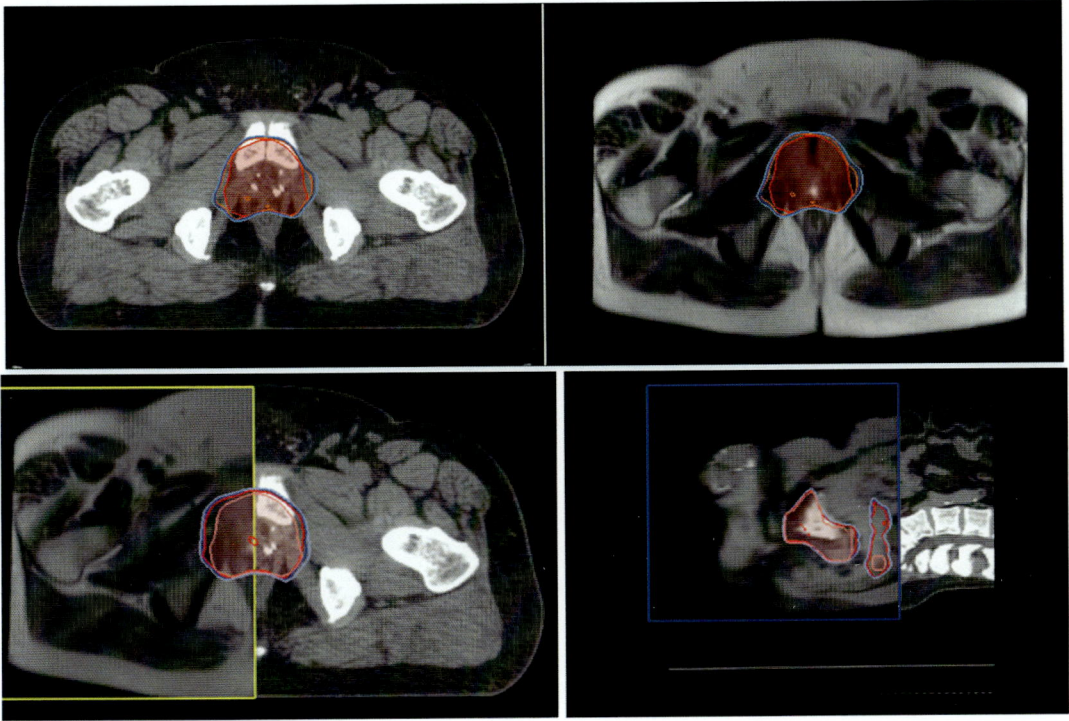

FIGURE 2 Demonstration of MRI to CT fusion used in delineating structures during treatment planning. Note the vesicourethral anastomosis or beak on MRI compared to CT imaging.

and constitutes the tissue volume at risk of subclinical microscopic and macroscopic tumor burden following prostatectomy. Cooperative consensus recommendations of treatment volumes have been published by Michalski et al. for treatment of the prostatic bed (78) and by Lawton et al. when additionally treating the pelvic lymph nodes (79). Both consensus statements are based on recurrence patterns following prostatectomy. These are published as a CT atlas on the RTOG Web site as well, for easy review.

To summarize briefly, the clinical target volume for the prostatic bed: in general, the superior border is defined at the level of the remnant of the vas deferens, which is typically easy to see on CT or MRI imaging. The genital urinary diaphragm, a structure not violated by retro pubic or laparoscopic surgical technique, defines the lower border. If an MRI is not available, this can be estimated by identifying the vesicourethral anastomosis on CT urethragram. The anterior border abuts the posterior pubis inferiorly and 1 to 2 cm behind the bladder, superiorly. The posterior border is defined by the mesorectal and rectal structures, which are best seen on MRI.

When the clinical target includes the pelvic lymph nodes, the target includes: distal common iliacs, presacral, external iliac, internal iliac, and obturator lymph nodes. An additional 7 mm is added as a clinical target expansion to vessels, omitting bone, bladder, rectum, and muscle, to approximate known radiographic and surgical location of the lymph nodes.

At Emory University, we use a pelvic MRI fused to a planning CT to best delineate clinical target volume (Figure 2). Patients are encouraged to have a moderately full bladder and use a rectal enema a few hours prior to simulation. The patient's legs are immobilized. If an MRI is not available, a urethrogram is performed. Once the clinical target volume is decided, it is expanded by 6 to 10 mm (generally 8 mm in all directions) to a PTV, to account for setup uncertainty and motion. We use on-board imaging to localize to bony landmarks daily. Some investigators have used fiducials markers placed by ultrasound. However, in treatment of the prostate bed after prostatectomy, the daily motion set up error and positioning error is within few millimeters for most sessions (80). Neither the motion nor the current dosage levels suggest the extra procedure is beneficial for routine use.

■ SINGLE-INSTITUTION TOXICITY/FIELD SIZE DATA

As described in the Toxicity section, toxicity data has been reported for adjuvant XRT trials, these data are limited to prostate-bed only treatment. It is unclear (a) whether pelvic nodal therapy adds to treatment toxicity in the postprostatectomy setting and (b) how toxicity rates of postprostatectomy XRT compare to treatment in the intact prostate setting. We describe single institution data on both of these issues:

Postprostatectomy—Prostate Bed Only Versus Whole-Pelvis Toxicity

At our institution, data on urinary and genitourinary (GU) and gastrointestinal (GI) toxicity in whole pelvis (WP) versus prostate bed only (PBO) radiation in prostate cancer patients following RP were compared. The records of consecutive prostate cancer patients at our institution who received post-RP radiation therapy (RT) for a persistently detectable or rising PSA were reviewed. The study group included 122 patients; 50 underwent WP RT (median 45 Gy

to pelvic lymph nodes) and 72 underwent PBO RT. RT was delivered at doses of 64.8 to 75.6 Gy. The two groups were balanced with respect to most major demographic, disease, and non-target volume (TV) treatment factors. RTOG morbidity scoring was used to chart GU and GI toxicity. Toxicity rates were compared using the chi-square test (Table 5). Ordered logit regression analyses for each toxicity endpoint were performed using treatment factors as covariates (Table 6). As shown in Table 5, in our study, TV was independently associated with late GU and acute GI toxicity. IMRT use independently lowers both GU and GI toxicity. In conclusion, GU and GI toxicity was lower in patients treated with PBO (versus WP) post-RP RT. IMRT was instrumental in decreasing toxicity in both groups. Although ongoing randomized trials will provide additional data on post-RP PLN RT efficacy and toxicity, our study was important in identifying IMRT as an independent variable in toxicity reduction.

Intact Prostate—Prostate Only Versus Whole-Pelvis Toxicity

Similar to the above effort in the postprostatectomy setting, toxicity outcomes between WP and prostate only (PO) were compared. Additionally, factors influencing toxicity outcomes were analyzed. The study group consisted of 205 men; 105 who received

TABLE 5 Single-institution toxicity data in postprostatectomy setting—Chi-square analysis

Grade	0	1	2	3	4	5	P
Acute GU							
WP	8 (16%)	32 (64%)	9 (18%)	0 (0%)	0 (0%)	0 (0%)	0.07
PBO	17 (24%)	45 (63%)	9 (13%)	0 (0%)	1 (1%)	0 (0%)	
Acute GI							
WP	1 (2%)	6 (12%)	42 (84%)	0 (0%)	0 (0%)	0 (0%)	<0.01
PBO	19 (26%)	12 (17%)	41 (57%)	0 (0%)	0 (0%)	0 (0%)	
Late GU							
WP	18 (36%)	16 (32%)	10 (20%)	3 (6%)	0 (0%)	0 (0%)	<0.01
PBO	53 (74%)	13 (18%)	3 (4%)	1 (1%)	2 (3%)	0 (0%)	
Late GI							
WP	30 (60%)	9 (18%)	8 (16%)	0 (0%)	0 (0%)	0 (0%)	0.18
PBO	52 (72%)	10 (14%)	9 (13%)	1 (1%)	0 (0%)	0 (0%)	

TABLE 6 Single-institution toxicity data in postprostatectomy setting—Multivariate analysis

Acute GU	Hormone Use	Target Volume	IMRT Use	RT Dose
Coefficient	0.482	0.158	1.215	−0.002
P	0.31	0.72	0.01	0.08
95% CI	−0.45to 1.41	−0.70 to 1.02	0.30 to 2.13	−0.004 to 0.0002
Acute GI				
Coefficient	−0.582	−1.105	1.275	−0.001
P	0.32	0.03	0.01	0.28
95% CI	−1.7288 to 0.5657	−2.1245 to −0.0862	0.3557 to 2.1942	−0.0033 to 0.0010
Late GU				
Coefficient	0.354	−0.898	1.132	−0.001
P	0.46	0.04	0.02	0.28
95% CI	−0.59 to 1.30	−1.76 to −0.03	0.17 to 2.09	−0.004 to 0.001
Late GI				
Coefficient	0.321	−0.087	0.636	0.001
P	0.53	0.85	0.18	0.51
95% CI	−0.6687 to 1.3108	−0.9610 to 0.7875	−0.3034 to 1.5763	−0.0014 to 0.0028

WP, whole pelvis; PBO, prostate bed only.

WP and 100 who received PO RT. The WP group had a higher percentage of high-risk patients (57% versus 12%), a lower percentage of IMRT use (47% versus 92%), and a higher percentage of hormone use (70% versus 34%); otherwise the groups were balanced (notably, mean final dose was 77.09 versus 77.8 Gy [WP versus PO]). Toxicity events (acute and late; GU and GI) were charted using RTOG morbidity scoring and compared using the chi-square test (Table 7). Ordered logit regression analyses were performed on each toxicity endpoint using all major demographic, disease, and treatment factors as covariates (Table 8). Median follow-up was 2.5 years. Toxicity analyses demonstrated that acute GI toxicity was significantly higher in the WP versus PO arm; other toxicity endpoints were not significantly different. Ordered logit regression analyses showed that age correlated with acute GU toxicity, IMRT use correlated with acute GI toxicity, and RT dose correlated with late GU toxicity; otherwise, no factors reached significance. In our study, WP did not independently influence GU or GI toxicity outcomes. IMRT use (rather than WP) strongly predicted for acute GI toxicity. Similarly, RT dose (rather than WP) correlated strongly with late GU toxicity. These findings suggest that treatment

technique and final dose are stronger predictors of toxicity outcomes than region treated.

The summary of the above reports suggests that (a) addition of pelvic nodal treatment to either prostate-bed or prostate radiation does contribute to additional toxicity, but in either case, treatment technique is a primary factor in reducing toxicity and (b) although not compared formally, the overall GU and GI toxicity rates of radiotherapy appear to be generally similar in the intact prostate and postprostatectomy settings (with lower acute GU toxicity rates in the post-RRP setting, perhaps due to the lower total dose typically used).

■ WORK UP AND NOVEL IMAGING

The work up of a patient prior to adjuvant or salvage radiotherapy includes laboratory studies and imaging. A great challenge to medicine at this time is to improve on diagnostic imaging. While approximately one-third of patients will have biochemical evidence of recurrence after prostatectomy and the resultant therapeutic approach depends not only on confirming recurrence but particularly in determining if

TABLE 7 Single-institution toxicity data in intact prostate setting—Chi-square analysis

	Grade 0	Grade 1	Grade 2	Grade 3	*P*
Acute GU: WP	7*	39	61	0	0.281
Acute GU: PO	3	36	62	0	
Acute GI: WP	5	21	81	0	<0.001
Acute GI: PO	15	30	56	0	
Late GU: WP	58	14	4	1	0.921
Late GU: PO	54	13	26	4	
Late GI: WP	73	16	12	0	0.321
Late GI: PO	72	17	7	1	

*Entries are numbers of patients.

TABLE 8 Single-institution toxicity data in intact prostate setting—Multivariate analysis

Factor	*P*-Value: Acute GU/Acute GI	*P*-Value: Late GU/Late GI
Age	0.008/0.409	0.125/0.084
T-stage	0.240/0.517	0.200/0.428
Gleason	0.518/0.375	0.297/0.793
PSA	0.382/0.725	0.695/0.479
RT dose	0.084/0.526	0.048/0.497
Region (WP versus PO)	0.925/0.364	0.432/0.384
IMRT use	0.290/0.001	0.558/0.256
Hormone use	0.327/0.878	0.073/0.246

the recurrence is confined to the prostate bed or is extra prostatic (81,82). We generally use a combination of bone scan, CT, and MRI to evaluate for disease extent (81,82). Most of the data known of these imaging techniques is in de novo patients, not after prostatectomy, but we also order these studies as a baseline prior to intervention.

ProstaScint received Food and Drug Administration approval in 1996 for use as an imaging agent for the restaging of postprostatectomy patients with a rising PSA level. A ProstaScint is 111Indium-capromab-pendetide and is a radiolabeled murine monoclonal antibody, which recognizes an intracellular epitope of prostate-specific membrane antigen (83). Reported sensitivity varies widely, ranging from 17% to 75% (83–88), likely reflecting study population and design, and Seltzer and coworkers compared ProstaScint imaging to biopsy sampled nodes and reported that ProstaScint was true positive in only one of six patients for proven nodal metastasis (87). Perhaps due to low sensitively and positive predictive value, the benefit of Prostascint on disease outcome remains controversial (89). However, several efforts have been undertaken to analyze the role of ProstaScint in clinical decision-making, in influencing toxicity outcomes, and in influencing PSA control (90–95).

Our current imaging techniques have limitations, but newer imaging studies do hold promise. An MRI with supermagnetic nanoparticles may be promising for lymph node assessment (96). Also, Anti 1-amino-3-[18F]fluorocyclobutane-1-carboxylic acid (anti-[18F]FACBC) is a synthetic l-leucine analog which has demonstrated promise in a pilot study for the staging and restaging of prostate carcinoma (97). A noninvasive method to guide pathologic confirmation is needed, especially one that has reasonable accuracy at low PSA levels.

■ CURRENT CLINICAL STUDIES

- *Within the RTOG*:
  - 0534: A phase III trial of short-term andro-gen therapy with pelvic lymph node or PBO radiotherapy in prostate cancer patients with a rising PSA after radical prostatectomy.
  - 0622: A phase II trial of samarium 153 fol-lowed by salvage radiotherapy in high-risk nonmetastatic prostate cancer patients after radical prostatectomy.
- *Other efforts Within the United States*:
  - PR06 at University of Florida, a proton ther-apy study for postoperative or salvage radio-therapy for node negative prostate cancer patients following radical prostatectomy
  - At University of Michigan: Salvage radiation therapy and Taxotere (chemotherapy) for PSA failure after radical prostatectomy
- *Outside of United States*:
  - Trans Tasmanian Radiation Oncology Group: Radiotherapy—Adjuvant Versus Early Salvage (RAVES).

■ CONCLUSIONS AND FUTURE DIRECTIONS

From the published experience of phase III clini-cal trials and large outcome series with significant follow-up, to greater understanding on selection of patients and the recent developments in mod-ern technique, radiotherapy after prostatectomy remains a standard of care, of significant benefit to our patients. Much work remains, including enroll-ment on clinical trials designed to address questions on the benefit of hormonal therapy, field size, dos-age, and timing of additional therapy. Further, bet-ter imaging techniques are needed to select patients for benefit, and better treatment technique may be needed to limit toxicity. Ultimately, though, we have level 1 evidence to support radiotherapy following prostatectomy, particularly in the adjuvant setting. Radiotherapy use improves biochemical survival, local control, metastases free survival, PCSS and overall survival. Similar to other solid tumor dis-ease sites, we note that when local disease control can be maximized, major oncologic endpoints can be affected. It is noteworthy that a modest dose of radiotherapy directed to the surgical bed following prostatectomy can have such a profound effect on

prostate outcome. We recommend that every patient in this clinical scenario be counseled on the benefits and risks of radiotherapy after prostatectomy. More work is needed with quality-controlled clinical trials and continued dialogue by practitioners across clin-ical specialties.

■ REFERENCES

1. Jani AB, Johnstone PA, Liauw SL, Master VA, Rossi PJ. Prostate cancer modality time trend analyses from 1973 to 2004: a Surveillance, Epidemiology, and End Results registry analysis. *Am J Clin Oncol.* 2010;33(2):168–172.
2. Litwin MS, Pasta DJ, Stoddard ML, Henning JM, Car-roll PR. Epidemiological trends and financial outcomes in radical prostatectomy among Medicare beneficiaries, 1991 to 1993. *J Urol.* 1998;160(2):445–448.
3. Makarov DV, Trock BJ, Humphreys EB, et al. Updated nomogram to predict pathologic stage of prostate cancer given prostate-specific antigen level, clinical stage, and biopsy Gleason score (Partin tables) based on cases from 2000 to 2005. *Urology.* 2007;69(6):1095–1101.
4. Kattan MW, Zelefsky MJ, Kupelian PA, et al. Pretreat-ment nomogram that predicts 5-year probability of metastasis following three-dimensional conformal radi-ation therapy for localized prostate cancer. *J Clin Oncol.* 2003;21(24):4568–4571.
5. Cooperberg MR, Pasta DJ, Elkin EP, et al. The University of California, San Francisco Cancer of the Prostate Risk Assessment score: a straightforward and reliable preoper-ative predictor of disease recurrence after radical prosta-tectomy. *J Urol.* 2005;173(6):1938–1942.
6. Partin AW, Mangold LA, Lamm DM, Walsh PC, Epstein JI, Pearson JD. Contemporary update of prostate cancer staging nomograms (Partin tables) for the new millen-nium. *Urology.* 2001;58(6):843–848.
7. Yu JB, Makarov DV, Sharma R, Peschel RE, Par-tin AW, Gross CP. Validation of the partin nomo-gram for prostate cancer in a national sample. *J Urol.* 2010;183(1):105–111.
8. Bhojani N, Salomon L, Capitanio U, et al. External validation of the updated partin tables in a cohort of French and Italian men. *Int J Radiat Oncol Biol Phys.* 2009;73(2):347–352.
9. Penson DF, Grossfeld GD, Li YP, Henning JM, Lubeck DP, Carroll PR. How well does the Partin nomogram predict pathological stage after radical prostatectomy in a community based population? Results of the cancer of the prostate strategic urological research endeavor. *J Urol.* 2002;167(4):1653–7; discussion 1657.
10. Epstein JI, Partin AW, Sauvageot J, Walsh PC. Prediction of progression following radical prostatectomy. A multi-variate analysis of 721 men with long-term follow-up. *Am J Surg Pathol.* 1996;20(3):286–292.
11. Kupelian PA, Katcher J, Levin HS, Klein EA. Stage T1–2 prostate cancer: a multivariate analysis of factors

affecting biochemical and clinical failures after radical prostatectomy. *Int J Radiat Oncol Biol Phys.* 1997;37(5):1043–1052.

12. Freedland SJ, Humphreys EB, Mangold LA, et al. Risk of prostate cancer-specific mortality following biochemical recurrence after radical prostatectomy. *JAMA.* 2005;294(4):433–439.

13. Yee DS, Lowrance WT, Eastham JA, Maschino AC, Cronin AM, Rabbani F. Long-term follow-up of 3-month neoadjuvant hormone therapy before radical prostatectomy in a randomized trial. *BJU Int.* 2010;105(2):185–190.

14. Giberti C, Chiono L, Gallo F, Schenone M, Gastaldi E. Radical retropubic prostatectomy versus brachytherapy for low-risk prostatic cancer: a prospective study. *World J Urol.* 2009;27(5):607–612.

15. Bill-Axelson A, Holmberg L, Filén F, et al. Radical prostatectomy versus watchful waiting in localized prostate cancer: the Scandinavian prostate cancer group-4 randomized trial. *J Natl Cancer Inst.* 2008;100(16):1144–1154.

16. Carver BS, Bianco FJ Jr, Scardino PT, Eastham JA. Long-term outcome following radical prostatectomy in men with clinical stage T3 prostate cancer. *J Urol.* 2006;176(2):564–568.

17. Mian BM, Troncoso P, Okihara K, et al. Outcome of patients with Gleason score 8 or higher prostate cancer following radical prostatectomy alone. *J Urol.* 2002;167(4):1675–1680.

18. Freedland SJ, Presti JC Jr, Amling CL, et al. Time trends in biochemical recurrence after radical prostatectomy: results of the SEARCH database. *Urology.* 2003;61(4):736–741.

19. Han M, Partin AW, Zahurak M, Piantadosi S, Epstein JI, Walsh PC. Biochemical (prostate specific antigen) recurrence probability following radical prostatectomy for clinically localized prostate cancer. *J Urol.* 2003;169(2):517–523.

20. Roehl KA, Han M, Ramos CG, Antenor JA, Catalona WJ. Cancer progression and survival rates following anatomical radical retropubic prostatectomy in 3,478 consecutive patients: long-term results. *J Urol.* 2004;172(3):910–914.

21. Bianco FJ Jr, Scardino PT, Eastham JA. Radical prostatectomy: long-term cancer control and recovery of sexual and urinary function ("trifecta"). *Urology.* 2005;66(5 suppl):83–94.

22. Porter CR, Kodama K, Gibbons RP, et al. 25-year prostate cancer control and survival outcomes: a 40-year radical prostatectomy single institution series. *J Urol.* 2006;176(2):569–574.

23. Berglund RK, Jones JS, Ulchaker JC, et al. Radical prostatectomy as primary treatment modality for locally advanced prostate cancer: a prospective analysis. *Urology.* 2006;67(6):1253–1256.

24. Zorn KC, Gofrit ON, Orvieto MA, Mikhail AA, Zagaja GP, Shalhav AL. Robotic-assisted laparoscopic prostatectomy: functional and pathologic outcomes with interfascial nerve preservation. *Eur Urol.* 2007;51(3):755–762; discussion 763.

25. White MA, De Haan AP, Stephens DD, Maatman TK, Maatman TJ. Comparative analysis of surgical margins between radical retropubic prostatectomy and RALP: are patients sacrificed during initiation of robotics program? *Urology.* 2009;73(3):567–571.

26. Menon M, Shrivastava A, Kaul S, et al. Vattikuti Institute prostatectomy: contemporary technique and analysis of results. *Eur Urol.* 2007;51(3):648–57; discussion 657.

27. Badani KK, Kaul S, Menon M. Evolution of robotic radical prostatectomy: assessment after 2766 procedures. *Cancer.* 2007;110(9):1951–1958.

28. Bill-Axelson A, Holmberg L, Ruutu M, et al. Radical prostatectomy versus watchful waiting in early prostate cancer. *N Engl J Med.* 2005;352(19):1977–1984.

29. Malcolm JB, Fabrizio MD, Barone BB, et al. Quality of life after open or robotic prostatectomy, cryoablation or brachytherapy for localized prostate cancer. *J Urol.* 2010;183(5):1822–1828.

30. Pound CR, Partin AW, Eisenberger MA, Chan DW, Pearson JD, Walsh PC. Natural history of progression after PSA elevation following radical prostatectomy. *JAMA.* 1999;281(17):1591–1597.

31. Trock BJ, Han M, Freedland SJ, et al. Prostate cancer-specific survival following salvage radiotherapy vs observation in men with biochemical recurrence after radical prostatectomy. *JAMA.* 2008;299(23):2760–2769.

32. Freedland SJ, Humphreys EB, Mangold LA, Eisenberger M, Partin AW. Time to prostate specific antigen recurrence after radical prostatectomy and risk of prostate cancer specific mortality. *J Urol.* 2006;176(4 Pt 1):1404–1408.

33. Han M, Partin AW. Nomograms for clinically localized prostate cancer. Part I: radical prostatectomy. *Semin Urol Oncol.* 2002;20(2):123–130.

34. Pound CR, Partin AW, Epstein JI, Walsh PC. Prostate-specific antigen after anatomic radical retropubic prostatectomy. Patterns of recurrence and cancer control. *Urol Clin North Am.* 1997;24(2):395–406.

35. Epstein JI, Carmichael M, Partin AW, Walsh PC. Is tumor volume an independent predictor of progression following radical prostatectomy? A multivariate analysis of 185 clinical stage B adenocarcinomas of the prostate with 5 years of followup. *J Urol.* 1993;149(6): 1478–1481.

36. Bastian PJ, Gonzalgo ML, Aronson WJ, et al. Clinical and pathologic outcome after radical prostatectomy for prostate cancer patients with a preoperative Gleason sum of 8 to 10. *Cancer.* 2006;107(6):1265–1272.

37. Thompson IM, Tangen CM, Paradelo J, et al. Adjuvant radiotherapy for pathological T3N0M0 prostate cancer significantly reduces risk of metastases and improves survival: long-term followup of a randomized clinical trial. *J Urol.* 2009;181(3):956–962.

38. Thompson IM Jr, Tangen CM, Paradelo J, et al. Adjuvant radiotherapy for pathologically advanced prostate cancer: a randomized clinical trial. *JAMA.* 2006;296(19):2329–2335.

39. Swanson GP, Hussey MA, Tangen CM, et al. Predominant treatment failure in postprostatectomy patients is local: analysis of patterns of treatment failure in SWOG 8794. *J Clin Oncol.* 2007;25(16):2225–2229.

40. Bolla M, van Poppel H, Collette L, et al. Postoperative radiotherapy after radical prostatectomy: a randomised controlled trial (EORTC trial 22911). *Lancet.* 2005;366(9485):572–578.

41. Wiegel T, Bottke D, Steiner U, et al. Phase III postoperative adjuvant radiotherapy after radical prostatectomy compared with radical prostatectomy alone in pT3 prostate cancer with postoperative undetectable prostate-specific antigen: ARO 96–02/AUO AP 09/95. *J Clin Oncol.* 2009;27(18):2924–2930.

42. Swindle P, Eastham JA, Ohori M, et al. Do margins matter? The prognostic significance of positive surgical margins in radical prostatectomy specimens. *J Urol.* 2005;174(3):903–907.

43. Kupelian P, Kuban D, Thames H, et al. Improved biochemical relapse-free survival with increased external radiation doses in patients with localized prostate cancer: the combined experience of nine institutions in patients treated in 1994 and 1995. *Int J Radiat Oncol Biol Phys.* 2005;61(2):415–419.

44. Kupelian P, Thames H, Levy L, et al. Year of treatment as independent predictor of relapse-free survival in patients with localized prostate cancer treated with definitive radiotherapy in the PSA era. *Int J Radiat Oncol Biol Phys.* 2005;63(3):795–799.

45. Hancock SL, Cox RS, Bagshaw MA. Prostate specific antigen after radiotherapy for prostate cancer: a reevaluation of long-term biochemical control and the kinetics of recurrence in patients treated at Stanford University. *J Urol.* 1995;154(4):1412–1417.

46. Schild SE, Wong WW, Grado GL, et al. Radiotherapy for isolated increases in serum prostate-specific antigen levels after radical prostatectomy. *Mayo Clin Proc.* 1994;69(7):613–619.

47. Hudson E, Kynaston H, Varma M, et al. Radiotherapy after radical prostatectomy for adenocarcinoma of the prostate: a UK institutional experience and review of published studies. *Clin Oncol (R Coll Radiol).* 2008;20(5):353–357.

48. Hudson MA, Catalona WJ. Effect of adjuvant radiation therapy on prostate specific antigen following radical prostatectomy. *J Urol.* 1990;143(6):1174–1177.

49. Lange PH. Prostate-specific antigen for staging prior to surgery and for early detection of recurrence after surgery. *Urol Clin North Am.* 1990;17(4):813–817.

50. Haab F, Meulemans A, Boccon-Gibod L, et al. Effect of radiation therapy after radical prostatectomy on serum prostate-specific antigen measured by an ultrasensitive assay. *Urology.* 1995;45(6):1022–1027.

51. Schild SE, Buskirk SJ, Wong WW, et al. The use of radiotherapy for patients with isolated elevation of serum prostate specific antigen following radical prostatectomy. *J Urol.* 1996;156(5):1725–1729.

52. Walsh PC, Partin AW, Epstein JI. Cancer control and quality of life following anatomical radical retropubic prostatectomy: results at 10 years. *J Urol.* 1994;152(5 Pt 2):1831–1836.

53. Cadeddu JA, Partin AW, DeWeese TL, Walsh PC. Long-term results of radiation therapy for prostate cancer recurrence following radical prostatectomy. *J Urol.* 1998;159(1):173–7; discussion 177.

54. Schild SE, Wong WW, Grado GL, et al. The result of radical retropubic prostatectomy and adjuvant therapy for pathologic stage C prostate cancer. *Int J Radiat Oncol Biol Phys.* 1996;34(3):535–541.

55. Wu JJ, King SC, Montana GS, McKinstry CA, Anscher MS. The efficacy of postprostatectomy radiotherapy in patients with an isolated elevation of serum prostate-specific antigen. *Int J Radiat Oncol Biol Phys.* 1995;32(2):317–323.

56. Kaplan ID, Bagshaw MA. Serum prostate-specific antigen after post-prostatectomy radiotherapy. *Urology.* 1992;39(5):401–406.

57. Morris MM, Dallow KC, Zietman AL, et al. Adjuvant and salvage irradiation following radical prostatectomy for prostate cancer. *Int J Radiat Oncol Biol Phys.* 1997;38(4):731–736.

58. Rogers R, Grossfeld GD, Roach M 3rd, Shinohara K, Presti JC Jr, Carroll PR. Radiation therapy for the management of biopsy proved local recurrence after radical prostatectomy. *J Urol.* 1998;160(5):1748–1753.

59. Stephenson AJ, Scardino PT, Kattan MW, et al. Predicting the outcome of salvage radiation therapy for recurrent prostate cancer after radical prostatectomy. *J Clin Oncol.* 2007;25(15):2035–2041.

60. Stephenson AJ, Scardino PT, Eastham JA, et al. Postoperative nomogram predicting the 10-year probability of prostate cancer recurrence after radical prostatectomy. *J Clin Oncol.* 2005;23(28):7005–7012.

61. Hugen CM, Polcari AJ, Quek ML, Garza RP, Fitzgerald MP, Flanigan RC. Long-term outcomes of salvage radiotherapy for PSA-recurrent prostate cancer: validation of the Stephenson nomogram. *World J Urol.* 2010;28(6):741–744.

62. Freedland SJ, Humphreys EB, Mangold LA, et al. Death in patients with recurrent prostate cancer after radical prostatectomy: prostate-specific antigen doubling time subgroups and their associated contributions to all-cause mortality. *J Clin Oncol.* 2007;25(13):1765–1771.

63. Moinpour CM, Hayden KA, Unger JM, et al. Health-related quality of life results in pathologic stage C prostate cancer from a Southwest Oncology Group trial comparing radical prostatectomy alone with radical prostatectomy plus radiation therapy. *J Clin Oncol.* 2008;26(1):112–120.

64. Swanson GP, Goldman B, Tangen CM, et al. The prognostic impact of seminal vesicle involvement found at prostatectomy and the effects of adjuvant radiation: data from Southwest Oncology Group 8794. *J Urol.* 2008;180(6):2453–2457; discussion 2458.

65. Pilepich MV, Winter K, John MJ, et al. Phase III radiation therapy oncology group (RTOG) trial 86–10 of androgen deprivation adjuvant to definitive radiotherapy in locally advanced carcinoma of the prostate. *Int J Radiat Oncol Biol Phys*. 2001;50(5):1243–1252.

66. D'Amico AV, Manola J, Loffredo M, Renshaw AA, DellaCroce A, Kantoff PW. 6-month androgen suppression plus radiation therapy vs radiation therapy alone for patients with clinically localized prostate cancer: a randomized controlled trial. *JAMA*. 2004;292(7):821–827.

67. Lawton CA, DeSilvio M, Roach M 3rd, et al. An update of the phase III trial comparing whole pelvic to prostate only radiotherapy and neoadjuvant to adjuvant total androgen suppression: updated analysis of RTOG 94–13, with emphasis on unexpected hormone/radiation interactions. *Int J Radiat Oncol Biol Phys*. 2007;69(3):646–655.

68. Jani AB, Sokoloff M, Shalhav A, Stadler W. Androgen ablation adjuvant to postprostatectomy radiotherapy: complication-adjusted number needed to treat analysis. *Urology*. 2004;64(5):976–981.

69. Spiotto MT, Hancock SL, King CR. Radiotherapy after prostatectomy: improved biochemical relapse-free survival with whole pelvic compared with prostate bed only for high-risk patients. *Int J Radiat Oncol Biol Phys*. 2007;69(1):54–61.

70. Jani AB, Kao J, Hellman S. Hormone therapy adjuvant to external beam radiotherapy for locally advanced prostate carcinoma: a complication-adjusted number-needed-to-treat analysis. *Cancer*. 2003;98(11):2351–2361.

71. Sanda MG, Dunn RL, Michalski J, et al. Quality of life and satisfaction with outcome among prostate-cancer survivors. *N Engl J Med*. 2008;358(12):1250–1261.

72. Pilepich MV, Winter K, Lawton CA, et al. Androgen suppression adjuvant to definitive radiotherapy in prostate carcinoma—long-term results of phase III RTOG 85–31. *Int J Radiat Oncol Biol Phys*. 2005;61(5):1285–1290.

73. Horwitz EM, Bae K, Hanks GE, et al. Ten-year follow-up of radiation therapy oncology group protocol 92–02: a phase III trial of the duration of elective androgen deprivation in locally advanced prostate cancer. *J Clin Oncol*. 2008;26(15):2497–2504.

74. Bolla M, de Reijke TM, Zurlo A, Collette L. Adjuvant hormone therapy in locally advanced and localized prostate cancer: three EORTC trials. *Front Radiat Ther Oncol*. 2002;36:81–86.

75. King CR, Spiotto MT. Improved outcomes with higher doses for salvage radiotherapy after prostatectomy. *Int J Radiat Oncol Biol Phys*. 2008;71(1):23–27.

76. Valicenti RK, Gomella LG, Ismail M, Mulholland SG, Petersen RO, Corn BW. Effect of higher radiation dose on biochemical control after radical prostatectomy for PT3N0 prostate cancer. *Int J Radiat Oncol Biol Phys*. 1998;42(3):501–506.

77. Valicenti RK, Gomella LG, Perez CA. Radiation therapy after radical prostatectomy: a review of the issues and options. *Semin Radiat Oncol*. 2003;13(2):130–140.

78. Michalski JM, Lawton C, El Naqa I, et al. Development of RTOG consensus guidelines for the definition of the clinical target volume for postoperative conformal radiation therapy for prostate cancer. *Int J Radiat Oncol Biol Phys*. 2010;76(2):361–368.

79. Lawton CA, Michalski J, El-Naqa I, et al. RTOG GU Radiation oncology specialists reach consensus on pelvic lymph node volumes for high-risk prostate cancer. *Int J Radiat Oncol Biol Phys*. 2009;74(2):383–387.

80. Schiffner DC, Gottschalk AR, Lometti M, et al. Daily electronic portal imaging of implanted gold seed fiducials in patients undergoing radiotherapy after radical prostatectomy. *Int J Radiat Oncol Biol Phys*. 2007;67(2):610–619.

81. Mohler JL. The 2010 NCCN clinical practice guidelines in oncology on prostate cancer. *J Natl Compr Canc Netw*. 2010;8(2):145.

82. Mohler J, Bahnson RR, Boston B, et al. NCCN clinical practice guidelines in oncology: prostate cancer. *J Natl Compr Canc Netw*. 2010;8(2):162–200.

83. Manyak MJ. Indium-111 capromab pendetide in the management of recurrent prostate cancer. *Expert Rev Anticancer Ther*. 2008;8(2):175–181.

84. Lange PH. PROSTASCINT scan for staging prostate cancer. *Urology*. 2001;57(3):402–406.

85. Kundra V, Silverman PM, Matin SF, Choi H. Imaging in oncology from the University of Texas M. D. Anderson Cancer Center: diagnosis, staging, and surveillance of prostate cancer. *AJR Am J Roentgenol*. 2007;189(4):830–844.

86. Brassell SA, Rosner IL, McLeod DG. Update on magnetic resonance imaging, ProstaScint, and novel imaging in prostate cancer. *Curr Opin Urol*. 2005;15(3):163–166.

87. Seltzer MA, Barbaric Z, Belldegrun A, et al. Comparison of helical computerized tomography, positron emission tomography and monoclonal antibody scans for evaluation of lymph node metastases in patients with prostate specific antigen relapse after treatment for localized prostate cancer. *J Urol*. 1999;162(4):1322–1328.

88. Kelloff GJ, Choyke P, Coffey DS. Challenges in clinical prostate cancer: role of imaging. *AJR Am J Roentgenol*. 2009;192(6):1455–1470.

89. Koontz BF, Mouraviev V, Johnson JL, et al. Use of local (111)in-capromab pendetide scan results to predict outcome after salvage radiotherapy for prostate cancer. *Int J Radiat Oncol Biol Phys*. 2008;71(2):358–361.

90. Liauw SL, Weichselbaum RR, Zagaja GP, Jani AB. Salvage radiotherapy after postprostatectomy biochemical failure: does pretreatment radioimmunoscintigraphy help select patients with locally confined disease? *Int J Radiat Oncol Biol Phys*. 2008;71(5):1316–1321.

91. Jani AB, Liauw SL, Blend MJ. The role of indium-111 radioimmunoscintigraphy in post-radical retropubic prostatectomy management of prostate cancer patients. *Clin Med Res*. 2007;5(2):123–131.

92. Su A, Blend MJ, Spelbring D, Hamilton RJ, Jani AB. Postprostatectomy target-normal structure overlap volume differences using computed tomography and radioimmunoscintigraphy images for radiotherapy treatment planning. *Clin Nucl Med*. 2006;31(3):139–144.

93. Jani AB, Blend MJ, Hamilton R, et al. Radioimmuno-scintigraphy for postprostatectomy radiotherapy: analysis of toxicity and biochemical control. *J Nucl Med.* 2004;45(8):1315–1322.

94. Jani AB, Blend MJ, Hamilton R, et al. Influence of radioimmunoscintigraphy on postprostatectomy radiotherapy treatment decision making. *J Nucl Med.* 2004;45(4):571–578.

95. Jani AB, Spelbring D, Hamilton R, et al. Impact of radioimmunoscintigraphy on definition of clinical target volume for radiotherapy after prostatectomy. *J Nucl Med.* 2004;45(2):238–246.

96. Harisinghani MG, Barentsz J, Hahn PF, et al. Noninvasive detection of clinically occult lymph-node metastases in prostate cancer. *N Engl J Med.* 2003;348(25):2491–2499.

97. Schuster DM, Nye JA, Nieh PT, et al. Initial experience with the radiotracer anti-1-amino-3-[18F]Fluorocyclobutane-1-carboxylic acid (anti-[18F]FACBC) with PET in renal carcinoma. *Mol Imaging Biol.* 2009;11(6):434–438.

Prostate Brachytherapy

Sean M. McBride* and Irving D. Kaplan

Beth-Israel Deaconess Medical Center, Boston, MA

■ ABSTRACT

Prostate brachytherapy, the temporary or permanent implantation of radioactive sources into the prostate parenchyma, has a storied and successful history in the treatment of localized prostate adenocarcinoma. Both high-dose-rate and low-dose-rate monotherapies have demonstrated impressive outcomes in low-risk patients. Increasingly, practitioners are looking upon prostate brachytherapy, in combination with androgen-deprivation therapy and external beam radiation, as a viable treatment option in intermediate and high-risk patients.

Keywords: prostate cancer, brachytherapy, low-dose, high-dose

■ INTRODUCTION

Prostate brachytherapy has evolved considerably since its introduction early in the 20th century and remains a staple of localized therapy for the disease. Modern *brachytherapy*, with its Greek etymological origin meaning "therapy at a short distance," is the placement of temporary or permanent radionuclide sources directly into the prostate parenchyma. In contrast to external beam radiotherapy, interstitial prostate brachytherapy allows for the deposition of the dose in close proximity to the source without it having to pass through normal tissue structures. Compared to its competitors in the local therapy

realm, brachytherapy achieves impressive recurrence-free survival with a tolerable side effect profile.

Interstitial prostate brachytherapy can be divided into two dominant techniques: 1) Low-dose-rate (LDR) brachytherapy, defined by the International Commission of Radiation Units and Measurements as using sources with dose rates of approximately 400 to 200 cGy/hour; LDR brachytherapy commonly involves the permanent placement of radionuclide sources. 2) High-dose-rate (HDR) brachytherapy, defined as using sources with activity greater than 1,200 cGy/hour, typically involves the temporary placement of its radionuclide sources.

Prostate brachytherapy has a substantial clinical history that dates back to the early part of the 20th century. The idea to use intracavitary or interstitial radioactive sources in the treatment of prostate cancer was almost coincident with the discovery of radiation itself. Hugh Hampton Young, a urologist at the Johns Hopkins Hospital, was the first

*Corresponding author, Harvard Radiation Oncology Program, Massachusetts General Hospital, Cox 3, 100 Blossom St, Boston, MA 02114

E-mail address: Javier.Torresroca@moffitt.org

Radiation Medicine Rounds 2:1 (2011) 81–94.
DOI: 10.5003/2151-4208.2.1.81

to experiment with intracavitary placement in the United States. Young's technique involved the temporary transurethral, transrectal, and transtrigonal placement of platinum and rubber encased radium sources into the aforementioned cavities for upwards of twenty sessions, over several months (1). Initial reports from Young included mention of dramatic results in cases of modern T3b disease, however, it soon became apparent that transurethral placement involved significant obstructive morbidity while, at the same time, failing to deliver an adequate dosage to the periphery of the prostate (2).

The first physician to experiment with interstitial (as opposed to Young's intracavitary) seed implants was Benjamin Barringer of the Memorial Hospital in New York. Initially, Barringer's technique involved the transrectal temporary implantation of radon tipped needles, left in place for 4 to 6 hours (3). These treatments were repeated over several months. Barringer was also the first to utilize permanent seed implants with gold-encapsulated radon seeds placed through a transperineal approach. The patients, placed in the lithotomy position with spinal anesthesia, had the transperineal placement of these seeds guided by the surgeon's finger, placed in the rectum. The implantation was then repeated until prostatic induration disappeared. Unfortunately, even in Barringer's experienced hands, largely owing to dosimetric issues and advanced presentation, only 6% of some 350 patients achieved local control for durations of 5 to 19 years (4). With the advent of surgical castration and the increasing popularity of external beam radiation, physicians largely abandoned brachytherapy as a radical or palliative technique in the years after World War II.

Perhaps the only significant innovation in technique until the 1980s involved the first use of Iodine 125 (I-125) as the radionuclide source by Whitmore et al. at Memorial Hospital in the early 1970s. Whitmore used an open, retropubic implantation technique for seed implantation. The more rapid dose fall off with I-125, as compared to Radon or colloidal Gold, allowed for increased conformality and reduced treatment sequelae (5). Unfortunately, the long-term outcomes were less than satisfactory, largely owing to poor seed distribution within the gland (6).

The problem of accurate seed placement and dose homogeneity was not solved until the publication of two seminal papers by H.H. Holm of the University of Copenhagen in the early 1980s. His work ushered in the modern era of prostate brachytherapy.

■ LDR INTERSTITIAL BRACHYTHERAPY

Technique

Modern LDR interstitial brachytherapy began with the introduction, by H.H. Holm, of transrectal ultrasound (TRUS) as a means of assuring accurate seed placement and improving dosage distribution (7). Holm's modification developed as a two-stage procedure: The first stage involved ultrasound visualization of the prostate with transverse images taken every 5 mm, from base to apex, with the patient in an extended lithotomy position. This formed the basis for volume calculation, which was then used to create a 3D plan for seed placement. In the second stage, the patient was brought to the OR and, while under anesthesia, positioned to mimic stage 1 placement. The TRUS was affixed to a stepping unit with an attached plexiglass template grid. A dot matrix pattern was superimposed on the ultra-sound image corresponding to the hole's locations on the template. Eighteen-gauge needles, preloaded with I-125 seeds separated by chromic catgut, were placed into the preplanned grid position; they were then passed, under ultrasound guidance, through the perineum into the prostate. Once the tip of the needle was in the correct transverse plane the seeds were deposited and the needle withdrawn.

Holm further modified this procedure with the introduction of the biplanar TRUS. This allowed for visualization of the prostate in both the transverse and sagittal planes, improving operator depth perception, and thus, seed placement (8). With the earlier procedure, superior displacement of the prostate likely occurred during needle implantation. Having only transverse images prevented correction for such intraoperative deviations. Sagittal imaging corrected this. As before, a planning procedure conducted weeks prior to implantation is necessary. The limitations to a two-step procedure are obvious, and include: 1) the need for two procedures requiring anesthesia; 2) a change in shape of the target volume between preplanning and actual implementation; and 3) difficulty in recapitulating patient positioning. Indeed, there is evidence that suggests that, in upwards of 70% of the cases, there is a discrepancy in recorded volume between the two procedures. While the volume alteration was small, to the order of 5.7%, this resulted in V100 degradation of up to 20.9%.

The next crucial step in the evolution of prostate brachytherapy involved the integration of planning and placement into a single procedure. This was first reported on by Richard Stock and Nelson Stone of Mt. Sinai Hospital in 1995 (9). They enrolled patients with clinical T1 or T2 disease, requiring a negative seminal vesicle biopsy and pelvic lymph node dissection. With the assurance of localized disease, the implants were preformed under general anesthesia. The patients were first placed in the extended dorsolithotomy position to ensure access to the anterior portion of the prostate. As part of this, a wedge shaped cushion was placed under the small of the back, improving alignment with the TRUS set-up and further maximizing anterior gland access. A Foley catheter was then placed, helping the radiation oncologist to visualize the urethra throughout the procedure. The scrotum was pulled both anterior and superiorly, giving unfettered access to the perineum. The ultrasound probe, attached to the stepper apparatus, itself secured either to the surgical bed or free moving, but braked in place, was placed into the rectum. The probe could move in the circumferential direction (the z-axis, giving serial sagittal images) or craniocaudally (the y-axis, giving serial transverse images). The probe was positioned so that the axial image of the prostate fell within the ultrasound unit's displayed grid. The grid appeared as small markings at 1 cm intervals in a rectangular pattern. Finally, a sterile template with holes at 0.5 cm increments was attached to the stepper apparatus and placed flush against the perineum, anterior to the ultrasound probe.

The authors then calculated the volume of the prostate by taking serial transverse images at 0.5 cm increments, outline the prostate in each image with a pen light. The authors then used either I-125 or Pd-103 seeds as the source material; they preferred Pd-103 for high-grade (Gleason 7 or lesions with any element of four disease) lesions, reasoning that the higher dose rate of Pd-103 may be more suitable to these, presumably, faster growing lesions. In order to determine the amount of radioactivity to implant, the authors referred to the Memorial Sloan-Kettering (MSKCC) nomograms with volume-based calculations designed to achieve peripheral dose goals of 160 Gy for I-125 and 115 Gy for Pd-103. The widest transverse image of the prostate was then determined, with all need insertions occurring with the probe set to display this image. Needles were first inserted into the template, then through the perineum into the

prostate. Stock and Stone would place two anchoring needles laterally and inferiorly to the urethra. For I-125 seeds, 70% of the activity was implanted in the periphery of the gland (this "rule of thumb" based dosimetry was derived from evaluation of prior plans). The periphery was where needles were first inserted, at approximately 1 cm intervals in a clockwise direction, with a distance of 0.5 cm from the anterior rectal wall for posterior peripheral insertions. Once confirming the individual needle's placement in the gland periphery, the ultrasound viewer was switched to a longitudinal view and the needle then advanced to the base of the gland. The craniocaudal length of the prostate along each needle tract was then calculated. With all peripheral needles placed as described, seeds were then inserted. The number of seeds per needle was calculated by dividing the activity by the number of needles placed, with longer needle tracts requiring more seeds. The seeds were then inserted at 0.5 and 1.0 cm intervals while retracting the needle. Real-time fluoroscopy was used to evaluate each seed row. This technique is referred to as "after loading," since the seeds are inserted into the needles subsequent to the placement of the needle into the gland. Once peripheral seed insertion was complete, the interior needles and seeds were placed in a similar manner. All needle placements were recorded on an implant record sheet. With the procedure completed, all instruments were withdrawn and a scintillation counter used to assure no extracorporeal seeds remained in the OR. The patient was to remain in hospital overnight and discharged once voiding.

The obvious limitation in Stock and Stone's one-step process was the reliance on operator experience and simple rules of thumb in determining needle placement and dose distribution, without the quantitative dosimetric evaluation that would occur with preplanning. This was corrected with the introduction of intraoperative, computer-based dosimetric planning and optimization. Several groups, including our own, began integrating intraoperative computer-based planning in the late 1990s and early 2000s. One of the first groups to report on this was at the University of Rochester (10). This group utilized the Prostate Implant Planning Engine for Radiotherapy (PIPER) software. Real-time, intraoperative image transfer from the TRUS to the PIPER software was achieved by video capture via direct cable connection and a frame-grabbing device. The patient positioning and set-up were similar to the Stock procedure. Here three anchoring needles were used, forming an inverted triangle. Again, transverse images of the prostate were obtained at 5 mm intervals from apex to base and stored as JPEG images on the computer. The TRUS overlaid coordinate system was precisely calibrated to match the physical template placed on the perineum. The planning target volume (PTV) and urethra were then manually delineated on grabbed transverse images. The computerized genetic algorithm then calculated the optimal needle distribution to achieve the desired peripheral dose. The quality of the plan was evaluated based upon the calculated mean peripheral dose, urethral and rectal doses, dose-volume histograms, and needle and seed placement as viewed on a computer generated 3D representation of the prostate. The dosimetric output gave the radiation oncologist precise information on needle template position, offset from the prostate base, and number of seeds for each needle. Needle placement was done according to the computer-generated plan and verified in real-time with TRUS. Seed placement was also verified, again in real-time, by TRUS. At the conclusion of the procedure, anterior-poster and lateral fluoroscopic radiographs were obtained and visually compared to the computer-generated 3D image of planned seed placement; the radiation oncologist could, if necessary, place additional seeds to compensate for any apparent cold spots. The authors found that, using this technique, only 18.2 minutes were added to the total operative time and that dosimetric evaluation compared favorably with the old two-stage procedure. A variety of different groups, including our own, adopted computer-based intraoperative dosimetric planning the late 1990s (11,12). The fundamental limitation to this initial technology was that plans were generated based on needle, not seed location.

The latest innovation in LDR technique involves what is termed intraoperative dynamic dose feedback. This involves recording seed location intraoperatively and adjusting dosimetry real-time to account for variations in seed placement. This technique was pioneered by Louis Potters at MSKCC in 2003 (13). Using an after-loading technique, Potters first placed needles in the prostate periphery and interior using a 3:1 peripheral:interior ratio. Varian software was then used to register needle positions. As with prior procedures, the PTV, rectum, and urethra were outlined on captured TRUS images spaced 5 mm apart. The software then tested thousands of permutations of seed numbers and positions within individual needles. The permutations were constrained by predefined minimum and maximum radiation doses to PTV and normal tissue. With modern processor speeds, an adequate plan could be devised within 45 to 60 seconds. Based upon the plan, seeds were then loaded into needles based on spacing defined by the plan. The position of seeds was visualized on sagittal TRUS imaging. The location of the seed was recorded and the dosimetry updated in real time. Future seed placement can thus be altered to account for any deviations in prior seed location. Postimplant dosimetry correlated well with intraoperative calculations.

Eligibility and Dose

Relative contraindications to LDR brachytherapy include patients with very large or very small prostates, patients with high International Prostate Symptom Score (IPSS), and patients with significant pubic arch interference. Current National Comprehensive Cancer Network (NCCN) Guidelines appropriately limit the eligibility of patients to receive prostate brachytherapy as monotherapy. In the latest iteration of these guidelines, it is recommended that practitioners limit monotherapy to those patients with low-risk disease (T1c/T2a and Gleason 6 and prostate-specific antigen [PSA] < 10) (14). Although combined modality regimens (CMT = EBRT + brachytherapy) were initially used in the low-risk setting, D'Amico's demonstration of the efficacy of brachytherapy alone in these patients caused these treatments to fall out of favor with these sub-groups (15). Additionally, several large retrospective studies did not demonstrate superiority of CMT versus brachy monotherapy in low-risk disease (16).

For intermediate-risk patients (Gleason 7 and/or PSA > 10 and/or T2b disease), brachy monotherapy may be used in conjunction with short course (4–6 months) androgen-deprivation therapy (ADT). In intermediate-risk patients with low volumes of Gleason 7 disease, we frequently order endorectal MRIs to evaluate the possibility of T3 disease before proceeding with brachytherapy. In the intermediate-risk setting, external beam radiation therapy (EBRT) may also be combined with reduced dose LDR brachytherapy, with or without the use of ADT. The primary rationale for combined EBRT and LDR treatment is the improved extraprostatic coverage that EBRT provides in patients who may have extracapsular extension or seminal vesicle invasion. Some authors argue that, given retrospective data that suggest ADT is of no benefit in intermediate-risk patients who get CMT, CMT, by avoiding the potential cardiac toxicity associated with ADT, should be the preferred radiation-based treatment for these patients (16).

Use of brachytherapy as a component of treatment for patients with high-risk disease is controversial. These patients, defined by the presence of PSA > 20 or Gleason 8–10 or T3 disease, have, traditionally, been treated with EBRT and 2 to 3 years of ADT. However, given the dose escalation that one can achieve with brachytherapy, the group at Mt Sinai has made a somewhat compelling argument for trimodal treatment (EBRT + brachy + ADT) in selected patients with high-risk disease.

Typical prescription doses for LDR monotherapy are 145 to 160 Gy for I-125 and 125 to 130 Gy for Pd-103. Initially, monotherapy doses were, in part, based upon early work by Hilaris at MSKCC (17). In the combined modality setting, a typical EBRT dose is at 45 Gy in 1.8 Gy fractions followed by a 110 Gy I-125 or 100 Gy Pd-103 boost. The parameters used to describe dosages vary between investigators. There is some consensus amongst brachytherapists on the importance of D90 (minimum dose received by 90% of the prostate) and V150 (volume of prostate receiving 150 Gy).

Although active debate continues, there does appear to be a dose response relationship when one examines biochemical recurrence and various D90s (18). Stock et al. reported retrospective data looking at T1-T2, Gleason 6 patients who received I-125 monotherapy without ADT (19); D90 in this population of patients ranged from 26 to 256 Gy. Biochemical failure was defined as two consecutive increases in PSA level or a nadir PSA that was above 1.0 ng/mL. When this group of patients was divided into groups with D90s less than or greater than 140 cGy, there was a clear relationship between dose and freedom-from-biochemical failure (FFBF); at 4 years, patients who had a D90 ≥ 140 cGy had an FFBF of 92% compared to 68% for those with D90s < 140 cGy. Furthermore, 2-year posttreatment biopsies were negative in 83% of patients with D90 ≥ 140 cGy, but in only 70% of the biopsies for those with lower doses. In multivariate analysis, the dosage was predictive of FFBF. The authors strongly recommended 140 cGy as a minimum dose for I-125 implants.

Zelefsky et al. also found a dose response relationship for patients treated with interstitial implants alone; either I-125 or Pd-103 (20). Here data from 2,693 patients with T1-T2 disease treated at 11 different institutions was aggregated in the hopes of identifying predictors of disease-free survival (DFS). The authors found that, in patients implanted with I-125, D90 ≥ 130 resulted in an 8-year relapse-free survival rate of 93% compared to 76% for those receiving lower doses. When looking only at patients with postimplant dosimetric evaluations, multivariate analysis found that D90 was a significant predictor of biochemical control.

Finally, more recently, Taira et al. reported on 463 low- and intermediate-risk patients treated with either I-125 or Pd-103 monotherapy alone, without either EBRT or ADT. On multivariate analysis, D90, as a percentage of the prescribed dose, was a significant predictor of biochemical control. Here the authors also used biologically effective dose (BED) in their analysis, assuming an alpha/beta of 2. For instance, in low-risk patients with a BED ≥ 116, the 12-year biochemical progression-free survival (bPFS) was 98.8% compared to 92.2% for those with lower BEDs. In intermediate-risk patients with BED ≥ 116 Gy, bPFS was 98% versus 86.4% for those with lower BEDs.

Fewer articles report on dose escalation and cancer control in patients treated with combined EBRT and LDR implant. Once again, Stock and colleagues have accrued a significant amount of data on this subject (21). As mentioned above, combined modality patients tend to have higher risk disease. The Mt. Sinai group looked at high-risk patients (defined as PSA > 20 ng/mL or Gleason 8–10 or T2c-T3 disease, or those patients with two intermediate-risk features) who were treated with 9 months of ADT (3 months neoadjuvant) and Pd-103 implant, followed 2 months later by 45 Gy of EBRT in 25 fractions. The dosimetric output used was BED, with the total BED being the sum of the BEDs for implant (D90) and external beam components. The "Phoenix" definition (PSA nadir + 2 ng/mL) was used to determine biochemical failure. Prostate biopsy was offered at 2 years after completion of therapy and was performed under ultrasound guidance with a minimum of six cores taken; results were scored as negative and positive only. Those patients with positive biopsies were then recommended to have biopsies yearly until negative or clear evidence of PSA progression.

The mean BED in the high-risk patients was 166 Gy2. There was a statistically significant relationship between total BED and the percentage of patients with positive biopsies in the high-risk group.

For BED ≤ 150 Gy2, BED >150–200 Gy2, and BED >200 Gy2, the percentage of patients with positive biopsies was 22%, 8.8%, and 2%, respectively. Using Cox regression analysis of cause-specific survival (CSS), the authors demonstrated that the only statistically significant variable associated with CSS was BED (as a continuous variable).

In summary, LDR brachytherapy, either combined with EBRT and ADT or as monotherapy, can play a role in the treatment of all prostate cancer risk sub-groups. While myriad data exists demonstrating a dose response relationship for EBRT and cancer control (22), there appears to be a similar relationship with LDR implants.

Outcomes

While no randomized trials exist that compare LDR brachytherapy to other modalities, most specifically EBRT and prostatectomy in low-risk patients, there are legions of retrospective and prospectively collected data looking at outcomes at a variety of institutions across multiple risk groups. Herein we focus upon the larger series, with many studies including admixtures of risk groupings and either adjuvant EBRT or ADT.

Zelefsky et al. reported the single largest experience with LDR monotherapy (20). Data was available on 2,693 patients treated at multiple institutions from 1988 to 1998, all with clinical stage T1-T2 prostate cancer with a median follow-up of 63 months; 68% of patients were treated with I-125, the remainder with Pd-103. PSA relapse was defined by either the ASTRO criteria of three successive PSA rises after posttreatment nadir, or the aforementioned "Phoenix" criteria. Risk groups were defined by NCCN criteria, with 1,444 patients in the low-risk group, 960 intermediate-risk patients, and 192 high-risk patients. We have already mentioned some of the results. The 8-year PSA relapse-free survival (PRFS) was 92%, 86%, 79%, and 67% for patients with PSA nadirs of 0 to 0.49, 0.5 to 0.99, 1.0 to 1.99, and >2.0 ng/mL, respectively. This trend was statistically significant. Interestingly, for patients who were relapse free after 8 years, the median PSA was 0.1 ng/mL, with 90% of patients having a nadir < 0.6 ng/mL. For the group as a whole, the 8-year metastases-free survival rate and clinical DFS rate were 74% and 69%, respectively. When examined by risk category, 8-year DMFS was 98%, 92%, and 85% for low-,

intermediate-, and high-risk patients, respectively. Overall survival (OS) at 8 years was 81%, 71%, and 63% for low-, intermediate-, and high-risk patients, respectively.

Stock et al. reported on their outcomes with 1,561 patients who received LDR monotherapy, or LDR implants supplemented with EBRT and/or ADT at Mt Sinai between 1990 and 2004, with a median follow-up of 3.8 years (23); 634 patients received brachytherapy alone, 420 received implants + ADT, and 507 received trimodal therapy (EBRT + implant + ADT). I-125 implants were used for patients with Gleason 6 disease, with Pd-103 used in patients with higher scores. ADT and EBRT tended to be used in intermediate- and high-risk patients, whereas low-risk patients generally received brachytherapy alone. Biochemical failure was defined using the ASTRO criteria. Posttreatment biopsies were recommended in all patients. For the study group as a whole, the prostate cancer–specific rate and OS rate at 10 years were 96% and 74%, respectively. On multivariate analysis, PSA status after treatment was most predictive of death from prostate cancer; at 10 years, prostate cancer–specific survival was 100%, 52%, and 98% for patients who had no PSA failure, patients with a PSA doubling time (DT) ≤ 10 months, and those with a DT ≥ 10 months, respectively.

More recently, the University of Washington reported outcomes on 1,656 patients treated with permanent interstitial brachytherapy between 1995 and 2006 (24). Median follow-up for these patients was 7.0 years. By risk grouping, 575 patients had low risk, 608 had intermediate risk, and 473 patients had high-risk disease. Approximately 38% received ADT and 50% had adjuvant EBRT either to the prostate and seminal vesicles alone or, if predicted to have a >10% risk of lymph node involvement, to the entire pelvis; patients receiving ADT or EBRT tended to have intermediate or high-risk disease. For implants, both I-125 and Pd-103 were used. The primary outcomes examined were CSS, bPFS, and OS. bPFS was oddly defined as patients failing to achieve a posttreat PSA nadir ≤ 0.40 ng/mL. Twelve-year bPFS was 98.6%, 96.5%, and 90.5% for men with low-, intermediate-, and high-risk disease, respectively. CSS was 99.8%, 99.3%, and 95.2% for the respective groups, and OS was 77.5%, 71.1%, and 69.2% for the same groups. On multivariate analysis, the strongest predictor of bPFS was percent positive cores and risk group; for CSS, the strongest predictor was OS. Also, signaling to the importance of comorbidities and the relative unimportance of prostate cancer in overall mortality, the strongest predictors of OS were age, smoking, and diabetes.

Because of data suggesting that prostate brachytherapy offers superior potency sparing in younger men with the disease, there is renewed interest in outcome data for younger patients. Pina et al. recently reported on their experience with 96 men, median age 53.0 years, treated with interstitial I-125 implants from May 1999 to November 2005 for clinical stage T1-T2 prostate cancer, without adjuvant ADT or EBRT (25). PSA relapse was defined using the "Phoenix" definition. Here the median D90 was 160.4 Gy. Median follow-up was 63 months, with all patients alive at the time of the last follow-up. One patient had a biochemical failure at 36 months. Overall, bPFS was 98.9% at 7 years, with 100% OS. The median PSA nadir for the entire group was 0.05 ng/mL; this nadir was reached at a median time of 48 months postimplant. The authors emphasized the excellent disease control in the young age cohort.

It is clear that the earlier technical revolution in LDR brachytherapy has led to a significant improvement in reported outcomes. Because of that, LDR monotherapy is an accepted and frequently sought after primary therapy for low-risk patients. Furthermore, many radiation oncologists are becoming increasingly convinced of the utility of LDR brachytherapy, often in combination with ADT or EBRT, in the treatment of their higher risk patients.

Morbidity

Any treatment decisions must take into account toxicities and the likely impact of the therapy on the patients' quality of life (QOL). Sanda et al. recently reported on a large, prospectively studied cohort of patients who had undergone prostatectomy, EBRT, or LDR brachytherapy alone (26). The authors utilized both patient reported and partner reported outcome measures to evaluate a variety of toxicity and satisfaction end-points; more specifically, sexual, urinary, and bowel function were examined. In total, 1,201 patients were enrolled on the study, including 306 patients who received LDR brachytherapy alone. Distress related to erectile function was reported in 44% of patients who underwent prostatectomy, 22% of patients who had EBRT, and only 13% who had brachytherapy. However, patients in the brachytherapy group complained of significant irritative and obstructive urinary symptoms. Overall urinary "moderate or big" bother at 24 months was 7% in the prostatectomy group, 11% in the EBRT group and 16% in the brachytherapy group; these differences were statistically significant. Additionally, patients who underwent either form of radiation therapy reported increased rates of bowel bother at 24 months, including 11% of EBRT patients and 8% of brachytherapy patients. The variable most associated with outcome satisfaction in the entire cohort of patients was sexual function, of which brachytherapy performed the best.

Another quite recent prospective study also reported on QOL outcomes associated with radical prostatectomy, EBRT, and brachytherapy in a cohort of 435 patients (27). As with the Sanda data, QOL was assessed before and after treatment with the Expanded Prostate Cancer Index Composite (EPIC) score. In the group of patients who reported no issues with sexual function prior to treatment, at 3 years approximately 40% of patients in the EBRT and brachytherapy groups had preserved sexual function compared with only 10% of patients undergoing radical prostatectomy. At 3 years, between 54% and 69% of the prostatectomy patients had issues with urinary incontinence, compared to 25% of those in the brachytherapy group. Contrary to the Sanda study, only patients in the EBRT group had a statistically significant moderate worsening of bowel symptoms; brachytherapy patients were generally spared.

Finally, Radiation Therapy Oncology Group (RTOG) 98–05 was a prospective study looking at health-related QOL outcomes in men who received prostate monotherapy in the form of I-125 seeds to a prescription dose of 145 Gy (28). For the 98 patients enrolled on this study who received brachytherapy, there was a statistically significant increase in the number of patients reporting urinary incontinence, between 3 and 6 months that resolved by the 9th month. Additionally, obstructive urinary symptoms were often present and persisted beyond 1 year. For 73% of men, erectile function was sufficient for sexual activity prior to treatment; this number dropped to 59% of patients after treatment.

Two phase II studies looking at the toxicity profile of combined EBRT and LDR brachytherapy have been reported upon. The first, RTOG 0019, enrolled men with cT1c and T2a disease and either Gleason scores of 6 or lower with PSA between 10 and 20 ng/mL or Gleason 7 patients with PSA levels up to 20 ng/mL. Overall, the 138 patients enrolled underwent EBRT to the prostate and seminal vesicles with a total dose of 45 Gy followed 2 to 6 weeks later by an LDR brachytherapy boost with I-125 at a dose of 108 Gy. ADT use was variable, with the decision left up to the treating physician. Toxicities were graded according to the Common Toxicity Criteria (CTC) Version 2.0. With a median follow-up of 19 months, acute grade 3 toxic events were seen in approximately 8% of patients. Specifically, grade 3 GU and GI toxic effects were seen in 10.8% and 3.1% of patients, respectively. Grade 3 or higher GI and GU toxicity at 4 years was estimated at 15%. These rates were higher than one would expect for either therapy alone.

CALGB 99809 also evaluated toxicity profiles in patients treated with EBRT and brachytherapy. Here, again, patients were treated with external beam at 45 Gy, with brachytherapy boost using either I-125 or Pd-103, 2 to 4 weeks after completion of EBRT. All patients received 6 months of ADT. The median follow-up of the 63 patients enrolled was 38 months. Toxicity grade was assigned based upon CTC V 2.0, as before. Short-term grade 2 toxicity included urinary frequency (16%), urinary retention (7%), and proctitis (7%). The most common long-term grade 2 toxicity was urinary frequency, seen in 5% of patients. The two above mentioned combined modality trials are limited by their exclusive use of physician-reported side effects.

■ HDR BRACHYTHERAPY

HDR prostate brachytherapy utilizes radio-isotopes whose rate of radiation deposition is on the order of 1,200 cGy/hour or higher. Compared to LDR brachytherapy, which involves the permanent implantation of radioactive sources, HDR prostate brachytherapy involves the temporary placement of radio-isotope sources, commonly, Iridium 192 (Ir-192). There are multiple putative advantages to HDR prostate brachytherapy compared to its more established LDR cousin: 1) the absence of permanent, live radioactive sources abrogates the need for significant radioprotective measures; 2) the implantation of catheters into the prostate capsule, periprostatic tissue, and seminal vesicles that are then after-loaded with sources, allows for the safe treatment of locally advanced disease; and 3) knowing the exact location of dwell positions prior to after-loaded delivery of Ir-192 seeds allows for very accurate dosimetric calculations. The radiobiologic benefit of HDR

compared to LDR resides with the assumed low alpha/beta ratio for prostate cancer. Assuming this to be the case, cancer control may be facilitated by the high dose-per-fraction that HDR can provide.

Technique

There are significant similarities between LDR and HDR techniques. HDR technique has evolved since its inception in the 1980s and 1990s, but includes several basic steps: 1) physician placement of after-loaded catheters into the prostate and surrounding region; 2) image acquisition after Catheters have been placed; 3) treatment planning using software capable of grabbing acquired images; and 4) placement of the HDR sources, and delivery of therapy (29). Slessinger, in describing the initiation of an HDR prostate brachytherapy program in his own hospital, gives an excellent overview of general technique (30).

The night prior to procedure, the patient undergoes adequate bowel preparation. On the day of procedure, with the patient under general or spinal anesthetic, the radiation oncologist generally inserts 12 to 22 catheters in and around the prostate through a template placed flush against the perineum, under TRUS guidance. One may also place TRUS-guided gold fiducial markers at the base and apex of the prostate to facilitate planning. Catheter placement is generally done with the largest cross-section of the prostate seen on TRUS as the reference point, starting first at the prostate periphery. Preliminary CT images are then obtained with slight adjustments to the needle position made as necessary to ensure adequate coverage. Once final positions are ensured, rectal contrast is introduced, obturators are removed from the catheters, and serial planning CT images are obtained; some centers may also use TRUS or MRIs for planning images. The radiation oncologist then contours out the CTV, and, generally, the urethra, bladder, and rectum. A peripheral dose is then prescribed, with the software calculating dwell times for the Ir-192 sources. The physician can then either alter the dwell times him/herself or pull in the isodose lines with the software then re-calculating dwell times. It is important to meet rectal and urethral dose constraints; the RTOG, in 0321, attempted to limit the volume of the urethra receiving 125% of prescription dose to 1 mL and the volume of the bladder and rectum receiving 75% of prescription dose to

1 mL. With the plan calculated, flexible needle transfer tubes are inserted into the appropriate catheter attached to the after-loaded device. Treatment is then delivered, with the physicist, at completion, ensuring that all sources have returned into the tungsten-shielded after-loader. Catheters may be re-inserted if treatment is over weeks. However, some institutions will leave catheters in place, have patients admitted to the floors, and treat over 2 to 4 days.

Eligibility and Dose

In 2008, The American Brachytherapy Society (ABS) Prostate High Dose Rate Task Group released its report, looking at a variety of issues related to prostate HDR. Specifically, they addressed patient eligibility. Patients eligible for HDR monotherapy include those with cT1b-T2b disease and Gleason ≤ 7, and PSA ≤ 10 ng/mL. The Task Force suggested that, in high-risk patients (those with cT3-T4 disease, Gleason 7–10, or PSA > 10), HDR may play an important role in boosting disease before or after EBRT treatment.

There is interinstitutional variability when it comes to HDR monotherapy doses. William Beaumont delivers 9.5 Gy × 4 fractions with a BID fractionation regimen. Here, a single catheter implant is used; the BED is 74 Gy2. In contrast, the California Endocurietherapy Cancer Center (CET) delivers 7 Gy × 6 fractions, given BID with two different catheter placements spaced 1-week apart. The ABS Task Force also mentions treatments of 10.5 Gy × 3 fractions (31).

In the high-risk patients, who often receive HDR treatment as a boost given in addition to external beam treatment, dose variability is even more significant. Generally, EBRT doses range from 36 to 50 Gy delivered in 20 to 28 fractions. The RTOG HDR boost trial used an HDR dose scheme of 9.5 Gy × 2 (32). William Beaumont, in their ongoing dose escalation trial, has used a variety of regimens including 5.5 to 6.5 Gy × 3 and 8.25 to 11.5 Gy × 2; these boosts are delivered on top of 46 Gy of EBRT (33).

Outcomes

Recently, Martinez et al. reported on the combined experience of William Beaumont and the CET in the treatment of favorable risk prostate cancer using HDR monotherapy (31). In this retrospective look,

they compared outcomes and toxicities between patients receiving HDR and LDR monotherapy. In total, 248 patients were treated with HDR Ir-192 therapy and 206 patients were treated with LDR Pd-103 therapy. All patients had cT1c-T2a disease, Gleason ≤ 7, and PSA ≤ 12. For LDR treatments, done entirely at Beaumont, PTV dose was 120 Gy. At CET, HDR dose was 7 Gy × 6 using two separate implants spaced 1-week apart. At Beaumont, HDR was given 9.5 Gy × 4 with BID dosing. The Phoenix Definition was used to determine biochemical failure. With a median follow-up of 4.8 years, LDR and HDR therapies were equivalent in terms of biochemical control; 5-year PFS for patients treated with HDR was 88%; LDR PFS was 89% at 5 years.

The Osaka Group, one of the earliest pioneers of HDR monotherapy, reported on 112 prostate cancer patients, 68 of whom had high-risk disease (34); ADT was used in 94 of the patients, which was neoadjuvant in the intermediate and high-risk groups with additional adjuvant therapy in the high-risk patients. The prostate, with a 5 mm margin along with all areas of seminal vesicle invasion or ECE, were included in the CTV. Patients were treated, between 1996 and 2005, with 54 Gy in nine fractions over 5 days. Median follow-up was 5.4 years. Again, the Phoenix definition was used to determine biochemical failure. PSA failure occurred in 19 patients, with 4 patients dead of disease, the latter all in the high-risk group. The 5-year local control, OS, DFS, and PSA failure-free rate was 97%, 96%, 87%, and 83%, respectively. Looking at the low-, intermediate-, and high-risk groups, 5-year PSA failure-free survival was 85%, 93%, and 79%, respectively. Multivariate analysis revealed that initial PSA and younger age were predictors of PSA failure.

Outcome data is more robust in the combined treatment setting. In 2005, Demanes et al. reported on CET's experience with HDR boost in concert with EBRT in 209 consecutive patients treated from 1991 to 1998 (35). Over 66% of patients were in the intermediate- or high-risk groupings. The total HDR dosage to the prostate, including any disease extension with margin, was 22 to 24 Gy in four fractions of 5.5 to 6.0 Gy. EBRT was given two weeks later at a total dose of 36 Gy in 20 fractions. The definition of general clinical failure (GCF) included positive exam or positive biopsy > 2 years after treatment, distant failure, hormonal therapy, or PSA > 25 ng/mL after treatment. Both the old ASTRO definition and the Phoenix definition were used to define biochemical failure. Median follow-up was 7.25 years; GCF was seen in 10% of patients. CSS was 97%, OS was 79%. Five-year biochemical PFS (using the Phoenix definition) was 93%, 93%, and 83% for the low-, intermediate-, and high-risk groups, respectively. Although beyond their median follow-up, with 18 patients still at-risk, the 8 year bPFS in the high-risk group was 66%. It did not change appreciably from the 5-year rates for the low- and intermediate-risk groups.

Vargas et al. reported on William Beaumont's Phase II experience with dose-escalated combined modality treatment in 197 patients treated between 1991 and 2003, all with intermediate and high-risk disease (33). All patients received EBRT at 46 Gy in 23 fractions, to the pelvis. HDR boost was given in either two or three treatments, with patients divided into low-dose (mean BED = 88.2 Gy) and high-dose (mean BED = 116.8 Gy) groups. The ASTRO definition was used to determine biochemical failure. Clinical failure was defined as local failure or distant metastasis. Prostate cancer events were defined as biochemical failure, salvage ADT, or clinical failure. At 5 years, the cumulative incidence of biochemical failure was 18.6%, of clinical failure was 9.8%. Clinical Event Free Survival (cEFS) was 84.8%, CSS was 98.3%, and OS was 92.9%. Five-year bPFS, cEFS, CSS, and OS were all statistically showing significant improvement in the high-dose group compared to the low-dose group. On multivariate analysis, high dose was predictive of OS.

Hoskin et al. reported on a randomized Phase III trial wherein 220 prostate cancer patients with no evidence of distant metastases and a PSA < 50 were randomized to EBRT alone or EBRT + HDR. In the EBRT alone group (111 patients), dosage was taken to 55 Gy in 20 fractions. In the combined modality group, EBRT dose was at 35.75 Gy in 13 fractions followed 6 days later by an HDR boost of 17 Gy in two fractions over 24 hours. PSA-failure was determined using the ASTRO definition. In the high-risk group, 93% of patients used ADT compared to 67% and 50% in the intermediate and low-risk groups, respectively. ADT use was balanced between both arms. At a median follow-up of only 30 months, there was a statistically significant advantage for combined modality treatment in terms of bPFS; mean PSA relapse-free survival was 5.1 years in the combined arm versus 4.3 years in the EBRT alone group. Improvement was seen regardless of PSA, Gleason Score, and T Stage. As expected, OS, given the median follow-up, was unchanged.

The above findings were corroborated by two recent retrospective studies. Deutsch et al. reported on the MSKCC experience, comparing 160 patients treated with IMRT + HDR to 470 patients treated with high-dose IMRT alone (36). The IMRT alone patients received dosage to the prostate and seminal vesicles of 86.4 Gy. In the combined modality group, HDR (7 Gy × 3) was followed by IMRT at 50.4 Gy. Biochemical failure was defined using the Phoenix definition of nadir + 2 ng/mL. Looking at all risk groups, PRFS at 5 years was 97.7% versus 82% for the combined versus IMRT-alone groups. There was no difference in PRFS in the low-risk group. In the intermediate-risk group, 5-year PFS favored the combined modality group 98% versus 84%; in the high-risk setting, adding HDR improved PRFS from 71% to 93%. On multivariate analysis, only combined modality treatment and risk group were associated with PRFS.

Zwahlen et al. retrospectively compared 196 patients treated with 3DCRT and HDR boost to those treated with 3DCRT alone (37). Approximately 42% of patients had NCCN-defined intermediate-risk disease and 42% had high-risk disease. ADT was given to 75% of patients. In the combined modality group, external beam dose was at 46 Gy to the prostate and SV with an 18 Gy, one-time HDR boost. In the 3DCRT group only, dose was 70 Gy to the prostate and SV in most cases (four patients received WPRT). The ASTRO definition was used to determine biochemical failure. The median follow-up was 5.5 years. The combined modality arm displayed more advanced disease. On multivariate analysis, the addition of HDR was associated with a 36% relative improvement in bPFS (HR = 0.64, $P = 0.047$).

Morbidity

In the monotherapy setting, HDR morbidity data is somewhat limited. Corner et al. recently published a Phase II trial of HDR monotherapy using three dose levels: 34 Gy in four fractions, 36 Gy in four fractions, and 31.5 Gy in three fractions (38). Acute and late toxicities were evaluated using the IPSS checklist. The RTOG/CTC score systems were also used to evaluate urologic and rectal events. Seven patients required catheterization acutely, with only three remaining catheterized at 12 weeks. RTOG Group 1 and 2 GI toxicity was seen in 61%, 68%, and 77% of patients in order of increasing dose escalation group. However, no significant overall differences were seen in toxicities between the dose-escalated groups.

In the aggregated data from Beaumont and CET, compared to LDR monotherapy, HDR monotherapy was associated with less acute grade 1 to 3 dysuria (60% vs. 39%), urinary frequency/urgency (90%–58%), and rectal pain (17%–6.5%) (31). Late term urinary side effects were also less frequent in the HDR group. Finally, impotence rates were decreased, although not significantly so, in the HDR group (30% vs. 20%).

The most significant study on toxicity related to combined EBRT with HDR boost is the recently published preliminary results from RTOG 0321 (32). Patients with locally confined, cT1c-T3b prostate cancer were eligible for enrollment. Treatment included EBRT at 45 Gy to the prostate and seminal vesicles or whole pelvis, depending on calculated risk of lymphatic involvement. HDR brachytherapy was delivered at 19 Gy over two fractions. All adverse events were graded according to the Common Terminology Criteria for Adverse Events. Adverse event data was available on 112 of the 129 enrolled patients, all of whom were treated from 2004 to 2006. The median follow-up was 29.6 months. The estimated rate of grade 3 to 5 GU and GI adverse events was on the order of 2.43%. In looking at GI/GU toxicity, three grade 3 acute events occurred, including two instances of urinary frequency and one of urinary retention. The median interval to these toxicities was 1.15 months. The rate of late grade 3 to 5 GU/GI events at 18 months was 2.56%. Four grade 3 or greater late GI/GU events occurred, including urinary retention, cystitis, urinary incontinence, and proctitis. All totaled, five patients developed grade 3 sexual dysfunction.

In Demanes' retrospective look at the CET combined EBRT and HDR experience, the rate of grade 3 and 4 late urinary toxicity was 6.7% and 1%, respectively (35). No patients experienced grade 3 or 4 rectal toxicity. Of the 76 patients with normal sexual function prior to treatment, 67% remained at baseline.

Overall, HDR, either alone or in combination with EBRT, was well tolerated in the populations studied. More mature follow-up will obviously be needed.

SALVAGE BRACHYTHERAPY

A not insignificant number of prostate cancer patients treated with EBRT will experience biochemical failure. Increasingly, repeat brachytherapy is playing a critical and successful role in salvaging those patients with local-only disease at relapse. Multiple, single institution studies have looked at salvage, mainly LDR, prostate implants after biopsy confirmed local-only recurrence. One of the larger case series is reported by Aaronson et al. from UCSF (39). Here 37 patients had a local recurrence after EBRT, a median of 49 months after initial treatment. MRI re-staging was used to localize the recurrent disease and allow for biopsy. The authors treated recurrent disease with I-125 implants at 144 Gy with 108 Gy going to the remaining gland. After a median follow-up of 30 months, biochemical relapse-free survival, as judged by the Phoenix criteria, was 88%. Within this small group of patients, three patients experience failure, two with distant and regional metastatic disease. The Mayo Clinic also reported on their salvage brachytherapy series in a cohort of patients who failed locally after EBRT (40). Patients were implanted with either Pd-103 or I-125 to a dose of 120 Gy and 160 Gy, respectively. Here biochemical failure was defined as two consecutive PSA increases above nadir. With a median follow-up of 64 months, 3- and 5-year bDFS rates were 48% and 34%, respectively. Nguyen and colleagues aggregated data on brachytherapy salvage and found grade 3 and 4 GU and GI toxicity rates of 17% and 5.6%, respectively (41). Brachytherapy treatment in patients who have failed, is a successful method of salvage treatment with an acceptable toxicity profile.

FUTURE DEVELOPMENTS

It is assumed that continued advances in intraoperative planning and imaging, including the increasing utilization of intraoperative MRI, will lead both to improved dose conformity and outcomes. Ultimately, the radiation oncology community will have to commit itself to conducting thorough Phase III trials in order to determine the optimal radiotherapeutic treatment of localized prostate cancer.

REFERENCES

1. Darget R. Treatment of carcinoma of the prostate with radium. *Urol Cutaneous Rev.* 1948;52(6):352–357.
2. Aronowitz JN. Dawn of prostate brachytherapy: 1915–1930. *Int J Radiat Oncol Biol Phys.* 2002;54(3):712–718.

3. Barringer BS. Radium in the treatment of prostatic carcinoma. *Ann Surg.* 1924;80(6):881–884.

4. Barringer BS. Treatment of prostatic carcinoma. *Bull N Y Acad Med.* 1943;19(6):417–422.

5. Whitmore WF Jr, Hilaris B, Grabstald H. Retropubic implantation to iodine 125 in the treatment of prostatic cancer. *J Urol.* 2002;167(2 Pt 2):981–983; discussion 984.

6. Zelefsky MJ, Whitmore WF Jr. Long-term results of retropubic permanent 125iodine implantation of the prostate for clinically localized prostatic cancer. *J Urol.* 1997;158(1):23–9; discussion 29.

7. Holm HH, Juul N, Pedersen JF, Hansen H, Strøyer I. Transperineal 125iodine seed implantation in prostatic cancer guided by transrectal ultrasonography. *J Urol.* 1983;130(2):283–286.

8. Holm HH, Torp-Pedersen S, Myschetzky P. Transperineal seed-implantation guided by biplanar transrectal ultrasound. *Urology.* 1990;36(3):249–252.

9. Stock RG, Stone NN, Wesson MF, DeWyngaert JK. A modified technique allowing interactive ultrasound-guided three-dimensional transperineal prostate implantation. *Int J Radiat Oncol Biol Phys.* 1995;32(1):219–225.

10. Messing EM, Zhang JB, Rubens DJ, et al. Intraoperative optimized inverse planning for prostate brachytherapy: early experience. *Int J Radiat Oncol Biol Phys.* 1999;44(4):801–808.

11. Kaplan ID, Holupka EJ, Meskell P, et al. Intraoperative treatment planning for radioactive seed implant therapy for prostate cancer. *Urology.* 2000;56(3):492–495.

12. Beyer DC, Shapiro RH, Puente F. Real-time optimized intraoperative dosimetry for prostate brachytherapy: a pilot study. *Int J Radiat Oncol Biol Phys.* 2000;48(5):1583–1589.

13. Potters L, Calguaru E, Thornton KB, Jackson T, Huang D. Toward a dynamic real-time intraoperative permanent prostate brachytherapy methodology. *Brachytherapy.* 2003;2(3):172–180.

14. Mohler JL. The 2010 NCCN clinical practice guidelines in oncology on prostate cancer. *J Natl Compr Canc Netw.* 2010;8(2):145.

15. D'Amico AV, Whittington R, Malkowicz SB, et al. Biochemical outcome after radical prostatectomy, external beam radiation therapy, or interstitial radiation therapy for clinically localized prostate cancer. *JAMA.* 1998;280(11):969–974.

16. Soto DE, McLaughlin PW. Combined permanent implant and external-beam radiation therapy for prostate cancer. *Semin Radiat Oncol.* 2008;18(1):23–34.

17. Hilaris BS, Whitmore WF Jr, Batata MA, Grabstald H. Radiation therapy and pelvic node dissection in the management of cancer of the prostate. *Am J Roentgenol Radium Ther Nucl Med.* 1974;121(4):832–838.

18. Morris WJ, Halperin R, Spadinger I. Point: the relationship between postimplant dose metrics and biochemical no evidence of disease following low dose rate prostate brachytherapy: is there an elephant in the room? *Brachytherapy.* 2010;9(4):289–292; discussion 297–298.

19. Stock RG, Stone NN, Tabert A, Iannuzzi C, DeWyngaert JK. A dose-response study for I-125 prostate implants. *Int J Radiat Oncol Biol Phys.* 1998;41(1):101–108.

20. Zelefsky MJ, Kuban DA, Levy LB, et al. Multi-institutional analysis of long-term outcome for stages T1-T2 prostate cancer treated with permanent seed implantation. *Int J Radiat Oncol Biol Phys.* 2007;67(2):327–333.

21. Stone NN, Stock RG, Cesaretti JA, Unger P. Local control following permanent prostate brachytherapy: effect of high biologically effective dose on biopsy results and oncologic outcomes. *Int J Radiat Oncol Biol Phys.* 2010;76(2):355–360.

22. Zietman AL, Bae K, Slater JD, et al. Randomized trial comparing conventional-dose with high-dose conformal radiation therapy in early-stage adenocarcinoma of the prostate: long-term results from proton Radiation Oncology Group/American College of Radiology 95–09. *J Clin Oncol.* 2010;28(7):1106–1111.

23. Stock RG, Cesaretti JA, Stone NN. Disease-specific survival following the brachytherapy management of prostate cancer. *Int J Radiat Oncol Biol Phys.* 2006;64(3):810–816.

24. Taira AV, Merrick GS, Butler WM, et al. Long-term outcome for clinically localized prostate cancer treated with permanent interstitial brachytherapy. *Int J Radiat Oncol Biol Phys.* 2010.

25. Gómez-Iturriaga Piña A, Crook J, Borg J, Lockwood G, Fleshner N. Median 5 year follow-up of 125iodine brachytherapy as monotherapy in men aged<or=55 years with favorable prostate cancer. *Urology.* 2010;75(6):1412–1416.

26. Sanda MG, Dunn RL, Michalski J, et al. Quality of life and satisfaction with outcome among prostate-cancer survivors. *N Engl J Med.* 2008;358(12):1250–1261.

27. Pardo Y, Guedea F, Aguiló F, et al. Quality-of-life impact of primary treatments for localized prostate cancer in patients without hormonal treatment. *J Clin Oncol.* 2010;28(31):4687–4696.

28. Feigenberg SJ, Lee WR, Desilvio ML, et al. Health-related quality of life in men receiving prostate brachytherapy on RTOG 98–05. *Int J Radiat Oncol Biol Phys.* 2005;62(4):956–964.

29. Morton GC. The emerging role of high-dose-rate brachytherapy for prostate cancer. *Clin Oncol (R Coll Radiol).* 2005;17(4):219–227.

30. Slessinger ED. Practical considerations for prostate HDR brachytherapy. *Brachytherapy.* 2010;9(3):282–287.

31. Martinez AA, Demanes J, Vargas C, Schour L, Ghilezan M, Gustafson GS. High-dose-rate prostate brachytherapy: an excellent accelerated-hypofractionated treatment for favorable prostate cancer. *Am J Clin Oncol.* 2010;33(5):481–488.

32. Hsu IC, Bae K, Shinohara K, et al. Phase II trial of combined high-dose-rate brachytherapy and external beam radiotherapy for adenocarcinoma of the prostate: preliminary results of RTOG 0321. *Int J Radiat Oncol Biol Phys.* 2010;78(3):751–758.

33. Vargas CE, Martinez AA, Boike TP, et al. High-dose irradiation for prostate cancer via a high-dose-rate

brachytherapy boost: results of a phase I to II study. *Int J Radiat Oncol Biol Phys.* 2006;66(2):416–423.

34. Yoshioka Y, Konishi K, Sumida I, et al. Monotherapeutic high-dose-rate brachytherapy for prostate cancer: five-year results of an extreme hypofractionation regimen with 54 Gy in nine fractions. *Int J Radiat Oncol Biol Phys.* 2010.

35. Demanes DJ, Rodriguez RR, Schour L, Brandt D, Altieri G. High-dose-rate intensity-modulated brachytherapy with external beam radiotherapy for prostate cancer: California endocurietherapy's 10-year results. *Int J Radiat Oncol Biol Phys.* 2005;61(5):1306–1316.

36. Deutsch I, Zelefsky MJ, Zhang Z, et al. Comparison of PSA relapse-free survival in patients treated with ultra-high-dose IMRT versus combination HDR brachytherapy and IMRT. *Brachytherapy.* 2010;9(4):313–318.

37. Zwahlen DR, Andrianopoulos N, Matheson B, Duchesne GM, Millar JL. High-dose-rate brachytherapy in combination with conformal external beam radiotherapy

in the treatment of prostate cancer. *Brachytherapy.* 2010;9(1):27–35.

38. Corner C, Rojas AM, Bryant L, Ostler P, Hoskin P. A phase II study of high-dose-rate afterloading brachytherapy as monotherapy for the treatment of localized prostate cancer. *Int J Radiat Oncol Biol Phys.* 2008;72(2):441–446.

39. Aaronson DS, Yamasaki I, Gottschalk A, et al. Salvage permanent perineal radioactive-seed implantation for treating recurrence of localized prostate adenocarcinoma after external beam radiotherapy. *BJU Int.* 2009;104(5):600–604.

40. Grado GL, Collins JM, Kriegshauser JS, et al. Salvage brachytherapy for localized prostate cancer after radiotherapy failure. *Urology.* 1999;53(1):2–10.

41. Nguyen PL, D'Amico AV, Lee AK, Suh WW. Patient selection, cancer control, and complications after salvage local therapy for postradiation prostate-specific antigen failure: a systematic review of the literature. *Cancer.* 2007;110(7):1417–1428.

Stereotactic Body Radiation Therapy for Prostate Cancer

Thomas P. Boike and Robert D. Timmerman*

University of Texas Southwestern Medical Center, Dallas, TX

■ ABSTRACT

Stereotactic body radiation therapy (SBRT) has been successfully used to treat tumors in the lung, liver, and spine. Advances in technology and increased understanding in radiation biology have lead to the investigation of SBRT for prostate cancer. This study reviews the current clinical experiences of SBRT for prostate cancer, highlighting insights as to the toxicity, quality of life, and early prostate-specific antigen response.

Keywords: stereotactic, ablative, image guidance, prostate cancer, outcomes

■ INTRODUCTION

Stereotactic body radiation therapy (SBRT) is a new therapeutic paradigm for treating tumors outside of the central nervous system and involves delivering very high doses of focused radiation using unique beam arrangements and special immobilization equipment. SBRT was defined by the American College of Radiology and American Society of Therapeutic Radiology and Oncology to involve the use of large doses per fraction delivered in 1 to 5 fractions (1). A system for SBRT was first described in 1994 by Blomgren and Lax (2). This system involved a custom-formed body pillow and a frame with imbedded fiducials.

Reproducibility was within 5 to 8 mm for tumors of the lung and liver, in 90% of their patients. Treatment was designed with eight individually shaped noncoplanar beams. One-year later, Hamilton and Lulu published on a second system for SBRT that was more invasive, employing spinal or skeletal osseous fixation to immobilize patients (3). These early treatment were cumbersome, but local control was greater than 80% and toxicity was minimal, making this an attractive treatment option (2–4). Experience in lung and liver has continued to grow with mature phase II studies reported with local control greater than 90% for metastatic and primary cancers with low toxicity rates (5–7). Large series of patients with spinal metastasis have also been treated with acceptable toxicity and high local control (8–10). Typically, doses of >8 Gy/fraction have been used for lung, liver, and spine treatments given in 1 to 5 fractions. To draw a line between reported experiences of hypofraction and SBRT in prostate cancer, 6 Gy or more will be required for SBRT.

*Corresponding author, Department of Radiation Oncology, University of Texas Southwestern Medical Center, 5801 Forest Park Rd, Dallas, TX 75390

E-mail address: robert.timmerman@utsouthwestern.edu

Radiation Medicine Rounds 2:1 (2011) 95–102.
DOI: 10.5003/2151-4208.2.1.95

■ RATIONALE

The radiobiologic argument for hypofractionation and SBRT in prostate cancer revolves around the growing body of evidence that the α/β for prostate cancer is lower than that for other cancers. Brenner et al. first described an α/β as low as 1.5 Gy (95% confidence interval [CI] 0.8–2.2) based on a review of 367 patients treated with either low dose rate brachytherapy or external beam radiation (11). This was in agreement with a larger retrospective analysis by Fowler et al., of 1,471 men treated at 10 different centers with either low dose rate brachytherapy or external beam radiation where an α/β of 1.49 Gy (12). Results from single arm and randomized trials of hypofractionated external beam radiation have shown prostate cancer α/β values of 1.12 to 2.4 Gy with wide CIs (13–15). The α/β for late rectal toxicity is suggested to be 2.3 to 5.4 Gy (16). With this evidence supporting a lower α/β for prostate cancer than the normal rectum, the linear quadratic (LQ) model would predict higher local control and lower toxicity from hypofractionated regimes including SBRT.

The LQ model accurately describes radiation effects for the low dose per fraction scheme used in conventionally fractionated radiation therapy (CFRT) and it potentially overestimates the radiation effect at higher dose per fraction. This effect is amplified with low α/β tissues. Many groups have proposed alternative models or alterations to the LQ model to better predict the effects of doses greater than 6 Gy (17).

SBRT employs daily treatment doses dramatically higher than typical for CFRT. In turn, it is incorrect to assume that SBRT radiobiology is similar to historical CFRT. Indeed, a unique biology of radiation response for very large dose per fraction treatments is being appreciated both in terms of tumor control as well as normal tissue consequences, translating into unique clinical outcomes. For example, local control with CFRT in early stage lung cancer is consistently reported below 50%, while several series using SBRT show local control around 90% (7,18). If not careful, toxicity that was rare with CFRT is seen more frequently with SBRT for lung tumors such as central airway necrosis, chest wall pain, and brachial plexopathies (19–21). Clinical data regarding control and toxicity is growing everyday and being integrated with our understanding.

The physics of external radiation treatment delivery has been improving rapidly with the incorporation of image guidance, intensity modulation, and image fusion. Image guidance has allowed for correction of daily set up errors and also monitoring of prostate motion during treatment delivery (22,23). This has facilitated smaller clinical target volume (CTV) to planning target volume (PTV) margins for SBRT targets, reducing the amount of normal rectum and bladder in the PTV. Steep dose gradients around the bladder and rectum are carved out with ease using intensity modulation. Heterogeneous dose distributions that spare the urethra and mimic high dose rate (HDR) brachytherapy can be delivered (24). MRI-CT fusion has been shown to aid in prostate contouring by reducing target size (25). Together, the stage has been set for clinical SBRT protocols.

■ CLINICAL EXPERIENCE

An extreme hypofractionated schedule, like SBRT, is not a new idea. Motivated by limited resources, a clinical program was started in the United Kingdom in the late 1960s. Patients were treated in six fractions to a total dose of 36 Gy over 3 weeks (26). A 22-year follow up that confirmed long-term safety and potential effectiveness of this treatment was reported. Interpretation of this experience is limited by the retrospective nature of the report, pre prostate-specific antigen (PSA) staging and follow up, and simple radiation techniques.

Modern clinical trials with SBRT for prostate cancer began in April of 2000 at Virginia Mason with their stereotactic hypofractionated accurate radiotherapy of the prostate (SHARP trial), but the first report did not come until 2007 from this same group. To date there are four clinical papers regarding SBRT for prostate cancer. Three of these are prospective phase I/II clinical trials with 30 to 41 patients (27–29) and the last is a large experience involving over 300 patients (30). The primary endpoint of these trials has been toxicity and feasibility leading to the small patient numbers. Table 1 outlines the many similarities and some differences amongst the trials.

■ TREATMENT

These reports focus on the treatment of low-risk patients but King et al. included several patients with low volume Gleason score 7 (3 + 4) disease and

TABLE 1   The similarities and differences amongst the trials

Author	Number of Patients	Risk Group	Total Dose (per fraction)	Schedule	PTV Margin	Technique
Madsen et al.	40	Low	33.5 Gy (6.7 Gy)	Consecutive days	4–5 mm	3D with six noncoplanar beams
Tang et al.	30	Low	35 Gy (7 Gy)	Once weekly	4 mm	IMRT with seven fields
King et al.	41	Low and intermediate	36.25 Gy (7.25 Gy)	Consecutive days; 21 patients Every other day; 20 patients	5 mm and 3 mm posteriorly	Cyberknife
Katz et al.	304	Low, intermediate, and high	35 Gy (7 Gy); 50 patients 36.25 Gy (7.25 Gy); 254 patients	Consecutive days	5 mm and 3 mm posteriorly*	Cyberknife

*For intermediate and high-risk patients the proximal half of the seminal vesicles was added. For high-risk patients the PTV was expanded 8 mm on the involved sides.

Katz et al. included even high-risk disease. Most patients had to have mild to no lower urinary tract symptoms, no history of TURP, and prostate glands less than 60 mL in size. These were adopted from prostate brachytherapy guidelines as SBRT was thought to mimic HDR brachytherapy. All patients had 3 to 4 gold fiducials placed for image guidance. Inter-fraction errors were corrected in all trials and King et al. and Katz et al. were able to monitor intra-fraction with periodic kV images. Patient set-up was most different in the SHARP trial as men were in a flex-prone position and radiation was delivered with noncoplanar 3D beams. Supine positioning was used by the rest of the groups with standard linac-based IMRT utilized by Tang et al., and Cyberknife treatment accounting for the rest. The CTV was defined in all groups with CT, however, MRI was available for some patients. Expansions from CTV to a PTV were 3 to 4 mm posteriorly and 4 to 8 mm elsewhere. Tang et al. treated patients once a week over 29 days, while more conventional SBRT schedules such as consecutive days or every other day were used for the rest. Dose per fraction ranged from 6.7 Gy to 7.25 Gy. All treatment was delivered in a total of five treatments. Hormone therapy was generally not allowed or just used for prostate downsizing, except in the Katz et al. experience, where hormonal therapy was at the discretion of the urologist and given for intermediate- and high-risk patients (30).

■ TOXICITY

All patients were followed closely for toxicity using the radiation therapy oncology group (RTOG) or common toxicity criteria version three (CTCv3) scoring systems. The median follow up for the studies ranged from 12 to 41 months. For the purpose of this discussion, acute toxicity was defined from the start of treatment until a one month follow up, then any new toxicity was considered late; but this definition varied within each study. There was a single grade 3 acute toxicity event across all the trials (28). Within the SHARP trial, urinary obstruction following the first fraction occurred in a patient with a 97 mL prostate and an initial AUA score of 11. He required catheterization but was managed conservatively with ibuprofen and tamsulosin. He went on to finish treatment. Table 2 shows a summary of toxicity across the trials. Two patients amongst all the trials experienced grade 3 late genitourinary (GU) toxicity (27) while there were no grade 3 or greater gastrointestinal (GI) toxicities reported. Grade 2 GI toxicity was observed in 2.9 to 50% and 0 to 15% of patients for acute and late reactions, respectively. While, grade 2 GU toxicity was present in 4 to 23% and 2 to 24% of patients for acute and late reactions, respectively.

Patient reported outcomes such as AUA scores, international prostate symptom scores (IPSS), and expanded prostate cancer index composite (EPIC)

TABLE 2   Summary of toxicity across the trials

Author	Median Follow-Up (Range)	Toxicity Scale	Grade 2 GI		Grade 2 GU		≥Grade 3 GI		≥Grade 3 GU	
			Acute (%)	Late* (%)	Acute (%)	Late (%)	Acute (%)	Late (%)	Acute (%)	Late (%)
Madsen et al.	41 months (12–60)	RTOG	13	7.5	20.5	20	0	0	2	0
Tang et al.	12 months (NA)	CTCv3	50	13	23	13	0	0	0	0
King et al.	33 months (6–45)	RTOG	NA	15	NA	24	NA	0	NA	5
Katz et al.	30 months (26–37); low dose	RTOG	2.9	0	5.8	2	0	0	0.5	0
	17 months (8–27); high dose		3.6	4	4.7	4	0	0	0	0

*Toxicity greater than 1 month posttreatment was considered late.

questionnaires were collected. Median AUA scores of patients treated in the SHARP trial increased at the 1-month follow up and then returned to baseline. Within this trial, 20 patients' AUA scores increased while 10 decreased at one month. After 12 months, 15 patients had slightly worse scores while 21 patients reported improved scores. This highlights the variability across patients in how they respond to stereotactic radiation doses (28). Likewise, King et al. reported worse urinary quality of life from IPSS at the three-month follow up, however, these improved over baseline scores at two years. EPIC bowel related scores decreased at 3 months and only slightly climbed at one and two years, never returning back to baseline (27). King et al. treated patients initially on consecutive days for the first 21 patients, but switched to every other day when an acceptable but high rate of acute GI toxicity was observed. With this change in treatment schedule, a significant difference in rectal quality of life was observed. This is interesting but was not part of the original design of the trial or an intended analysis at the outset.

The largest amount of quality of life data for prostate cancer patients treated with SBRT comes from Katz et al. (30). They used the EPIC questionnaire and reported results for bowel, urinary, and sexual domains. Compliance with obtaining questionnaires was good with all patients completing baseline evaluations and 87%, 67%, 64%, and 76% of questionnaires were available at 3 weeks, 5 months, 11 months, and 17 months, respectively. Bowel and urinary scores declined significantly from baseline at three weeks, but returned to baseline at 5 months and held throughout follow up. Patients

were questioned regarding sexual potency. Nearly 228 patients out of 304 were potent at baseline and of these, 198 patients remained potent at a median of 18 months follow up. This was consistent with a small 10% drop in the EPIC sexual domain that was persistent over follow up. Wiegner et al. looked at sexual function in the Stanford clinical trial. They had a baseline potency rate of 62% that decreased to 29% at a median follow up of 4 years (31). Mean EPIC sexual domain scores progressively decline over follow up. At last follow up, more than half of the men <70 years old remained potent, but only 15% of men over 70 years old remained potent. This is consistent with other reports of men treated with various radiation modalities and dependant on age (32–34).

■   PROSTATE-SPECIFIC ANTIGEN

The median follow up on these studies ranges from 12 months to 41 months making it difficult to gauge efficacy from these studies. The report from Tang et al. had only 12 month median follow ups and thus PSA nadir was not yet reached in many patients. King et al. reported no biochemical failures with a median of 33 months. A total of three biochemical failures, two low-risk patients and one high-risk patient, were observed by Katz et al. All three were in the high dose group with a median follow up of 17 months, range 8 to 27 months. These patients all underwent a 12 core transrectal biopsy which was negative in the two low-risk patients but 4/12 cores revealed Gleason score 10 in the high-risk patient. Thus only one of these was a local failure. Madsen et al. has the longest median follow up at 41 months and they have reported 90% biochemical control by nadir +2 and 70% biochemical control by the old ASTRO three consecutive rises definition. This was attributed to late PSA bounces, but further follow up is needed to confirm these were just bounces. PSA bounces have been seen in 16% to 29% of patients with a median time to bounce of 18 months (27,30). PSA nadir has been promising also, with most patients reaching nadir below 1 ng/dL and over half of the patients with nadirs below 0.5 ng/dL.

■ DISCUSSION

New technology is often met with enthusiasm which can be magnified based on initial reports of success. External forces such as industry, hospitals, physicians, or patient advocacy groups can amplify this excitement prior to a through evaluation. Prostate cancer is particularly prone to the introduction of new treatments due to the high prevalence of the disease, indolent nature of many tumors, and long survival associated with even observation (35). Certainly hypofractionation for prostate cancer is not a new idea in radiation therapy. St. Thomas' Hospital in London, England, started treating patients in the late 1960s with a five fraction course. Their updated report shows a low rate of death from disease with little toxicity, given crude radiation techniques by todays standards (26). The use of SBRT in prostate cancer is rooted in the compelling radiobiology evidence of a low α/β ratio and made possible by advancements in treatment delivery.

Using clinical data along with the LQ model most suggest the α/β for prostate cancer to be low, between 1 and 4 Gy (36). This translates to equivalent doses of 78 Gy to 90 Gy delivered to the prostate in the above four SBRT prostate experiences, assuming an α/β of 1.5 Gy. There is less clinical data to support the α/β of the rectum but it appears to be between 2.3 and 5.4 Gy (16), which is in agreement with previously done animal studies. This translates into an equivalent dose of 65 Gy to 75 Gy delivered to the small volumes of the rectum in the reported SBRT experiences. The high rates of initial control and low toxicity in these early SBRT reports support this model. However, further follow up and additional trials are needed to verify this.

Conventionally fractionated dose escalation is widely practiced for low and intermediate-risk prostate cancer patients. The current SBRT reports for prostate cancer compare favorably with the toxicity profile of 78 Gy and 79.2 Gy on the MD Anderson and PROG dose escalation trial. Grade 2 or greater acute GI toxicity was 57% to 64% and grade 2 or greater GU toxicity was 49% to 62% in the MD Anderson and PROG dose escalation trials compared with 2.9% to 50% and 4.7% to 23%, respectively, for the current SBRT experiences (37–39). Late toxicity is not fully appreciated at this point. From the MD Anderson dose escalation trial, there was not a plateau in toxicity up to a five-year follow up (37). The median follow up on these SBRT studies ranges from 12 to 41 months. These SBRT experiences have thus far shown an encouraging low rate of grade 2 or grater GI/GU toxicity of 0% to 15%/2% to 24% to date.

Early conventional dose escalation trials did not have a great understanding of DVH parameters that may lead to increased toxicity. These have been developed and analyzed as we gain more follow up. The same is true for SBRT experiences. King et al. notes that steering high dose within the prostate away from the urethra may improve GU symptoms similar to brachytherapy. Katz et al. premedicated patients with rectal amifostine added to each SBRT treatment, which possibly led to their very low rates of toxicity (30). Rectal amifostine has proven to be beneficial in conventionally fractionated patients, but is inconvenient for the small gains seen there (40). However, when patients are only receiving five treatments, they may be more willing to undergo this additional procedure.

Follow up for these initial SBRT reports is again a problem when gauging the efficacy of this treatment. Early PSA results are promising, with nadirs often reaching below 0.5 ng/dL (27,30). PSA bounces have been observed, similar to brachytherapy and conventional radiation (27,30). In lung cancer, SBRT failures occur later compared with conventionally treated patients. This will most likely be true in prostate cancer as well, with its slow growth rate and the initial potency of SBRT.

At the time of this review, there are ten trials registered with the U.S. National Institutes of Health related to SBRT for prostate cancer. The University of Texas Southwestern has completed a multi-institutional phase I, dose escalation trial in low and intermediate-risk prostate cancer that has only been reported in abstract form. The MTD was not reached and the final dose of 50 Gy in five fractions

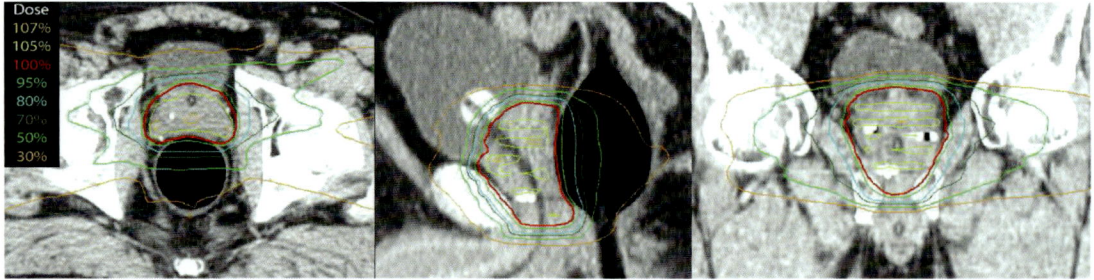

FIGURE 1   SBRT treatment planning dosimetry for a patient enrolled to the University of Texas dose escalation trial in the axial, sagittal, and coronal planes. The red line is the prescription isodose. A large balloon is positioned within the rectum (also used for treatment) and a Foley catheter defining the position of the urethra is in place for the simulation (not the treatment). Intensity modulation is used to steer dose higher than the prescription away from the urethra.

is now being expanded for phase II. An example isodose plan from a patient on this trial is shown in Figure 1. The RTOG is planning on opening their own multi-institutional randomized phase II trial in low-risk prostate cancer patients with one of the arms being SBRT and the other a less aggressive hypofractionation. These trials will help define what doses are possible to give and how SBRT compares with hypofractionation, helping to shape future trials as SBRT could expand into intermediate- and high-risk patients.

One central difficulty in these trials is defining clinically relevant end points. Treatment outcomes such as survival and freedom from distant metastasis for low-risk prostate cancer are currently excellent. Therapy is thus aimed at decreasing side effects, improving quality of life, and making treatment more convenient. Current trials are generally designed with toxicity and quality of life end points. However, eventually there will need to be true comparative effectiveness research related not only to toxicity and quality of life but also to survival, distant metastasis, individual cost and societal health care cost related to treatment. Data for cost of SBRT treatment has been scarce at this point, but Katz et al. points out that SBRT in his clinic is approximately US$15,000 less than conventional IMRT (30).

■ CONCLUSIONS

Initial trials in SBRT are promising for both toxicity and PSA response. Further follow up and investigation is needed to assure SBRT's safety, efficacy, and overall role in prostate cancer therapy.

■ REFERENCES

1. Potters L, Kavanagh B, Galvin JM, et al. American Society for Therapeutic Radiology and Oncology (ASTRO) and American College of Radiology (ACR) practice guideline for the performance of stereotactic body radiation therapy. *Int J Radiat Oncol Biol Phys*. 2010;76(2):326–332.

2. Lax I, Blomgren H, Näslund I, Svanström R. Stereotactic radiotherapy of malignancies in the abdomen. Methodological aspects. *Acta Oncol*. 1994;33(6):677–683.

3. Hamilton AJ, Lulu BA. A prototype device for linear accelerator-based extracranial radiosurgery. *Acta Neurochir Suppl*. 1995;63:40–43.

4. Blomgren H, Lax I, Goranson H, et al. Radiosurgery for tumors in the body: clinical experience using a new method. *J Radiosurg*. 1998;1(1):63–74.

5. Rusthoven KE, Kavanagh BD, Burri SH, et al. Multi-institutional phase I/II trial of stereotactic body radiation therapy for lung metastases. *J Clin Oncol*. 2009;27(10):1579–1584.

6. Rusthoven KE, Kavanagh BD, Cardenes H, et al. Multi-institutional phase I/II trial of stereotactic body radiation therapy for liver metastases. *J Clin Oncol*. 2009;27(10):1572–1578.

7. Timmerman R, Paulus R, Galvin J, et al. Stereotactic body radiation therapy for inoperable early stage lung cancer. *JAMA*. 2010;303(11):1070–1076.

8. Gerszten PC, Burton SA, Ozhasoglu C, Welch WC. Radiosurgery for spinal metastases: clinical experience in 500 cases from a single institution. *Spine*. 2007;32(2):193–199.

9. Ryu S, Rock J, Jain R, et al. Single fraction radiosurgery of epidural spinal cord compression: tumor control and neurologic outcome. *Proc Am Soc Clin Oncol*, 2007;25:2041.

10. Yamada Y, Bilsky MH, Lovelock DM, et al. High-dose, single-fraction image-guided intensity-modulated radiotherapy for metastatic spinal lesions. *Int J Radiat Oncol Biol Phys*. 2008;71(2):484–490.

11. Brenner DJ, Hall EJ. Fractionation and protraction for radiotherapy of prostate carcinoma. *Int J Radiat Oncol Biol Phys*. 1999;43(5):1095–1101.

12. Fowler J, Chappell R, Ritter M. Is alpha/beta for prostate tumors really low? *Int J Radiat Oncol Biol Phys.* 2001;50(4):1021–1031.

13. Bentzen SM, Ritter MA. The alpha/beta ratio for prostate cancer: what is it, really? *Radiother Oncol.* 2005;76(1):1–3.

14. Kupelian PA, Thakkar VV, Khuntia D, Reddy CA, Klein EA, Mahadevan A. Hypofractionated intensity-modulated radiotherapy (70 Gy at 2.5 Gy per fraction) for localized prostate cancer: long-term outcomes. *Int J Radiat Oncol Biol Phys.* 2005;63(5):1463–1468.

15. Yeoh EE, Holloway RH, Fraser RJ, et al. Hypofractionated versus conventionally fractionated radiation therapy for prostate carcinoma: updated results of a phase III randomized trial. *Int J Radiat Oncol Biol Phys.* 2006;66(4):1072–1083.

16. Brenner DJ. Fractionation and late rectal toxicity. *Int J Radiat Oncol Biol Phys.* 2004;60(4):1013–1015.

17. Park C, Papiez L, Zhang S, Story M, Timmerman RD. Universal survival curve and single fraction equivalent dose: useful tools in understanding potency of ablative radiotherapy. *Int J Radiat Oncol Biol Phys.* 2008;70(3):847–852.

18. Wulf J, Haedinger U, Oppitz U, Thiele W, Mueller G, Flentje M. Stereotactic radiotherapy for primary lung cancer and pulmonary metastases: a noninvasive treatment approach in medically inoperable patients. *Int J Radiat Oncol Biol Phys.* 2004;60(1):186–196.

19. Dunlap NE, Cai J, Biedermann GB, et al. Chest wall volume receiving >30 Gy predicts risk of severe pain and/or rib fracture after lung stereotactic body radiotherapy. *Int J Radiat Oncol Biol Phys.* 2010;76(3):796–801.

20. Forquer JA, Fakiris AJ, Timmerman RD, et al. Brachial plexopathy from stereotactic body radiotherapy in early-stage NSCLC: dose-limiting toxicity in apical tumor sites. *Radiother Oncol.* 2009;93(3):408–413.

21. Timmerman R, Papiez L, McGarry R, et al. Extracranial stereotactic radioablation: results of a phase I study in medically inoperable stage I non-small cell lung cancer. *Chest.* 2003;124(5):1946–1955.

22. Kupelian P, Willoughby T, Mahadevan A, et al. Multi-institutional clinical experience with the Calypso System in localization and continuous, real-time monitoring of the prostate gland during external radiotherapy. *Int J Radiat Oncol Biol Phys.* 2007;67(4):1088–1098.

23. Xie Y, Djajaputra D, King CR, Hossain S, Ma L, Xing L. Intrafractional motion of the prostate during hypofractionated radiotherapy. *Int J Radiat Oncol Biol Phys.* 2008;72(1):236–246.

24. Fuller DB, Naitoh J, Lee C, Hardy S, Jin H. Virtual HDR CyberKnife treatment for localized prostatic carcinoma: dosimetry comparison with HDR brachytherapy and preliminary clinical observations. *Int J Radiat Oncol Biol Phys.* 2008;70(5):1588–1597.

25. McLaughlin PW, Evans C, Feng M, Narayana V. Radiographic and anatomic basis for prostate contouring errors and methods to improve prostate contouring accuracy. *Int J Radiat Oncol Biol Phys.* 2010;76(2):369–378.

26. Lloyd-Davies RW, Collins CD, Swan AV. Carcinoma of prostate treated by radical external beam radiotherapy using hypofractionation. Twenty-two years' experience (1962–1984). *Urology.* 1990;36(2):107–111.

27. King CR, Brooks JD, Gill H, Pawlicki T, Cotrutz C, Presti JC Jr. Stereotactic body radiotherapy for localized prostate cancer: interim results of a prospective phase II clinical trial. *Int J Radiat Oncol Biol Phys.* 2009;73(4):1043–1048.

28. Madsen BL, Hsi RA, Pham HT, Fowler JF, Esagui L, Corman J. Stereotactic hypofractionated accurate radiotherapy of the prostate (SHARP), 33.5 Gy in five fractions for localized disease: first clinical trial results. *Int J Radiat Oncol Biol Phys.* 2007;67(4):1099–1105.

29. Tang CI, Loblaw DA, Cheung P, et al. Phase I/II study of a five-fraction hypofractionated accelerated radiotherapy treatment for low-risk localised prostate cancer: early results of pHART3. *Clin Oncol (R Coll Radiol).* 2008;20(10):729–737.

30. Katz AJ, Santoro M, Ashley R, Diblasio F, Witten M. Stereotactic body radiotherapy for organ-confined prostate cancer. *BMC Urol.* 2010;10:1.

31. Wiegner EA, King CR. Sexual function after stereotactic body radiotherapy for prostate cancer: results of a prospective clinical trial. *Int J Radiat Oncol Biol Phys.* 2010;78(2):442–448.

32. Beard CJ, Propert KJ, Rieker PP, et al. Complications after treatment with external-beam irradiation in early-stage prostate cancer patients: a prospective multiinstitutional outcomes study. *J Clin Oncol.* 1997;15(1):223–229.

33. Hamilton AS, Stanford JL, Gilliland FD, et al. Health outcomes after external-beam radiation therapy for clinically localized prostate cancer: results from the Prostate Cancer Outcomes Study. *J Clin Oncol.* 2001;19(9):2517–2526.

34. Penson DF, Feng Z, Kuniyuki A, et al. General quality of life 2 years following treatment for prostate cancer: what influences outcomes? Results from the prostate cancer outcomes study. *J Clin Oncol.* 2003;21(6):1147–1154.

35. Albertsen PC, Hanley JA, Fine J. 20-year outcomes following conservative management of clinically localized prostate cancer. *JAMA.* 2005;293(17):2095–2101.

36. Dasu A. Is the alpha/beta value for prostate tumours low enough to be safely used in clinical trials? *Clin Oncol (R Coll Radiol).* 2007;19(5):289–301.

37. Kuban DA, Tucker SL, Dong L, et al. Long-term results of the M. D. Anderson randomized dose-escalation trial for prostate cancer. *Int J Radiat Oncol Biol Phys.* 2008;70(1):67–74.

38. Zietman AL, Bae K, Slater JD, et al. Randomized trial comparing conventional-dose with high-dose conformal radiation therapy in early-stage adenocarcinoma of the prostate: long-term results from proton radiation oncology group/American College of Radiology 95–09. *J Clin Oncol.* 2010;28(7):1106–1111.

39. Zietman AL, DeSilvio ML, Slater JD, et al. Comparison of conventional-dose vs high-dose conformal radiation therapy in clinically localized adenocarcinoma of the prostate: a randomized controlled trial. *JAMA.* 2005;294(10):1233–1239.

40. Athanassiou H, Antonadou D, Coliarakis N, et al. Protective effect of amifostine during fractionated radiotherapy in patients with pelvic carcinomas: results of a randomized trial. *Int J Radiat Oncol Biol Phys.* 2003;56(4):1154–1160.

Proton Therapy for the Treatment of Prostate Cancer

Quynh-Nhu Nguyen*, Seungtaek Choi, and Andrew K. Lee
The University of Texas MD Anderson Cancer Center, Houston, TX

■ ABSTRACT

The use of proton therapy for therapeutic purposes was first proposed by Robert Wilson; since then there has been a resurgence of interest in this treatment modality. It is its physical characteristic that makes its use attractive in therapeutic radiation oncology. The attraction for proton beam radiotherapy is the potential to increase dose delivery to the tumor while minimizing dose to the surrounding normal tissue. In this article, we will review the technical aspects of proton therapy, summarize the clinical trials, and describe recent technologic advances in the use of proton beam therapy for localized prostate cancer.

Keywords: proton therapy, prostate cancer

■ INTRODUCTION

The use of protons for therapeutic purposes was first proposed by Robert Wilson in 1946; since then there has been a resurgence of interest, with several new facilities under operation and future centers proposed worldwide (1). The radiobiologic properties of protons do not differ significantly from photons (x-rays). It is the physical characteristic that makes its use attractive in therapeutic radiation oncology. The attraction for proton beam radiotherapy is the physical ability to improve dose distribution. Specifically to increase dose delivery to the tumor while minimizing dose to the surrounding normal tissue. Multiple dose escalation studies have demonstrated that increasing the radiation dose used for prostate cancer treatment leads to an improved biochemical disease-free survival and freedom from clinical failure rates (2–4). The sharp drop-off in dose after energy deposition characteristic of proton beam radiation (PBT) results in almost no dose delivered to normal tissue beyond the Bragg-peak. Thus, proton beam therapy offers the potential to safely escalate the radiation dose to the tumor because of the reduced scatter and exit dose compared with photons. This paper will review the technical aspects of proton therapy, summarize the clinical trials, and describe recent technologic advances in the use of proton beam therapy for localized prostate cancer.

■ PHYSICAL AND TECHNICAL ASPECTS OF PROTON BEAM THERAPY

Protons and other heavy charged particles have the unique physical property of depositing most of their dose at the narrow Bragg peak at a fixed depth in tissue (Figure 1), with very little dose deposited beyond that peak. The range of the proton beam is

---

*Corresponding author, Department of Radiation Oncology, The University of Texas MD Anderson Cancer Center, Unit 1202, 1515 Holcombe Blvd, Houston, TX 77030
E-mail address: qnnguyen@mdanderson.org

Radiation Medicine Rounds 2:1 (2011) 103–112.
DOI: 10.5003/2151–4208.2.1.103

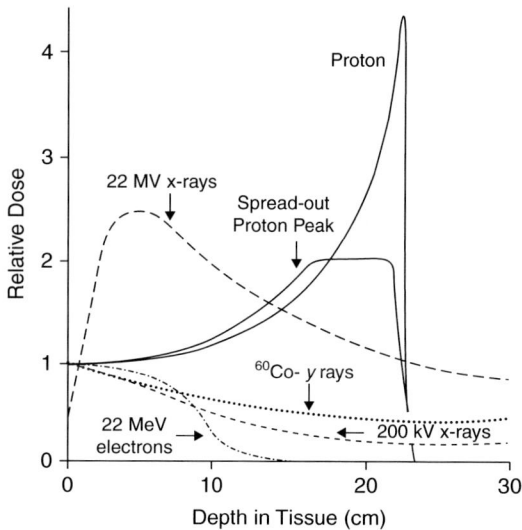

FIGURE 1 Diagram of Bragg Peak and x-rays.

determined by the energy of the charged particle. To treat tumors adequately with uniform dose requires that the width of the Bragg peak be spread out in depth to cover the entire target volume (5). The most common beam delivery method is the passive scattering system, which utilizes a scatterer to expand the pencil beam laterally and a range modulation device to create a spread-out Bragg peak (SOBP) in the proximal to distal direction. Customized apertures shape the field lateral to the beam path and compensators then shape the distal edge of the beam to conform to the shape of the target volume. The treatment planning and quality assurance for the passive scattering beam system is generally less intricate compared to the actively scanned beam.

Another method to deliver proton therapy involves the use of actively scanned proton beams. This technique is typically known as pencil-beam scanning or spot-scanning proton therapy. A scanning pencil beam delivers the protons with sequential superposition of multiple pristine pencil beams. A pencil beam (spot) is magnetically scanned in both directions perpendicular to the beam direction to irradiate a target volume without scattering devices or hardware introduced in the beam path (6–8). Multiple monoenergetic pencil beams with different energies are used to create the planned dose distribution in the distal and proximal directions. This technique allows the radiation dose to conform both the proximal as well as distal edge of the target volume, and therefore, minimizes dose to normal tissue. The scanning beam also has the

ability to achieve nonplanar dose distributions using a single gantry angle. The advantages of the scanning beam include reduction in manpower for creating customized apertures and compensators in addition to changing the field-specific equipment for each patient (9). Without the interaction of the protons with the collimators, apertures, range modulators, and other field-specific devices, the neutron dose to the patient is also decreased with the scanning beam. Since no patient-specific hardware is required in the snout, multiple gantry angles may be employed more efficiently for a daily fraction than in a passive-scattered system. Furthermore, pencil-beam scanning is the precursor technology in the development of multifield optimized intensity-modulated proton therapy (IMPT).

■ CLINICAL STUDIES

Increasing the radiation dose delivered to patients with localized prostate cancer has been shown to improve local control in addition to lower positive rebiopsy rates. Zelefsky et al. from their dose escalation study demonstrated lower rates of positive biopsy when higher radiation doses were delivered with photons. They showed that the positive rebiopsy rate was 7% when 81 Gy was delivered, 48% when 75.6 Gy was delivered, 45% when 70.2 Gy was delivered, and 57% when 64.8 Gy was delivered (10). Massachusetts General Hospital (MGH) also showed in a randomized study a local control advantage and lower positive rebiopsy rate for patients with poorly differentiated tumors when receiving a higher dose with a proton boost of 77 Gy compared to 67 Gy (11). At MD Anderson Cancer Center (MDACC), Pollack and colleagues randomized 301 patients with clinical stage T1-T3 prostate cancer to receive 70 Gy or 78 Gy. At a median follow up of 8.7 years, there was a significant improvement in freedom from biochemical failure rate of 78% for the 78 Gy arm compared to 59% in the 70 Gy arm ($P = .004$). The rate of clinical failure was also reduced from 15% in the lower dose arm to 7% for those receiving the higher radiation dose ($P = .014$) (2,3). The Dutch Multicenter dose escalation trial randomized 669 men diagnosed with localized prostate cancer to receive 68 Gy or 78 Gy. After a median of 70 months, the freedom from biochemical failure rate was superior in those receiving 78 Gy compared to 68 Gy. The freedom from biochemical failure rate was 56% compared to 45% ($P = .03$), respectively, with similar genitourinary toxicities observed in both treatment arms at long-term follow up. However, there was an increased incidence of late GI grade ≥2 in the 78 Gy arm (39% vs 25%, P = 0.04) (12).

Proton beam therapy was the earliest method utilized for dose escalation therapy for the treatment of patients with localized prostate cancer (13). In 1982, an initial dose escalation study was performed at MGH where 202 patients diagnosed with stage T3 and T4 prostate cancer received 50.4 Gy initially with a four field photon technique. These patients were then randomized to receive an additional 25.2 CGE conformal proton boost (arm 1) or an additional 16.8 Gy photon boost (arm 2). For arm 1, the proton boost of 25.2 CGE was hypofractionated, delivered at 2.1 CGE per fraction 4 days per week begun 7 to 14 days after completion of the 50.4 Gy. This was to allow healing of any radiation proctitis for placement of the rectal probe for the delivery of the proton boost. Due to the time period these patients were treated, PSA screening was not available and older treatment techniques such as a perineal boost were utilized. With a median follow up of 61 months, there was no significant difference in overall survival (OS), or disease-specific survival (DSS). However, among those completing treatment, the local control rate at 5 and 8 years for arm 1 was significantly improved at 92% and 77% compared to 80% and 60% for arm 2 (P = .0014) (11). Gardner et al. reported that the long-term rate of grade 3 or greater hematuria was 3% and 8% at 5 and 15 years, the rate of grade 2 or greater gastrointestinal morbidity was 13% at 5 and 15 years, and the rate of grade 1 rectal bleeding occurred in 41% for those receiving 77.4 CGE to the prostate in this randomized trial (14).

In 1991, Slater and colleagues published their experience on patients with localized prostate cancer stage Ia-III treated with conformal PBT alone or with a combination of photon-PBT therapy at the Loma Linda Medical Center (LLUMC). A total of 1,255 patients with no prior surgery or hormone therapy received 74 to 75 CGE. Patients with a >15% risk or higher for nodal metastasis based on the Partin tables received 45 Gy to the pelvis with photons followed by a conformal proton boost of 30 CGE to the prostate and seminal vesicles. The other group of patients received 74 CGE with proton therapy alone prescribed to the isocenter. Patients were treated daily with rectal balloons filled with water. These patients were treated with only a single proton field per day, which can increase dose heterogeneity compared to delivering

two fields per day. With a median follow up of 62 months, the 5- and 8-year biochemical disease-free survival rate was 75% and 73% (using the 1996 ASTRO consensus definition of three consecutive rises). Patients whose PSA levels reached a nadir ≤0.5 ng/mL had the highest 5- and 8-year bNED rates of 88% and 87%, respectively. The LLUMC group reported 5- and 10-year rates of freedom from grade 3 and 4 GI toxicity in both treatment groups to be 99%, respectively. The rates for freedom of GU grade 3 and 4 toxicity were also both 99%, with the most common toxicity reported as urethral strictures and hematuria (15).

Beginning in the mid-late 1990s, investigators at LLUMC and MGH began enrolling patients on Proton Radiation Oncology Group (PROG) protocol 95–09. A total of 393 patients with localized prostate cancer stage T1b-T2b with serum PSA <15 ng/mL were enrolled at one of two radiation oncology centers, LLUMC or MGH. All patients received conformal photon therapy to a fixed dose of 50.4 Gy to the prostate and seminal vesicles. The difference between the arms was in the boost dose which was delivered using proton beam. Patients were randomized to receive protons to 19.8 CGE followed by 3D photons to an additional 50.4Gy (total dose 70.2 Gy) or 28.8 CGE followed by 50.4 Gy of photons (total dose 79.2 Gy). No upfront hormone therapy was allowed. At LLUMC, patients were treated in the supine position using opposed lateral 250 MV proton beams. At the MGH, patients were treated in the lithotomy position using a single 160 MeV proton beam directed through the perineum. They reported no difference in overall survival between the two treatment arms. However, at 5 years, there was a significantly higher freedom from biochemical failure in those patients treated in the high dose arm of 91.3% compared to 78.8% in the conventional dose arm (P < .001). Only 1% of patients receiving conventional dose and 2% receiving high dose experienced acute GU or GI morbidity of grade 3 or greater. The authors reported only 2% of patients in the conventional dose arm and 1% of patients in the high dose arm experiencing late grade 3 or greater toxicity (4) (Figure 2).

After 10 years of follow up, men receiving the high-dose radiation therapy were significantly less likely to experience a local failure with a hazard ratio of 0.57. The 10-year biochemical failure rates were 32.4% for the conventional dose treatment arm compared to 16.7% for the high-dose radiation treatment arm (P < .0001) (16). With a median follow up of

9.4 years, there was no observed difference in rates of urinary obstruction (P = .36), urinary incontinence (P = .99), bowel problems (P = .7), or sexual dysfunction (P = .65) between those patients receiving conventional-dose compared to high-dose (17). Eleven percent of patients in the standard dose arm have required subsequent androgen deprivation for recurrence as compared to only 6% of men in the high dose arm.

Coen et al. reported both acute and late toxicity after dose escalation to 82 CGE using conformal proton radiation for localized prostate cancer in a subsequent phase II study American College of Radiology (ACR) 03–12. The ACR 03–12 phase II trial tested the safety and efficacy of delivering 82 CGE with conformal proton radiation without

androgen-deprivation therapy for patients with localized prostate cancer. The prostate and caudal seminal vesicles received 50 CGE followed by an additional 32 CGE boost to the prostate at 2 CGE per fraction. All treatments were delivered with an opposed lateral field arrangement without daily image guidance techniques. Therefore, the posterior coverage to the PTV was often limited by rectal constraints. At their initial report of a median follow up of 31.6 months, the rate of acute grade 3 GU/GI toxicity was 2%. The rate of late grade 3 GU/GI toxicity was 7% and late grade 4 GI/GU toxicity was 1% (18). Table 1 summarizes the late GI or GU toxicities from the randomized trials.

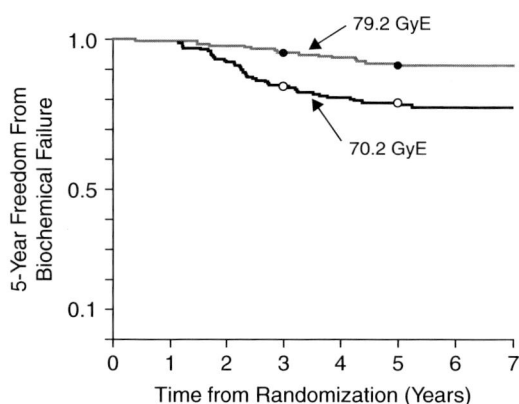

FIGURE 2 Freedom from biochemical failure (increasing PSA level) following either conventional-dose (70.2 GyE) or high-dose (79.2 GyE) conformal radiation therapy (Gray test P < .001). Adapted from Zietman et al., *JAMA.* 2008;299(8):899.

■ THE MD ANDERSON PROTON THERAPY SYSTEM

At the MDACC, patients have been treated with the Hitachi proton therapy system since May 2006. The Proton Therapy Center in Houston (PTC-H) consists of four treatment rooms, three equipped with isocentric gantries and one with two fixed horizontal beamlines (Figure 3). The passive scattering proton beams are delivered in three treatment rooms, and the pencil-scanning beam is delivered in one treatment room. A synchrotron accelerates the protons at ranges of 100 to 250 MeV for the passive system and 72.5 to 221.8 MeV for the scanning beam into three gantries and two horizontal fixed beam lines. The beam transport system is composed of magnets, which bend and control the position of the beam as it enters each treatment room. After entering each treatment room, the beamline travels through the

TABLE 1 Summary of late GI or GU toxicities from randomized trials

Trial	≥ Grade 2 GI	≥ Grade 3 GI	≥ Grade 3 GU
MDACC: Photon			
Pollack et al: 70 Gy vs. 78 Gy	13% vs. 26%	1% vs. 7%	5% vs. 4%
DUTCH: Photon			
Al-Mamgani et al: 68 Gy vs. 78 Gy	25% vs. 35%	4% vs. 6%	12% vs. 13%
PROG: Proton			
Zietman et al: 70.2 Gy vs. 79.2 Gy	8% vs. 17%	1% vs. 2%	1% vs. 2%
ACR 03-12: Proton			
Coen et al: 78-82 GyE	N/A	7%	7%

Proton Therapy Center-Houston

PTC-H
3 Rotating Gantries
1 Fixed Port
1 Eye Port
1 Experimental Port

Pencil Beam Scanning Port

Passive Scattering Port

Experimental Port

Accelerator System
(slow cycle synchrotron)

Large Fixed Port   Eye Port

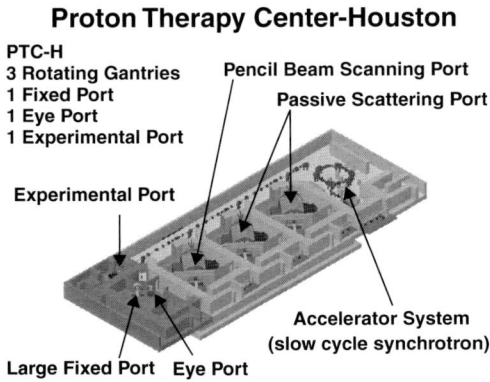

FIGURE 3   Diagram of MDACC PTC.

treatment delivery nozzle. Devices in the nozzle that include the control and safety components shape various physical parameters of the treatment beam for the passive or active scanning proton beam to ensure accurate beam delivery. The nozzle also includes lasers and x-ray tubes used for patient setup, alignment, and verification with daily image-guided radiation therapy (19).

For the passive scattering beam system, the narrow proton beam entering the nozzle is spread out laterally by a double scattering system. The rotating range modulating wheel scatters and produces a uniform SOBP. The apertures are used to shape the field laterally and the range compensator shapes the distal edge of the beam to the target volume. The compensators and apertures are manually changed for each treatment field.

The spot scanning nozzle at the PTC-H can treat patients with 94 different energies ranging from 72.5 to 221.8 MeV. In general, proton scanning beam systems may employ one of several different methods such as dynamic spot scanning, raster scanning, or discrete spot scanning. In dynamic scanning, the beam is scanned continuously across a target volume, while in discrete scanning the beam is turned off during the change of parameters for the delivery of the next spot to a new location (7,20,21). The discrete spot scanning method is currently being used at MDACC. This delivery system utilizes 2D spot scanning in the beam's transverse plane to deposit proton dose to the target volume (22). The scanning beam has the capability of better dose conformality without collimators, apertures, and compensators. This can also lower the neutron contamination compared to the passive scattering technique (23).

The risk of secondary malignancies secondary to intensity-modulated radiation therapy (IMRT) and proton therapy has been a topic of debate. IMRT utilizes multiple treatment fields and delivers low dose to a larger volume of normal tissue compared to 3D conformal photon therapy or proton therapy. Hall estimated that for men treated with IMRT for prostate cancer their risk of secondary malignancy rate was 1.75% at 10 years compared to 1% for those treated with conventional 3D conformal therapy (24). In a separate study, Hall hypothesized that the passive scattering system resulted in high rates of neutron scatter from the beam interaction with the scattering foils, apertures, and compensators resulting in a greater incidence of secondary malignancy than IMRT (25). Paganetti et al. reported that the neutron dose was overestimated by Hall in calculating for the risk of secondary malignancy. Both the pencil and passive scanning beam result in lower integral dose than IMRT and potentially decrease rates of secondary malignancies (26).

There is limited literature regarding secondary neutron exposure to proton therapy patients, and even more sparse quantitative measures of neutron dose. Experiments reveal that the neutron dose equivalent value from neutrons per therapeutic absorbed dose (H/D) varies significantly with the treatment technique, patient orientation, proton beam energy, range modulation, field size, and beam delivery system (passive or scanning beam). The relative uncertainty in H/D values is approximately 40% (27). The risk of secondary malignant neoplasm (SMN) after the treatment for prostate cancer from proton therapy relative to IMRT was assessed at MDACC. The risk of a SMN was estimated from primary and secondary doses on an organ-by-organ basis using risk models from the Committee on the Biological Effects of Ionizing Radiation. Contrary to Hall's estimates, the authors concluded that proton therapy actually reduced the risk of an SMN by 26% to 39% compared to IMRT. The risk from the in-field organs were lower with proton therapy mostly due to the sparing of dose to the rectum and bladder (28).

■ TREATMENT OF PROSTATE CANCER WITH PBT

The superior dose-depth distribution of protons can be advantageous; however, due to the physical characteristic of the Bragg-peak there can be uncertainties in the particle range when treating patients with prostate cancer. In addition to the uncertainty of the dose at the distal edge of the Bragg-peak and the RBE, this could be further magnified by variations in patient's positioning and rotation. Customized brass apertures shape the desired treatment fields. The distal dose distribution and range of the beam is conformed by the specific milled compensators made out of plastic material. To account for the daily motion of the prostate and patient rotational movements, smearing is applied to prevent under-dosing of the distal target volume. Smearing ensures target coverage accounting for setup misalignments by applying a calculated algorithm to enlarge the milled compensator (Figure 4). When treating prostate cancer, opposed lateral proton beams are designed to reproduce the beam range compared to other beam angles. Opposed lateral beams also pro-vide adequate proximal and distal coverage of the

planning target volume while minimizing the dose to the rectum and bladder.

To evaluate changes in dose distribution to the target volume and critical structures from rotational setup errors in prostate cancer patients treated with PBT using the passive scanning system, Sejpal and colleagues analyzed 70 prostate plans using par-allel opposed beams delivering a total dose of 76 Cobalt-60 Gy equivalent (CGE). With the intention of simulating the pelvic tilt, rotational setup errors of $+3^\circ$, -3°, $+5^\circ$, -5° angles and horizontal couch shifts of $+3^\circ$ and -3° were generated. They reported mean changes in clinical target volume (CTV) dose of only ≤ 2 CGE (range of 77.2–78.4 CGE) for all shifts, and <5% change to the critical structures in the worse case scenario for all shifts. When treating with opposed lateral beams, patient rotational movements of 3°, 5°, and horizontal couch shifts of 3° did not result in clin-ically significant dose changes to the target volumes

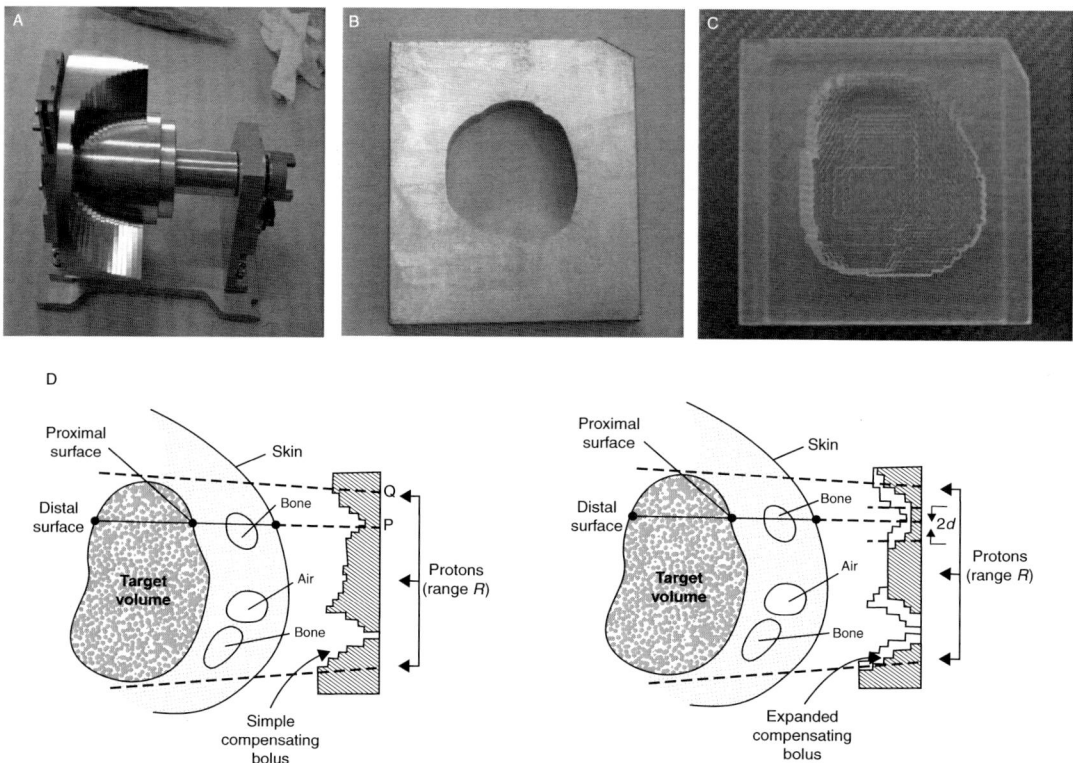

FIGURE 4   Proton beam modifiers. (A) The Bragg peak is spread out by introducing extra absorbing material rotating stepped absorber, called the range modulator wheel (RMW). (B) A metal aperture shapes the treat-ment field. (C) A compensator shapes the distal surface of the target volume and modifies the proton range. (D) Compensator smearing is applied to maintain distal coverage of the target for shifts in the relative position of anatomy, and thus changes in the radiological path length, along the beam path. Part D adapted from Urie et al., *Phys Med Biol.* 1983;29(5):553.

or critical structures (29) (Figures 5 and 6). Meyer et al. followed this dosimetric analysis associated with patient alignment errors and studied it with using opposed lateral scanning proton fields. After delineation of the clinical target volume, a small expansion was used to create a scanning target volume (STV) to ensure adequate coverage because of the lack of range compensators and smearing used with passive scattered protons for organ motion and patient setup error. The mean dose to the CTV with rotational, yaw, and translational errors was almost identical between the control and test cases (30). Like photon therapy, dose

reductions due to target movements in proton therapy showed strong directional dependency, studied by Yoon et al. (31). They compared movement induced dose reduction during photon and proton beam treatment in a scanned phantom. To decrease the effect of movement-induced uncertainty, a target with sufficient margins should be delineated. The transverse margins should be accounted in the smearing factor and the longitudinal margins with the thickness of

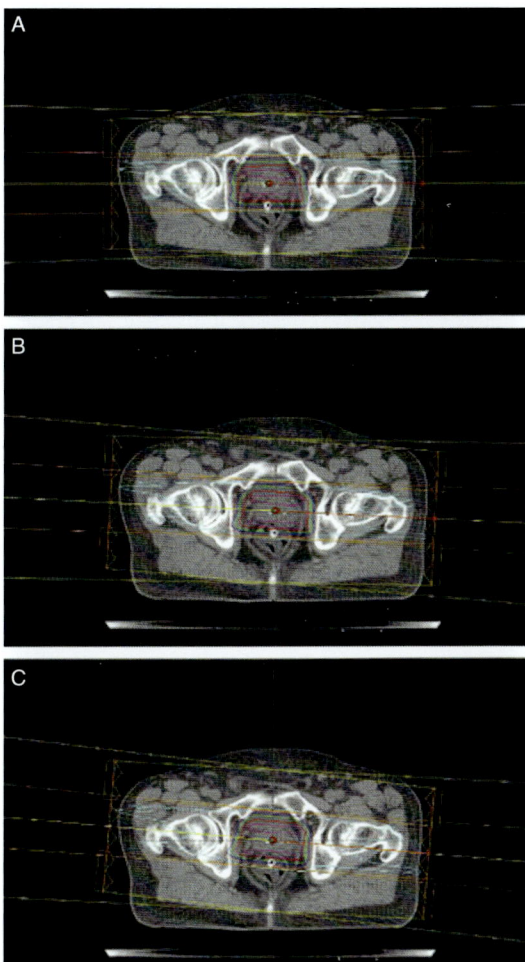

FIGURE 5 Axial CT images of parallel opposed lateral beams demonstrating rotational setup errors achieved with gantry rotations (A) 0° (control), (B) 3° (gantry at 273° and 93°), and (C) 5° (gantry at 275° and 95°).

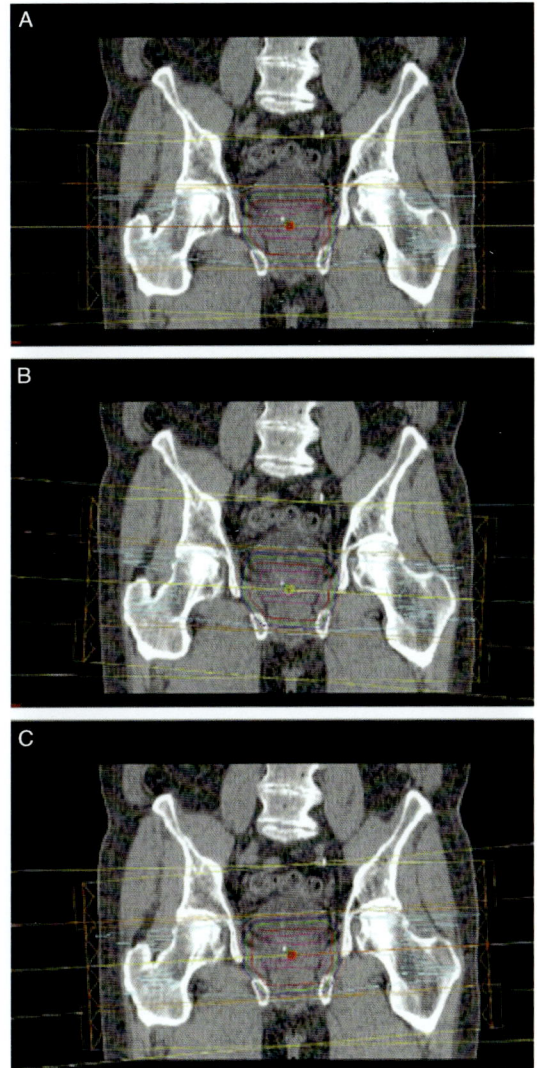

FIGURE 6 Coronal CT images of parallel opposed lateral beams demonstrating rotational setup errors achieved with gantry rotations (A) 0° (control), (B) 3° (gantry at 273° and 93°), and (C) 5° (gantry at 275° and 95°).

the SOBP. Small target movements may reduce the target dose; therefore sufficient distal margin is necessary to avoid dose reduction in proton therapy.

There are no randomized studies demonstrating that proton therapy confers a clear improvement in efficacy and toxicities compared to IMRT. However, there have been dose-volume comparison studies between proton therapy and IMRT plans for prostate cancer. Vargas et al. at the University of Florida compared the proton plans of ten prostate cancer patients with a generated and optimized IMRT plan. The bladder and rectal doses were reduced with proton therapy compared with IMRT while maintaining excellent planning target volume coverage (32). We are currently enrolling prostate cancer patients treated with IMRT or PBT (Figure 7) into quality of life protocols to evaluate whether low doses to large volumes of normal tissues increase treatment-related morbidity or late side effects. This may be important to study with the increasing interest for hypofractionated radiation regimens in localized prostate cancer.

There is an increasing volume of studies exploring the efficacy of delivering a hypofractionated course of radiation for patients with prostate cancer. This is largely due to the hypothesized low α/β ratio associated with slowly proliferating prostate tumors. Tumors usually have a high α/β ratio, whereas low α/β ratios are typical of late responding normal tissue. The α/β ratio of prostate tumors have been postulated to be between 1.5 and 3, making them preferentially sensitive to larger fractionational doses compared to surrounding normal tissue that may have a slightly higher α/β ratio (33,34). Therefore, with standard fractionation schemes, prostate tumor cells could have a greater capacity to repair radiation

damages and suffer less cell kill at small daily fraction sizes. With larger doses delivered per fraction, there could be an increase in the therapeutic ratio for tumors with low α/β ratio, conferring a biologic advantage.

Kupelian et al. showed trends of increased bNED with decreased late complications in their preliminary nonrandomized study comparing 70 Gy at 2.5 Gy per fraction to 78 Gy at 2 Gy per fraction (35,36). Pollack report their acute toxicity in the first 100 men treated for prostate cancer in a randomized dose escalation trial. The trial compared 76 Gy in 38 fractions to 70.2 Gy delivered in 26 fractions. They found no differences in acute GI or GU toxicity between the treatment arms and concluded the hypofractionated regimen of 2.7 Gy per fraction was well tolerated using the treatment planning parameters defined in the protocol (37). In another study, patients treated at the Regina Elena National Cancer Institute were randomized to receive 62 Gy at 3.1 Gy per fraction compared to 80 Gy at 2 Gy per fraction. With a median follow up of almost 3 years, there was no difference in acute GI or GU toxicities. The authors concluded that the hypofractionation regimen was safe with no statistical difference in grade 2 or greater late GI or GU toxicities between the two treatment arms (38). RTOG 04–15 randomized patients to receive 73.8 Gy in 1.8 Gy fractions versus 70 Gy in 2.5 Gy fractions. This protocol has closed to accrual and is currently being analyzed for efficacy and toxicity with hypofractionated regimens compared to standard fractionation for patients with favorable risk prostate cancer.

Studies of ultra-hyofractionated dose regimens began to evaluate the feasibility and toxicity of

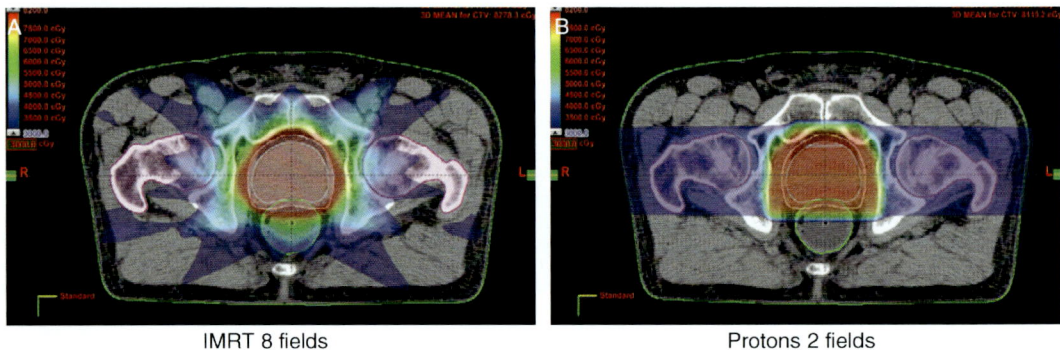

IMRT 8 fields   Protons 2 fields

FIGURE 7   Comparison treatment plan with (A) IMRT and (B) PBT.

delivering stereotactic regimens for treating patients with localized prostate cancer. A phase I/II trial of stereotactic hypofractionated accurate radiotherapy (SHARP) was performed using 33.5 Gy in five fractions using noncoplanar fields and implanted fiducials to treat 40 men with localized prostate cancer. The rate of late grade 1-2 GU toxicity was 45%, grade 1-2 GI toxicity was 37%, and there were no grade ≥3 GI or GU toxicity reported with a median follow-up of 41 months. The actuarial 48-month biochemical freedom from relapse was 90% using the Phoenix definition (nadir +2 ng/mL) (39). Forty-one low-risk prostate cancer patients were treated at Stanford University with a dose regimen of 36.25 Gy also delivered in five fractions using image-guided SBRT with cyberknife. At a median follow-up of 33 months, the rate of late grade 2 GU toxicity was 24%, grade 2 GI was 15%, grade 3 GU was 5%, and there were no grade ≥3 GI toxicity reported. Their preliminary results report that no PSA failures were observed in their last follow up (40). These two studies have demonstrated the feasibility of treating patients with localized prostate cancer with large ultra-hypofractionated regimens. These preliminary results from higher hypofractionated regimens demonstrate both the acute and late toxicities to be similar to those observed with conventional fractionation.

CONCLUSION

As we move toward larger hypofractionated regimens, it will be more critical to incorporate daily techniques to improve patient positioning and image guidance for better target delineation to safely dose escalate. Utilizing a lower density carbon fiducial improves target accuracy without causing large dose perturbations in patients receiving proton therapy when they are oriented perpendicular to the beam axis (41). Modification of treatment apparatus such as adding bulk shields near the patient, substituting the brass apertures for a tungsten alloy material, or adding an upstream proton collimator near the range sifter assembly can reduce stray doses to the patients. In addition, a more technologically advanced beam delivery system with IMPT with the scanning beam will allow us to deliver a higher tumor dose resulting in potential for increased tumor control. IMPT delivers multiple individually weighted narrow pencil beams superpositioned to conform to the treatment field results in similar target dose conformality

and homogeneity as IMRT but with decrease dose to the organs at risk. As the proton treatment delivery system evolves, future improvements may allow us to safely deliver even higher doses of conformal radiation therapy limited by photons.

REFERENCES

1. Wilson RR. Radiological use of fast protons. *Radiology*. 1946;47(5):487–491.
2. Pollack A, Zagars GK, Starkschall G, et al. Prostate cancer radiation dose response: results of the M. D. Anderson phase III randomized trial. *Int J Radiat Oncol Biol Phys*. 2002;53(5):1097–1105.
3. Kuban DA, Tucker SL, Dong L, et al. Long-term results of the M. D. Anderson randomized dose-escalation trial for prostate cancer. *Int J Radiat Oncol Biol Phys*. 2008;70(1):67–74.
4. Zietman AL, DeSilvio ML, Slater JD, et al. Comparison of conventional-dose vs high-dose conformal radiation therapy in clinically localized adenocarcinoma of the prostate: a randomized controlled trial. *JAMA*. 2005;294(10):1233–1239.
5. Bragg WH, Kleeman R. On the ionization curves of radium. *Phil Mag A*. 1904;8:726–738.
6. Zhu XR, Sahoo N, Zhang X, et al. Intensity modulated proton therapy treatment planning using single-field optimization: the impact of monitor unit constraints on plan quality. *Med Phys*. 2010;37(3):1210–1219.
7. Pedroni E, Bacher R, Blattmann H, et al. The 200-MeV proton therapy project at the Paul Scherrer Institute: conceptual design and practical realization. *Med Phys*. 1995;22(1):37–53.
8. Haberer T, Becher W, Schardt D, et al. Magnetic scanning system for heavy ion therapy. *Nucl Instrum Methods Phys Res A*. 1993;330:296–305.
9. Delaney TF, Kooy HM. *Proton and Charged Particle Radiotherapy*. Lippincott Williams and Wilkins. 2009; Chapter 5B, p. 41.
10. Zelefsky MJ, Leibel SA, Gaudin PB, et al. Dose escalation with three-dimensional conformal radiation therapy affects the outcome in prostate cancer. *Int J Radiat Oncol Biol Phys*. 1998;41(3):491–500.
11. Shipley WU, Verhey LJ, Munzenrider JE, et al. Advanced prostate cancer: the results of a randomized comparative trial of high dose irradiation boosting with conformal protons compared with conventional dose irradiation using photons alone. *Int J Radiat Oncol Biol Phys*. 1995;32(1):3–12.
12. Al-Mamgani A, van Putten WL, Heemsbergen WD, et al. Update of Dutch multicenter dose-escalation trial of radiotherapy for localized prostate cancer. *Int J Radiat Oncol Biol Phys*. 2008;72(4):980–988.
13. Coen JJ, Zietman AL. Proton radiation for localized prostate cancer. *Nat Rev Urol*. 2009;6(6):324–330.
14. Gardner BG, Zietman AL, Shipley WU, Skowronski UE, McManus P. Late normal tissue sequelae in the second

decade after high dose radiation therapy with combined photons and conformal protons for locally advanced prostate cancer. *J Urol.* 2002;167(1):123–126.

15. Slater JD, Rossi CJ Jr, Yonemoto LT, et al. Proton therapy for prostate cancer: the initial Loma Linda University experience. *Int J Radiat Oncol Biol Phys.* 2004;59(2):348–352.

16. Zietman AL, Bae K, Slater JD, et al. Randomized trial comparing conventional-dose with high-dose conformal radiation therapy in early-stage adenocarcinoma of the prostate: long-term results from proton radiation oncology group/American College of Radiology 95–09. *J Clin Oncol.* 2010;28(7):1106–1111.

17. Talcott JA, Rossi C, Shipley WU, et al. Patient-reported long-term outcomes after conventional and high-dose combined proton and photon radiation for early prostate cancer. *JAMA.* 2010;303(11):1046–1053.

18. Coen JJ, Kyounghwa B, Zietman AL, et al. Acute and Late toxicity after dose escalation to 82 CGE using conformal proton radiation for localized prostate cancer: initial report of American College of Radiology phase II Study 03–12. *Int J Radiat Oncol Biol Phys.* 2010. Article in press.

19. Smith A, Gillin M, Bues M, et al. The M.D. Anderson proton therapy system. *Med Phys.* 2009;36(9):1–16.

20. Paganetti H, Bortfield. *New Technologies in Radiation Oncology,* edited by T.B. W. Schlegel and A.L. Grosu. Berlin: Springer-Verlag. 2006, p. 345.

21. Farr JB, Mascia AE, Hsi WC, et al. Clinical characterization of a proton beam continuous uniform scanning system with dose layer stacking. *Med Phys.* 2008;35(11):4945–4954.

22. Gillin MT, Sahoo N, Bues M, et al. Commissioning of the discrete spot scanning proton beam delivery system at the University of Texas M.D. Anderson Cancer Center, Proton Therapy Center, Houston. *Med Phys.* 2010;37(1):154–163.

23. Lomax AJ, Boehringer T, Coray A, et al. Intensity modulated proton therapy: a clinical example. *Med Phys.* 2001;28(3):317–324.

24. Hall EJ, Wuu CS. Radiation-induced second cancers: the impact of 3D-CRT and IMRT. *Int J Radiat Oncol Biol Phys.* 2003;56(1):83–88.

25. Hall EJ. Intensity-modulated radiation therapy, protons, and the risk of second cancers. *Int J Radiat Oncol Biol Phys.* 2006;65(1):1–7.

26. Paganetti H, Bortfeld T, Delaney TF. Neutron dose in proton radiation therapy: in regard to Eric J. Hall (*Int J Radiat Oncol Biol Phys.* 2006;65:1–7). *Int J Radiat Oncol Biol Phys.* 2006;66(5):1594–5; author reply 1595.

27. Yan X, Titt U, Koehler AM, Newhauser WD. Measurement of neutron dose equivalent to proton therapy patients outside of the proton radiation field. Nuclear Instrum Methods Phys Res. 2002;A 476:429–434.

28. Fontenot JD, Lee AK, Newhauser WD. Risk of secondary malignant neoplasms from proton therapy and intensity-modulated x-ray therapy for early-stage prostate cancer. *Int J Radiat Oncol Biol Phys.* 2009;74(2):616–622.

29. Sejpal SV, Amos RA, Bluett JB, et al. Dosimetric changes resulting from patient rotational setup errors in proton therapy prostate plans. *Int J Radiat Oncol Biol Phys.* 2009;75(1):40–48.

30. Meyer J, Bluett J, Amos RA, et al. Spot scanning proton beam therapy for prostate cancer: treatment planning technique and analysis of consequences of rotational and translational alignment errors. *Int J Radiat Oncol Biol Phys.* 2010;78(2):428–434.

31. Yoon M, Shin D, Kwak J, et al. Characteristics of movement-induced dose reduction in target volume: a comparison between photon and proton beam treatment. *Med Dosim.* 2009;34(3):191–201.

32. Vargas C, Fryer A, Mahajan C, et al. Dose-volume comparison of proton therapy and intensity-modulated radiotherapy for prostate cancer. *Int J Radiat Oncol Biol Phys.* 2008;70(3):744–751.

33. Brenner DJ, Hall EJ. Fractionation and protraction for radiotherapy of prostate carcinoma. *Int J Radiat Oncol Biol Phys.* 1999;43(5):1095–1101.

34. Fowler J, Chappell R, Ritter M. Is alpha/beta for prostate tumors really low? *Int J Radiat Oncol Biol Phys.* 2001;50(4):1021–1031.

35. Kupelian PA, Reddy CA, Carlson TP, Altsman KA, Willoughby TR. Preliminary observations on biochemical relapse-free survival rates after short-course intensity-modulated radiotherapy (70 Gy at 2.5 Gy/fraction) for localized prostate cancer. *Int J Radiat Oncol Biol Phys.* 2002;53(4):904–912.

36. Reuther AM, Willoughby TR, Kupelian PA. Toxicity after hypofractionated external beam radiotherapy versus standard fractionation radiotherapy for localized prostate cancer. *Int J Radiat Oncol Biol Phys.* 2002;3(suppl 2):187–188.

37. Pollack A, Hanlon AL, Horwitz EM, et al. Dosimetry and preliminary acute toxicity in the first 100 men treated for prostate cancer on a randomized hypofractionation dose escalation trial. *Int J Radiat Oncol Biol Phys.* 2006;64(2):518–526.

38. Arcangeli G, Fowler J, Gomelini et al. Acute and Late toxicity in a randomized trial of conventional versus hypofractionated three-dimensional conformal radiotherapy for prostate cancer. *Int J Radiat Oncol Phys.* 2011;79(4):1013–1021.

39. Madsen BL, Hsi RA, Pham HT, Fowler JF, Esagui L, Corman J. Stereotactic hypofractionated accurate radiotherapy of the prostate (SHARP), 33.5 Gy in five fractions for localized disease: first clinical trial results. *Int J Radiat Oncol Biol Phys.* 2007;67(4):1099–1105.

40. King CR, Brooks JD, Gill H, Pawlicki T, Cotrutz C, Presti JC Jr. Stereotactic body radiotherapy for localized prostate cancer: interim results of a prospective phase II clinical trial. *Int J Radiat Oncol Biol Phys.* 2009;73(4):1043–1048.

41. Cheung J, Kudchadker RJ, Zhu XR, Lee AK, Newhauser WD. Dose perturbations and image artifacts caused by carbon-coated ceramic and stainless steel fiducials used in proton therapy for prostate cancer. *Phys Med Biol.* 2010;55(23):7135–7147.

Image-Guided Strategies for Prostate Cancer

Matthew H. Stenmark and Daniel A. Hamstra*

The University of Michigan Medical Center, Ann Arbor, MI

■ ABSTRACT

The success of highly conformal radiation therapy techniques in the treatment of clinically localized prostate cancer relies on the accurate delivery of radiation dose. Treatment delivery is complicated by geometric uncertainties such as set-up error and prostate motion, which can compromise tumor control and impact normal tissue toxicity. Image-guided radiation therapy (IGRT) has recently emerged as a crucial component in optimizing treatment accuracy and minimizing treatment related uncertainties. A wide variety of IGRT techniques have been implemented ranging from daily pretreatment imaging of implanted prostate fiducial markers to daily soft tissue imaging to continuous intrafraction motion assessment with implanted electromagnetic transponders. Each localization modality has varying degrees of spatial and temporal resolution resulting in distinct residual errors and dosimetric impacts that must be accounted for in the treatment planning margins. Ultimately, IGRT is paramount in enhancing the therapeutic ratio by allowing the delivery of dose-escalated radiation therapy with margins small enough to minimize normal tissue toxicity but large enough to avoid geographic misses.

Keywords: image-guided radiotherapy, prostate, motion, localization, tracking

■ INTRODUCTION

The Case for Dose Escalation in Prostate Cancer

Prostate cancer is very prevalent with an estimated >200,000 new cases and >25,000 deaths attributable to prostate cancer in the United States in 2009 (1). Radiation treatment represents a commonly utilized method of treating prostate cancer with an excellent chance of controlling disease with biochemical control at 5 years in excess of 90% in men with low-risk disease and 85% in men with locally confined but intermediate to high-risk disease (2). However, despite impressive biochemical control, local control remains a problem (2,3) with long-term relapse occurring within the prostate in up to 50% of men treated with conventional radiation doses of 70.2 Gy (4). Four randomized controlled trials performed in the United States and Europe demonstrated an increase in biochemical control with increased radiation dose (3–6). Dose escalation may decrease this local recurrence rate to <10%, which also serves to decrease a source of late metastatic failure (7,8). This was confirmed in the recent 10-year update of the MD Anderson dose-escalation study where metastases were observed in 19% of high risk patients treated

*Corresponding author, Department of Radiation Oncology, The University of Michigan Medical Center, 1500 East Medical Center Dr, Ann Arbor, MI 48109

E-mail address: stenmark@med.umich.edu and dhamm@med.umich.edu

Radiation Medicine Rounds 2:1 (2011) 113–130.
DOI: 10.5003/2151–4208.2.1.113

to 70 Gy as compared to 4% in those treated to 78 Gy ($P < .05$) (9).

The Toxicity of Dose Escalation

Although radiation dose escalation for prostate cancer has been achieved with generally acceptable increases in both acute and late toxicity, normal tissues in close proximity to the prostate remain the main dose-limiting factors (10). The Fox Chase Cancer Center initially described the influence of the volume of rectum irradiated on the rate of late rectal toxicity. A direct correlation was found between the ability to spare the rectum from higher doses of radiation and the ability to limit late rectal toxicity (11). In addition, the MD Anderson randomized dose-escalation trial reported an increase in grade 2 and higher rectal toxicity from 12% to 26% between the 70 Gy and 78 Gy arms. Further analysis demonstrated that both the volume of rectum treated to high doses (≥70 Gy) and to moderate doses (40–60 Gy) contributes to late rectal toxicity (5). To date, there have now been >12 retrospective reviews that support a correlation between late rectal toxicity and the volume of rectum treated between 50 and 75 Gy (12). Mathematical toxicity models using the Lyman-Kutcher methodology have also been derived to predict rectal and bladder toxicity and validated across multiple institutions (13). Therefore, the ability to provide dose-escalated radiation therapy while limiting dose to surrounding normal tissues is paramount, and image-guided radiation therapy (IGRT) represents a key component of this process.

Technologic Improvements in Radiation Therapy

Given that the improved outcomes with dose escalation came at the expense of increased toxicity, advances in external beam radiation treatment techniques, such as three-dimensional conformal radiation therapy (3D-CRT) and intensity-modulated radiation therapy (IMRT), were pursued in order to permit the delivery of higher doses of radiation to the prostate gland while constraining dose to normal tissue. The prospective trials performed for dose escalation were conducted relatively early in the clinical implementation of conformal radiotherapy when planning target volume (PTV) margins

were larger than current standards to compensate for variations in patient movement and internal organ motion. Improvements in imaging and target localization techniques have allowed for margin reductions leading to smaller radiation field sizes and a significant reduction in the overall rectal volume receiving high dose. Thus, recent toxicity data from series using either highly conformal IMRT techniques or improved targeting with IGRT show substantial improvements in rectal toxicity rates (14,15). For instance, Zelefsky et al. reported an actuarial rate of grade 2 or greater rectal toxicity at 10-years of 13% in patients using 3D-CRT and 5% using IMRT ($P < .0001$) (16). Of note, IMRT patients received higher doses of RT than 3D-conformal patients, but IGRT was also used with much greater frequency in the IMRT group, which makes it impossible to sort-out the influence of these two techniques.

The success of highly conformal radiation therapy techniques for both improved tumor control and reduced toxicity relies on the accurate delivery of radiation. It is, therefore, essential that the daily treatment setup replicates the patient position and anatomy at the time of treatment planning. Failure to account for positional variations of the prostate gland as well as surrounding normal tissue during the course of radiation therapy, may compromise tumor control and or lead to increased normal tissue toxicity. Retrospective analyses of two of the dose-escalation trials (17,18) found rectal distension at the time of treatment planning to be associated with a decreased probability of biochemical control, implying that rectal decompression over the course treatment shifted the prostate out of the treatment field and resulted in a geographical miss. These studies highlight the balance between margin reduction and target coverage that must be achieved for radiation dose escalation for prostate cancer. In other words, smaller margins are a vital component of toxicity reduction, yet they make accurate dosage delivery to the prostate, which is required for effective biochemical control, more difficult.

■ GEOMETRIC UNCERTAINTY

Treatment optimization in prostate cancer radiation therapy necessitates an understanding of the primary sources of geometric uncertainty in radiation treatment planning and delivery. These include target delineation error, patient setup uncertainty, and target position variation (primarily interfraction and intrafraction motion). IGRT aims to reduce geometric uncertainty by evaluating patient and target geometry at the time of each treatment and either altering the patient position or adapting the treatment plan with respect to anatomical changes that occur during the course of therapy.

In prostate cancer radiation therapy, the posterior margin creates an inherent optimization problem because of the high incidence of tumors located within the peripheral zone of the prostate and the proximity of the anterior rectal wall to the prostate gland. Thus, one of the primary objectives of image guidance is to optimize the PTV margin by reducing geometrical uncertainty. Since the prostate, seminal vesicles, and adjacent normal tissues are mobile structures, identification and appropriate correction of target positional variability is of critical importance. Uncertainties in target localization can occur either in the pretreatment stage or in the delivery stage. Pretreatment uncertainties are systematically reproduced during treatment while uncertainties in the delivery stage will vary on a daily basis. A review of the primary sources of geometric uncertainty, including target delineation error, setup uncertainty, and target position variation, will yield a better understanding of the advantages and limitations of the imaging and localization techniques in practice.

Target Delineation Error

Target delineation uncertainty relates to both the quality and resolution of the imaging modality as well as interobserver and intraobserver variation in target definition. Errors in target contouring generate systematic errors as they remain constant during the course of radiation therapy. Thus, these errors can have a large impact on the dose to the tumor and surrounding structures which no level of image guidance will eliminate. The unifying feature of 3D-conformal radiation and IMRT is their near uniform use of computed tomography (CT) based imaging for radiation planning. However, CT scans result in relatively poor discrimination of the prostate gland. Compared with CT, magnetic resonance (MR) imaging provides better definition of the prostate gland with respect to the surrounding tissues (19). The majority of contouring errors on CT occur at the apex and base of the gland and result in overestimation of prostate gland volumes (20–22). As a result,

the systematic discrepancy for prostate definition between expert observers on CT versus MR is greatest at the apex (3.0–3.6 mm) and at the base of the prostate and seminal vesicles (2.8–3.5 mm) (19,21). Despite the superior spatial resolution of MRI, the vast majority of prostate cancer radiation treatment planning in the modern era continues to be CT based. Inclusion of MRI information in the treatment planning process requires both the additional cost for an MRI scanner as well as the acquisition of the scans. In addition, the MRI volumes must be registered to the CT which itself introduces errors that may potentially negate the advantage of MRI (23).

Setup Error

An additional source of positional uncertainty is the variation in the daily setup of the patient and the prostate gland. Errors occur when the position and the anatomy of the patient at the time of planning are not accurately reproduced at the time of each treatment. Like all sources of error, setup error has both a systematic and random component. Systematic errors are reproducible consistent errors, occurring in the same direction and of similar magnitude over the course of treatment. Individual systematic errors represent the difference in the mean irradiation geometry from the treatment plan to each treatment fraction and arise predominately in the simulation and planning stages of treatment. Random errors represent positional variations in both direction and magnitude from fraction to fraction, which arise mostly during the daily delivery of treatment.

Prior to the implementation of image guidance, many studies examined pelvic immobilization techniques with the goal of improving the day to day reproducibility of treatment setup to the skeletal anatomy. Although there is controversy about the optimal device, pelvic immobilization has been shown to significantly reduce daily setup variations on the order of 3 to 6 mm without immobilization, to 1 to 3 mm with immobilization (24–27). Fiorino et al. randomized 52 patients undergoing definitive prostate radiation in the supine position to pelvic immobilization only versus pelvic and leg immobilization with an alpha-cradle system. Leg immobilization improved both the accuracy and reproducibility of treatment positioning with reductions in posterior-anterior shifts (2.6 vs. 4.4 mm), left-right shifts (2.4 vs. 3.6 mm), and craniocaudal shifts (2.7 vs. 3.3 mm) (28). Importantly, the rate of shifts of greater than 5 mm was reduced from 21.6% to 4% with leg immobilization. Nutting et al. randomized patients to standard foam immobilization at the ankles versus customized vacuum pelvic immobilization and found no difference between the two immobilization techniques (29). The reproducibility of both techniques was excellent with a median isocenter displacement from simulation to treatment of less than 2 mm in all directions.

Target Position Uncertainty

Although pelvic immobilization to align skeletal anatomy is widely utilized in prostate radiation therapy, its utility is limited by anatomical variations in the position, shape, and size of internal target organs, which move independently of the bony pelvis. Numerous studies have shown that normal bladder and rectal physiology as well as breathing lead to positional variability of the prostate. This occurs both between treatments as well as during radiation delivery. Thus, target localization during prostate radiation therapy has two aspects. The first aspect is the initial setup before the delivery of radiation, which deals predominately with interfraction variations of prostate position and is associated with the PTV margin. The second aspect is real-time target position monitoring during the actually delivery of radiation, which more recently has been associated with an internal target volume margin. However, in general, both interfraction and intrafraction motion have been included in one overall PTV margin.

Prior to the routine implementation of image guidance, PTV margins were typically on the order of 10 to 15 mm to account for unmeasured prostate motion (3–6). Given that an average prostate is between 30 and 50 cm^3 and presuming that it is spheroidal in shape, a 10 mm margin results in >3-fold increase in PTV volume. A reduction in PTV margin from 10 to 5 mm would result in a 1.6- to 1.8-fold decrease in the high-dose radiation volume, while a reduction from 10 to 3 mm would result in a 2.0- to 2.3-fold decrease. Since toxicity is closely associated with the volume of normal tissue receiving high dose, the use of IGRT alone may be the best opportunity to improve upon the therapeutic index of prostate radiation. However, in order to safely deliver treatment to the prostate with smaller PTV

margins, translation, rotation, and deformation of the prostate must all be accounted for in radiation treatment planning and delivery.

Interfraction Motion

The positional variability of the prostate gland has been recognized since the early 1990s (30) with multiple subsequent studies demonstrating that its movement is independent of the pelvic skeleton (31–33). A variety of techniques have been used to study interfraction prostate positional variability including, intraprostatic fiducial markers with portal imaging, transabdominal ultrasound, and periodic CT scans. Prostate and seminal vesicle positional variability during treatment has been shown to be largest in the anterior-posterior (AP) direction followed by the superior-inferior (SI), and mediolateral (ML) directions (31–33). The base of the prostate and seminal vesicles tend to exhibit larger variability than the apex, presumably due to tethering at the apex of the gland (34) while movement in the lateral plane is limited by the pelvic floor musculature. Overall, these positional changes are highly correlated with rectal filling and, to a lesser extent, with bladder filling and respiratory motion (32,35,36). The average interfractional deviations due to positional variability are typically within 5 mm of the initial target position although deviations of >10 mm have been observed in up to 30% of cases with maximal deviations of 18 mm (37). Figure 1 depicts the positional variations observed during the course of treatment and the resulting dosimetric impact.

Intrafraction Motion

Intrafraction motion characterizes the positional variability of the target that occurs from the completion of patient setup through the delivery of the treatment fraction. In other words, it represents the real-time motion of the target. With the increasing use of advanced treatment techniques, such as IMRT, that extend the radiation delivery process to an average of 15 to 20 minutes, the effect of intrafraction motion on positional variation becomes more important. Early studies of intrafaction motion using cinefluoroscopy of intraprostatic fiducial markers and cine-MRI reported relatively small mean displacements of the prostate and seminal vesicles compared to those reported in interfraction studies (35,39–41). However, similar to the interfraction studies, large displacements of the prostate in both the AP and SI

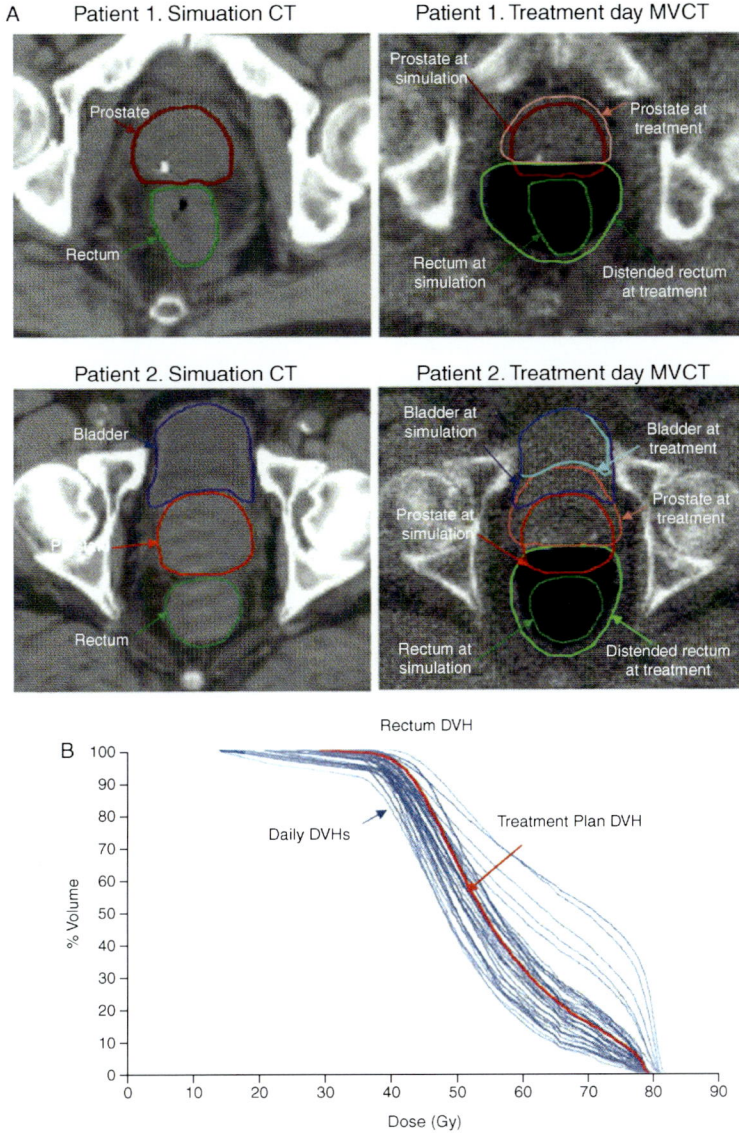

FIGURE 1 (A) Comparison of pelvic anatomy in two separate patients between the time of simulation and treatment. These CT scans show the deformation of the prostate, rectum, and bladder that would result in variations in delivered doses. (B) Rectal dose–volume histogram (DVH) for all 39 treatment fractions in 1 patient. Red line represents the planning CT DVH; thinner blue lines represent daily DVHs. From Ref. (38).

axes can be observed at low frequency. Using cine-MRI, Mah et al. reported prostate displacements (mean ± SD) of 0.26 ± 3.3 mm and 0.02 ± 3.36 mm, in the AP and SI dimensions respectively, with maximal displacements up to 1.2 cm anteriorly and superiorly (41). In another cine-MRI series, Padhani et al. observed AP displacements of greater than 5 mm in 29% of patients (40). Although these early studies

characterize the extent and variation of intrafraction motion, the duration of individual displacements is less clear. This is relevant as some displacement might be short-lived and clinically inconsequential.

Similar to the interfraction studies, the most significant predictor for intrafraction prostate motion is the status of rectal filling with distended rectums translating into greater prostate motion.

Furthermore, intrafraction prostate motion appears to be driven primarily by rectal peristalsis and to a lesser extent breathing patterns and variation in pelvic muscular tension. The influence of breathing is minimized when the patient is comfortable and in the supine position, as opposed to in the prone position or breathing deeply (36).

Although ultrasound and cine-MRI provide detailed anatomic information, their overall clinical utility is limited because they only provide short snapshots of prostate position and are unavailable during treatment delivery. The recent introduction of implantable electromagnetic transponders within the prostate allows for continuous, real-time positional monitoring of the target throughout treatment. The transponders act as a surrogate for prostate position and the system utilizes an external electromagnetic array to localize and continuously track the target isocenter of three implanted transponders at a frequency of 10 Hz. The technical details of the system are described in detail elsewhere in this report. At present, this is the only practical method for evaluating prostate motion in real-time, thereby greatly decreasing positional uncertainty during treatment.

Using electromagnetic transponders as a surrogate for prostate motion, Kupelian et al. continuously tracked the position of the prostate during radiation delivery in 35 prostate cancer patients for a total of 1,157 fractions (28–45 per patient) (42). Displacements exceeding 3 mm and 5 mm for cumulative durations of at least 30 seconds were observed in 41% and 15% of fractions, respectively. Significant variation was present within individual patients, with displacements ≥3 mm observed in 3% to 87% of fractions and displacements ≥5 mm in 0% to 56% of fractions. Additionally, the motion of the prostate was found to be irregular and unpredictable. This lack of a specific pattern makes it difficult to implement predictive approaches to deal with real-time intrafraction motion.

In a subsequent analysis, Noel et al. used the same continuous tracking data set as a reference to model the ability of pre- and posttreatment imaging to account for prostate motion (43). Orthogonoal images, pre- and posttreatment, demonstrated poor sensitivity to prostate motion unless sampled at a frequency of greater than two times per minute. These results support the value of continuous prostate tracking in reducing positional uncertainty during the delivery of radiation. However, the dosimetric

and clinical implications of such motion during treatment delivery are unclear.

Rotation and Deformation

In addition to translational movement in the -x, -y, and -z planes, it is also now recognized that deformation of the prostate, bladder, and/or rectum can occur both between and within an individual fraction which would alter radiation dose delivery to both the target and the organs at risk (44,45). For instance, one study found that large shifts in rectal shape and volume could result in a >15 Gy increase in mean rectal dose (46). In addition, even in cases where minimal deformation of the prostate occurs relative to implanted fiducial markers, the seminal vesicles have been demonstrated to have a larger propensity for motion and/or deformation, which might necessitate a larger PTV margin on the seminal vesicles (47). Finally, rotation about the axis of the prostate without overt displacement of the prostate has been observed which also might result in either increased dose to the organs at risk or decreased dose to the prostate (48). The real-time imaging, evaluation, and adaptive radiotherapy planning for the issues of deformation and rotation are at this time still be elucidated and have not entered routine clinical practice (49,50).

■ PLANNING VOLUME CONSIDERATIONS

To compensate for daily setup error and internal organ motion, a treatment margin is added to the clinical target volume (CTV) to form the PTV. The PTV margin ensures that the planned dose to the PTV represents the delivered dose to the CTV in the presence of all the possible geometrical uncertainties. Historically, site-specific PTV margins have been derived from studies of populations of patients that estimate the range of geometrical uncertainties for a given site. The most widely utilized population-based margin model differentially weights the systemic (Σ) and random (σ) components ($2.5\Sigma + 0.7\sigma$) to ensure that 90% of patients receive a minimum of 95% of the prescribed dose to the CTV (51). This model, by definition, will lead to underdosing of some patients and larger margins than necessary in others.

Over the past decade, the introduction of image guidance has led to a reduction in systematic positioning uncertainty and allowed for the optimization of treatment margins. Two general approaches, online and offline, have emerged for using the localization information provided by image guidance. Online approaches aim to localize the target volume on a daily basis, allowing for a reduction in both systematic and random target positioning errors for every patient from treatment to treatment. This improvement in precision and accuracy comes at the expense of increased treatment time and effort from the daily analysis and correction process. Offline approaches aim at eliminating systematic errors in individual target positioning, by retrospectively analyzing pretreatment images, to construct corrective offsets on the days imaging is not performed. For instance, offline adaptive radiation therapy uses daily portal imaging in conjunction with serial soft-tissue imaging in the early part of the treatment course to measure the positional uncertainties for a given patient. After approximately one week, the treatment plan is modified based upon the creation of a patient-specific PTV (52–54). The addition of daily adaptive therapy to the offline approach accounts for both systematic and random setup error.

Although online and offline IGRT approaches allow for improved dose conformality through margin optimization, both approaches neglect intrafractional motion. The offline approach also assumes that the target and surrounding normal tissues remain relatively stable following construction of the customized PTV. In a motion analysis, Litzenberg et al. demonstrated that random variations in prostate position during the course of therapy often violate the gaussian assumptions of adaptive and off-line correction models (55). Furthermore, Kupelian et al. found no specific pattern in the continuous motion behaviors of the prostate making it difficult to implement predictive approaches to deal with real-time intrafraction motion (42).

With the current limitations on image-guided adaptive radiation therapy, a method utilizing continuous target tracking for incorporation of intrafraction motion has proven advantageous. Using implanted electromagnetic transponders, Litzenberg et al. measured the deviations of the prostate from isocenter continuously during 1,157 treatment fractions (56). PTV margins were then estimated with van Herk's formula (51) for situations of skin-based positioning, prefraction marker positioning alone, and prefraction marker positioning with inclusion of corrective action levels. As shown in Table 1, prefraction target alignment based on the implanted

transponders produces significant reductions in PTV margins along all three axes. The additional implementation of action levels of 3 mm or 5 mm, for interventional correction during treatment, allow margins that are 1 to 2 mm smaller than prefraction alignment alone. Thus, continuous tracking can have a significant impact on the population margins required for prostate treatment. Increasing the degrees of corrective intervention offers the opportunity to reduce PTV margins while simultaneously allowing a larger percentage of patients to receive a minimum dose which is a higher percentage of the prescription dose. It should be noted, however, that the aforementioned measurements do not take prostate rotation or deformation into account, both of which may play a larger role as PTV margins decline.

■ TECHNIQUES

Historically, standard clinical practice in prostate external beam radiation therapy has been to perform PTV setup by aligning external skin marks to room-based lasers daily and using weekly portal imaging to align pelvic bony anatomy to digitally reconstructed radiographs (DRRs) derived from the planning CT. Reproducible misalignments on portal imaging are corrected by shifting the isocenter, relative to the position of the pelvic bony anatomy. However, as described above, both external skin marks and skeletal anatomy are poor surrogates for prostate position. Thus, these alignment approaches require large treatment margins (>10 mm), which are incompatible with the delivery of the high radiation doses (>70 Gy) that are currently employed in clinical practice.

The implementation of a wide variety of IGRT techniques has improved treatment accuracy allowing for both treatment margin optimization and dose escalation. These approaches range from daily imaging of implanted prostate fiducial markers to daily soft tissue imaging. Volumetric imaging techniques such as cone-beam CT (CBCT) provide excellent spatial resolution for daily positioning as well as for identifying anatomical changes concerning the target volume and organs at risk during the course of treatment. This technique provides a detailed snapshot of the anatomy prior to treatment, but is unable to provide information during the course of a treatment fraction. On the other hand, implanted electromagnetic transponders (Calypso 4D Localization System), provide superior temporal resolution but do

TABLE 1 PTV margins required for various setup and correction techniques, including real-time correction strategies

Target Volume Alignment Technique	Margins (mm)		
	LR	AP	SI
Prefraction skin markers without intrafraction motion	13.2	14.8	8.2
Prefraction skin markers with intrafraction motion	14.7	15.9	10.3
Prefraction implanted transponder alignment	2.0	4.5	4.6
Prefraction implanted transponder alignment with 5-mm threshold	2.0	3.5	3.5
Prefraction implanted transponder alignment with 3-mm threshold	2.0	2.6	2.5

TABLE 2 Comparison of image-guided localization techniques

Device	Efficient Localization	Noninvasive	Anatomic Information	Deformation	Intrafraction Tracking	Minimal Interobserver Variability	No Body Habitus Limitations	Expense
Endorectal balloon	✓					✓	✓	$
Transabdominal ultrasound	✓	✓	✓					$$
Radiopaque markers and EPID	✓					✓	✓	$
Electromagnetic transponders	✓				✓	✓		$$$
CT-based imaging alone		✓	✓	✓			✓	$$$$
CT-based imaging with markers			✓	✓		✓	✓	$$$$

not provide any information about prostate deformation, seminal vesicle motion, or critical normal tissue motion and deformation. Currently there is no available technique that comprehensively addresses both spatial and temporal resolution. The characteristics of the various localization techniques are summarized in Table 2.

Of note, advanced localization modalities should not be relied upon to overcome poor simulation technique. The goal of simulation is to replicate the conditions that will be used during therapy. Many institutions require an empty rectum during the time of simulation and treatment to minimize daily variation in position and motion. Significant rectal distension on the initial planning CT is often a strong indication of prostate deformation and rotation about its typical configuration. In these cases, the condition should be relieved and the planning CT repeated. Additionally, the supine position has been shown to reduce the intrafraction breathing motion observed compared to the prone position (36,39,41).

Rectal Balloon

Endorectal balloons are small air- or water-inflated balloons that are inserted into the rectum prior to daily treatment. The goals are to internally immobilize the prostate by compressing it anteriorly against the pubic symphysis and improve rectal dosimetry by reducing the volume of posterior rectal wall in the high dose region. Contrary to the belief of many radiation oncologists, endorectal balloons are relatively well tolerated. In a review of 3,561 patients undergoing conformal radiation at Loma Linda University, 97% of patients tolerated the balloon throughout the entire course of treatment (57). There is conflicting data, however, on the true effectiveness of endorectal balloons in reducing the positional variation of the prostate. In early reports, D'Amico et al. demonstrated a reduction in intra-fractional prostate motion with the use of an endorectal balloon during a measured 2-minute time interval and Wachter et al. showed significant reductions in maximum AP displacements of the prostate (58,59). Conversely, a more recent and comprehensive report by van Lin et al. showed no benefit from the endorectal balloon in reducing interfraction prostate motion (60).

There are multiple reports demonstrating improved rectal dosimetry when using an endorectal balloon in conjunction with 3D-CRT (59,61–63). This dosimetric improvement has been correlated clinically with a significant reduction in late rectal toxicity and late mucosal changes in the high dose regions as evaluated by interval rectosigmoidoscopy (63). The advantage of the endorectal balloon appears to be lost when including large portions of the seminal vesicles in the target as the balloon displaces the seminal vesicles laterally between the rectum and prostate (59). Although endorectal balloons yield more favorable rectal dosimetry, their clinical utility has been questioned in the era of IMRT as this highly conformal delivery technique permits dose to be wrapped around the rectum, thereby, achieving low rectal doses. Furthermore, positional uncertainty of the target from changes in rectal filling is minimized with the use of daily image guidance.

Transabdominal Ultrasound

Ultrasound-based localization systems utilize suprapubic transducers to acquire 2D or 3D images of the target region on a daily basis while the patient is in the treatment position. These images are overlaid on the treatment planning CT dataset and a shift correction is calculated in three orthogonal directions to correctly align the prostate with reference to the treatment field isocenter. The entire process of patient positioning, imaging, and alignment can usually be accomplished in 5 to 7 minutes.

The low cost and clinical efficiency of the transabdominal ultrasound in performing daily interfraction prostate localization have resulted in its widespread adaptation in radiation oncology departments. However, the accuracy and operator dependence of ultrasound have been questioned (64–67).

Using alignments based on radiographic images of implanted fiducial markers, Langen et al. found directed differences in the means (± SD) between ultrasound and marker alignments of 0.2 (± 3.7), 2.7 (± 3.9), and 1.6 (± 3.1) mm in the AP, SI, and lateral directions (65). The measurable differences between ultrasound and other prostate localization techniques suggest that ultrasound has residual uncertainties that must be accounted for with appropriate PTV margins. The uncertainties associated with ultrasound have been attributed to interobserver variability, image quality, operator-induced displacement of the prostate by probe pressure, and alignment uncertainty from contour volume differences between daily ultrasound and the planning CT. Factors negatively impacting image quality include obese patients, inadequate bladder filling and shadowing of the prostate by the pubic symphysis which leads to a reliance on the prostate-bladder interface for alignment in the SI axis. Newer ultrasound technologies that permit 3D visualization of the prostate may resolve some of the inaccuracies associated with ultrasound localization.

Radiopaque Intraprostatic Markers

The use of intraprostatic radiopaque markers with daily in-room imaging has gained significant popularity due the ease of use, limited interobserver variability, and low cost. Typically, three radiopaque markers, such as gold seeds or coils, are implanted into the periphery of the prostate via a transrectal or transperineal approach. Two are placed at the posterior base of the prostate and one at the apex. The stability of these fiducial markers within the prostate is well documented (33,68–70). Since the markers serve as a surrogate for prostate position, this arrangement helps ensure that the prostate/rectal interface is reproducibly identified even with prostate rotation and deformation. The markers are visualized on a daily basis with either portal or volumetric imaging. With portal imaging, corrections are made by matching marker locations to the DRRs while with volumetric imaging, a center of mass shift based on the 3D marker locations is most commonly used. When used with volumetric imaging, fiducial markers reduce interobserver variability (71). Although extensive research has been conducted on automating the fiducial registration process, the majority of systems rely on manual alignment by a radiation therapist. A disadvantage of fiducial markers is that implantation requires an invasive procedure, the risks of which are similar to a prostate biopsy, and include discomfort and possible bleeding and infection. Additionally, markers only track the prostate. They do not provide information on prostate deformation, seminal vesicle localization, or changes in the surrounding normal structures. Overall, intraprostatic markers are a reliable and cost-effective method to accurately localize the prostate gland. Although markers provide little information on deformation of the target, the dosimetric implications are likely minimal except in rare cases of extreme prostate deformation; in addition, it appears that the use of two or more markers decreases the impact of deformation which can be missed if a single fiducial marker is utilized (72).

Electromagnetic Transponders

The Calypso 4D Localization System (Calypso Medical Technologies, Seattle, WA, Figure 2), allows both pretreatment localization of the prostate as well as real-time evaluation of intra-treatment motion (73). This system consists of a tracking console in the radiation therapy control room while within the treatment room there are ceiling mounted infra-red cameras that localize an electromagnetic array which is placed over the patient before and during treatment. Finally, using resonant radio-frequencies, the array excites and localizes transponders which are implanted in the prostate. Each transponder (or beacon) (8.8 mm long × 1.85 mm in diameter) contains a capacitor and an inductor coil sealed in glass. Prior to treatment planning, three beacons are implanted at the apex, and right- and left-base of the prostate under ultrasound guidance. They then "echo" back to the electromagnetic array at distinct resonant radio frequencies with real-time tracking of their location 10 times per second. Thus, the array determines the real-time location of the prostate which is then aligned to the position of the room (and the treatment unit)

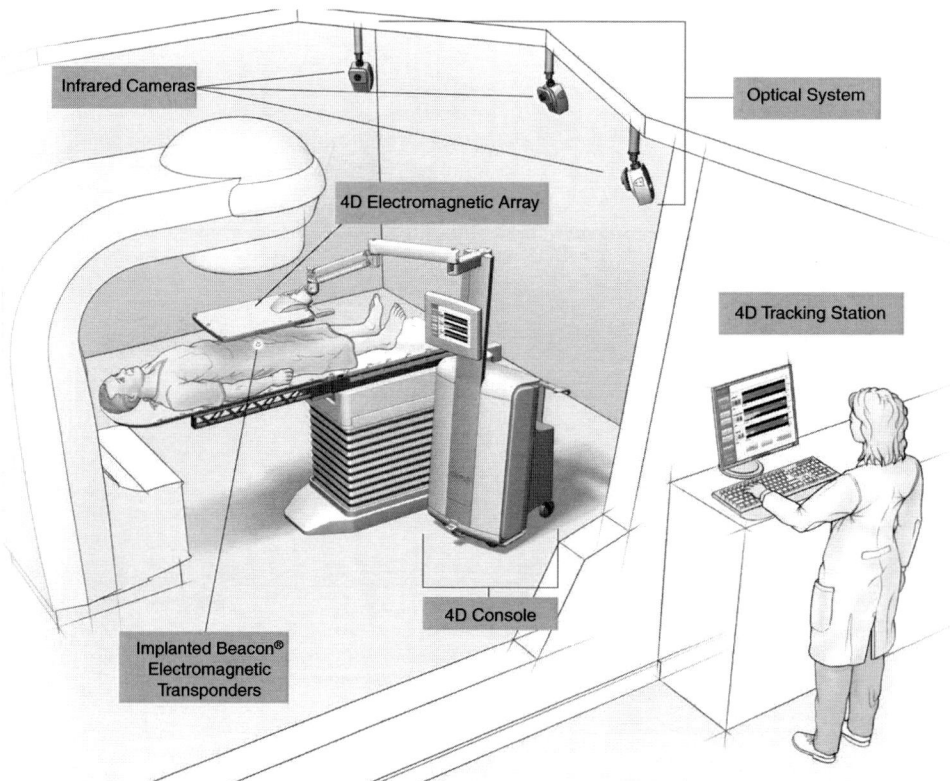

FIGURE 2   Components of the Calypso system include the implanted transponders, the 4D Console with attached 4D electromagnetic array, ceiling mounted infrared cameras, and the 4D tracking station.

using the camera system. The Calypso system can localize the prostate within 1 mm at the start of therapy; in addition, it also allows real-time evaluation of prostate motion, to monitor and account for motion during the course of treatment (74). At present this is the only practical method for evaluating prostate motion in real-time and even if the prostate is precisely aligned at the start of treatment, significant motion can occur, as shown in Figure 3. Using the transponders as surrogates for prostate motion, it has been demonstrated for a population of patients that after localization to the isocenter prior to the start of treatment, 13.6% of the time the prostate had deviated from isocenter by >3 mm. In addition, this intra-treatment motion is not uniform across patients, with some having very little while in others, this >3 mm deviation may occur as much as 36.2% of the time (75). Thus, the Calypso system allows a radiation plan to be developed taking into account an appropriate margin around the prostate (PTV margin) and an action level (AL) at which treatment is gated or interrupted to re-position the patient. Without the ability to actively monitor prostate motion (both translation and rotation) PTV margins would by definition have to be larger because they would have to account both for daily set-up uncertainty and for intra-treatment prostate motion. Limitations of the Calypso system include cost for a system that is largely limited to use in patients with prostate cancer, an inability to use the system in those with significant amounts of metal in the pelvis (such as an artificial hip), and the inability

to utilize the system in those with either a cardiac pacemaker or automatic implanted cardiac defibrillator. Additional limitations include the incompatibility of the Calypso system with MRI assessments of the prostate and limitations in the range of the signal such that in patients with larger body mass index (BMI), the system may be able to localize but not track the prostate. However, treatment in the prone position with a belly-board may minimize this limitation as patients with larger BMI are able to localized and tracked in this position (76). In addition, the Calypso system has been recently FDA approved for use in the postprostatectomy setting, although clear clinical data in this context is still pending.

CT-Based Image Guidance

In-room CT systems can be classified by beam quality, megavoltage (MV) or kilovoltage (kV), and beam collimation, fan-beam or cone-beam. Fan-beam systems use a linear array of detectors in conjunction with a rotating fan beam X-ray source. The fan-beam system can either exist as a peripheral CT-gantry (simulation CT) or be integrated with a linear accelerator resulting in a 2-in-1 concept that generates X-rays for both treatment and imaging. CBCT systems use an open beam X-ray source and large flat-panel detector mounted on the accelerator gantry perpendicular to the primary treatment axis, allowing for an entire image volume to be reconstructed

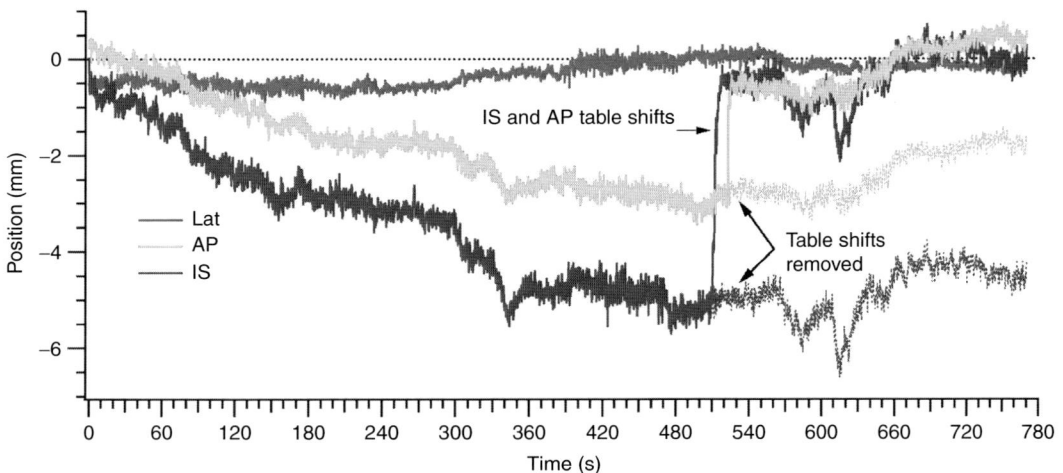

FIGURE 3 Raw tracking data with corrective table shifts toward isocenter in an individual patient using the Calypso system. Intrafraction prostate displacement is seen in the IS and AP directions.

from a single gantry rotation. The aforementioned combinations of beam quality and collimation yield four volumetric imaging methods all of which are commercially available. Varian and Elekta offer gantry-mounted kV CBCT systems (Elekta Synergy and Varian On-Board Imager) while Siemens offers an integrated MV CBCT system (MVision). Other systems include integrated helical fan-beam MV CT (TomoTherapy) and peripheral fan-beam kV CT (CT-on-rails). The main advantage of kV-imaging techniques compared to MV-imaging is the enhanced soft-tissue image contrast secondary to the prevalence of photoelectric interactions at low energies. However, the achievable image quality of the integrated kV systems still remains inferior to conventional CT. CT-on-rails offers the highest image quality of the available in-room imaging systems, but this system has largely been replaced by the advent of onboard imaging systems.

CT-based localization methods permit daily visualization of the prostate, thereby, enabling direct soft tissue alignment. However, given the limited resolution of onboard imaging systems, determining the precise location of the prostate can be challenging. Alternative techniques to soft tissue registration include intraprostatic fiducial marker alignment, planning CT contour alignment, and automatic 3D gray-value registration. Langen et al. evaluated three manual registration techniques using an onboard MV CT system: fiducial markers, soft tissue anatomy, and planning kV CT contours (77). Two radiation therapists and one physician retrospectively registered daily MV CT images with the planning kV CT images based on each of the three techniques. For each image pair, a reference alignment was computed from the center-of-mass of the fiducial markers. Overall, the contour-based results were significantly worse than the soft tissue anatomy-based registration results for both the physician and the radiation therapists. Misalignments of ≥5 mm occurred in <5% of all cases using soft tissue registration but were present in up to 25% of therapist cases and 13% of physician cases when only using the contours from simulation. When a 3 mm threshold was set, the frequency of misalignments with the soft tissue method increased, occurring in 24% and 33% of the therapists' registrations and 7% and 13% of the physician registrations in the AP and SI directions. The use of fiducial markers significantly reduced the inter-user variability associated with both of the nonmarker-based methods. In a similar study using kV CBCT imaging,

Moseley et al. reported misalignments in excess of 3 mm in 35% of registrations in both the AP and SI directions for the soft tissue based method (71). The observed deviations in the AP and SI directions highlight the uncertainties associated with prostate definition on CBCT and are concordant with the target delineation errors at the prostate apex and prostate-bladder interface reported in the literature. In clinical practice, the increase in precision gained with fiducial marker placement must be weighed against the inconvenience of invasive fiducial marker placement. Additionally, prostate rotation and deformation introduces uncertainties in marker-based alignment, the impact of which needs to be further explored. As documented above, soft tissue registration in the absence of markers is feasible but the residual uncertainties associated with this method must be accounted for in PTV margins. The accuracy of soft tissue alignment is likely to improve with continued advancement in on-board image quality.

In addition to daily visualization and localization of the target, CT-based methods permit characterization of soft tissue changes such as prostate deformation, rectal distension, and bladder filling. This accompanying anatomic information allows for real-time re-planning as well as the calculation of daily dose-volume-histograms for both the target and adjacent organs-at-risk. Although work is being performed to create the deformable registration algorithms that are required to account for daily anatomic changes, these are not yet universally available. Disadvantages of volumetric imaging include inter-observer variability, lack of continuous tracking, and increased machine time for image acquisition and processing.

Postprostatectomy

Image guidance has a clear place in the treatment of prostate cancer in the definitive setting with dozens of reports and more than 10-years of accumulated data attesting to the translation, deformation, and rotation of the prostate both between and during radiation treatments. The extent and impact of prostate bed motion following radical prostatectomy is far less clear at this time. However, a number of reports have attested to the use of IGRT to localize the prostate bed and reduce daily set-up error, including Calypso beacon localization (78), daily portal imaging with implanted gold seed fiducials

(79), ultrasound (80), and daily cone-beam imaging or kilovoltage imaging (81). The fundamental reason to use IGRT remains the same as in the definitive setting although the overall impact of motion and the amount of benefit in the postoperative setting at this time is unclear. Use of both IGRT and IMRT may allow dose escalation in the postoperative setting which some have suggested will correlate with improvements in outcome just as it has in the definitive RT setting (82).

Clinical Outcomes

Many studies have shown that image guidance strategies are feasible in terms of treatment accuracy and margin reduction. It is uncertain, however, if these geometric and dosimetric gains lead to improved clinical outcomes. Although no randomized studies assessing the clinical impact of image guidance are available, the clinical impact of anatomic variations in the pre-IGRT era was clearly demonstrated by de Crevoisier in 2005 (17). This study examined the effect of rectal distension at the time of simulation on biochemical control in 127 prostate cancer patients treated with high dose 3D-CRT. Patients with distended rectums, defined as a cross sectional area (CSA) >11.2 cm^2, on the planning CT scan had a 29% decrease in biochemical control at 5 years (63% for CSA >11.2 cm^2 and 92% for CSA ≤11.2 cm^2). Heemsbergen et al. confirmed this observation in patients treated without image guidance on the Dutch randomized dose-escalation study (18). The increase in biochemical failure in these studies is presumably due to systematic posterior displacement of the prostate during treatment relative to its perceived position at the time of planning; thereby, leading to geographic misses. Using a similar patient cohort, Kupelian et al. examined the impact of rectal distension in 488 patients treated with daily ultrasound guidance. In this retrospective study, rectal distension at the time of simulation was not found to impact biochemical control when daily image guidance was implemented. This can be attributed to a reduction in targeting errors through the correction of daily anatomic variations with image guidance. The study is one of few reports that show an actual improvement in clinical outcomes with image guidance.

Although image guidance was implemented largely in concert with IMRT, IMRT became the minimum standard for the treatment of prostate cancer at many centers by achieving dose escalation with acceptable toxicity (83). However, without image guidance, the highly conformal dose distributions and steep dose gradients produced with IMRT might be inadequate for a moving target such as the prostate. Image guidance not only minimizes the threat of a geographic miss, but also permits PTV margin reduction and dose-painting through improved setup accuracy and reproducibility. The impact of margin reduction on doses to surrounding structures may be just as critical as the steep IMRT dose gradients in translating to treatment-related toxicity. Ultimately, it is difficult to discern which technologic advance affords the greatest gain since they are most often utilized concurrently.

Given the excellent clinical control obtained for localized prostate cancer, recent emphasis has been placed on the impact of treatment on the overall health-related quality of life (QOL). Studies of patient-reported outcomes following prostatectomy or conventional radiotherapy found concern for urinary incontinence, bowel function, and sexual activity following treatment (84). However, the impact of newer treatment, modalities such as image guided therapy upon patient QOL have not been adequately addressed. The multi-institutional AIM trial (Assessing the Impact of Margin Reduction) recently reported a decrease in the acute reduction in patient reported QOL in patients treated with a reduced PTV margin (3 mm) using IMRT and electromagnetic tracking (85). As part of the AIM study QOL data was obtained prior to and after the completion of treatment and compared to the recently published PROST-QA results (84). For the PROST-QA group, IMRT was used with conventional PTV margins of 5 to 10 mm to deliver radiation doses of 75.6 to 79.2 Gy, while the AIM study utilized IMRT and electromagnetic tracking with 3 mm PTV margins to deliver 81 Gy. At the end of treatment there were significantly less detrimental impacts upon QOL when measured for the bowel/rectal, urinary obstructive and urinary incontinence domains in the AIM study. This was most pronounced for the bowel/rectal domain where despite a lower baseline QOL score (on a scale from 1 to 100) there was only a 1.5 point median decline (95% confidence interval [CI]: -7.6 to +4.5) observed on the AIM study as compared to a median 16 point decline in the PROST-QA study. Overall, the percentage of patients reporting a bowel problem increased from

4% to 20% in the PROST-QA group but did not increase in the AIM group. This change in acute effects of radiation therapy may be of particular importance, since it has recently been demonstrated that patients who exhibit acute toxicity to prostate radiation therapy are seven times more likely to have late toxicity (14). Therefore, there is the potential for real clinical benefit in terms of acute and long-term toxicity to be gained by further PTV margin reductions. While PTV margin reduction is an attractive option to further decrease toxicity, one must proceed with caution. In a study by Engels et al., the outcomes of patients treated with daily bony alignment and asymmetric PTV margins of 6 mm LR and 10 mm AP and CC were compared to patients treated with daily fiducial markers and asymmetric PTV margins of 3 to 5 mm (86). Surprisingly, the use of markers had a negative impact on biochemical control (5-year freedom from biochemical failure of 58% vs. 91%, P = .02). This study shows that margins for IGRT cannot be arbitrarily set and must account for the residual error for the given image guidance technique. Furthermore, small PTV margins may not be reliably utilized without actively taking into account intrafraction motion, including both translation and rotation of the prostate.

CONCLUSIONS

The treatment of prostate cancer with external beam radiation therapy has improved over the last twenty years with 3D dose distributions and inverse planning of radiation therapy allowing tailoring of the radiation dose to pretreatment planning images. Despite this improvement in dose conformality, planning margins are still needed to account for geometrical uncertainties such as interfractional and intrafractional prostate motion. The posterior treatment margin poses the main optimization problem because of the proximity of the anterior rectal wall to the prostate gland, and is further compounded by the fact that higher radiation doses are needed for improved biochemical control. The relatively recent implementation of daily image guidance techniques has helped mitigate the impact of prostate motion. Image guidance has not only led to improved targeting by minimizing the uncertainty associated with the positional variability of the prostate, but has also allowed for margin reductions and an improved toxicity profile.

Targeting the prostate has been performed with gold markers, CT scans, and ultrasound. These techniques, however, do not address the motion of the prostate (both translations and rotations) during the course of a single treatment. Over an 8-week course of radiation it has been suggested that the impact of positional changes are lessened by random variations which may offset daily variations. Recently, however, shorter treatment regimens (hypofractionation) have been evaluated in prostate cancer treatment due to theoretic improvements in the therapeutic index as well as dramatic reductions in time and cost of delivery. When using these hypofractionated regimens, errors in delivery on any given day would potentially have a much larger overall impact since each treatment represent a much larger proportion of the whole treatment. As a result IGRT may have an even greater role in both maintaining treatment efficacy and decreasing toxicity if treatment shifts towards the use of a smaller number of treatments.

Regardless of the image guidance technique utilized, a comprehensive quality assurance (QA) program must be implemented and integrated with standard treatment machine QA, including daily, monthly, and annual tests. As the use of advanced image guidance techniques becomes more widely available in the coming years, the uncertainties in dosimetric delivery of treatment plans due to inter- and intra-fraction positioning errors will be greatly reduced. As always, caution must be exercised when reducing treatment margins, taking care to account for the residual error for the given image guidance technique.

REFERENCES

1. Jemal A, Siegel R, Ward E, et al. Cancer statistics, 2007. *CA Cancer J Clin.* 2007;57(1):43–66.
2. Lee I, Sandler H. Hormone therapy and radiotherapy for intermediate risk prostate cancer. *Semin Radiat Oncol.* 2008;18(1):7–14.
3. Cahlon O, Hunt M, Zelefsky MJ. Intensity-modulated radiation therapy: supportive data for prostate cancer. *Semin Radiat Oncol.* 2008;18(1):48–57.
4. Zietman AL, DeSilvio ML, Slater JD, et al. Comparison of conventional-dose vs high-dose conformal radiation therapy in clinically localized adenocarcinoma of the prostate: a randomized controlled trial. *JAMA.* 2005;294(10):1233–1239.
5. Kuban DA, Tucker SL, Dong L, et al. Long-term results of the M. D. Anderson randomized dose-escalation trial

for prostate cancer. *Int J Radiat Oncol Biol Phys.* 2008;70(1):67–74.

6. Eade TN, Hanlon AL, Horwitz EM, et al. What dose of external-beam radiation is high enough for prostate cancer? *Int J Radiat Oncol Biol Phys.* 2007;68(3):682–689.

7. Jacob R, Hanlon AL, Horwitz EM, et al. The relationship of increasing radiotherapy dose to reduced distant metastases and mortality in men with prostate cancer. *Cancer.* 2004;100(3):538–543.

8. Coen JJ, Zietman AL, Thakral H, et al. Radical radiation for localized prostate cancer: local persistence of disease results in a late wave of metastases. *J Clin Oncol.* 2002;20(15):3199–3205.

9. Kuban DA, Levy LB, Cheung MR, et al. Long-term failure patterns and survival in a randomized dose-escalation trial for prostate cancer. Who dies of disease? *Int J Radiat Oncol Biol Phys.* 2010; In press, corrected proof, available online.

10. Peeters ST, Hoogeman MS, Heemsbergen WD, et al. Rectal bleeding, fecal incontinence, and high stool frequency after conformal radiotherapy for prostate cancer: normal tissue complication probability modeling. *Int J Radiat Oncol Biol Phys.* 2006;66(1):11–19.

11. Hanks GE, Schultheiss TE, Hunt MA, et al. Factors influencing incidence of acute grade 2 morbidity in conformal and standard radiation treatment of prostate cancer. *Int J Radiat Oncol Biol Phys.* 1995;31(1):25–29.

12. Vargas C, Yan D, Kestin LL, et al. Phase II dose escalation study of image-guided adaptive radiotherapy for prostate cancer: use of dose-volume constraints to achieve rectal isotoxicity. *Int J Radiat Oncol Biol Phys.* 2005;63(1):141–149.

13. Tucker SL, Dong L, Bosch W, et al. Fit of a generalized Lyman normal-tissue complication probability (NTCP) model to grade ≥ 2 late rectal toxicity data from patients treated on protocol RTOG 94–06 [abstract]. *Int J Radiat Oncol Biol Phys.* 2007;69(suppl 1):8–9.

14. Zelefsky MJ, Levin EJ, Hunt M, et al. Incidence of late rectal and urinary toxicities after three-dimensional conformal radiotherapy and intensity-modulated radiotherapy for localized prostate cancer. *Int J Radiat Oncol Biol Phys.* 2008;70(4):1124–1129.

15. Skala M, Rosewall T, Dawson L, et al. Patient-assessed late toxicity rates and principal component analysis after image-guided radiation therapy for prostate cancer. *Int J Radiat Oncol Biol Phys.* 2007;68(3):690–698.

16. Zelefsky MJ, Levin EJ, Hunt M, et al. Incidence of late rectal and urinary toxicities after three-dimensional conformal radiotherapy and intensity-modulated radiotherapy for localized prostate cancer. *Int J Radiat Oncol Biol Phys.* 2008;70(4):1124–1129.

17. de Crevoisier R, Tucker SL, Dong L, et al. Increased risk of biochemical and local failure in patients with distended rectum on the planning CT for prostate cancer radiotherapy. *Int J Radiat Oncol Biol Phys.* 2005;62(4):965–973.

18. Heemsbergen WD, Hoogeman MS, Witte MG, et al. Increased risk of biochemical and clinical failure for prostate patients with a large rectum at radiotherapy planning: results from the Dutch trial of 68 GY versus 78 Gy. *Int J Radiat Oncol Biol Phys.* 2007;67(5):1418–1424.

19. Parker CC, Damyanovich A, Haycocks T, et al. Magnetic resonance imaging in the radiation treatment planning of localized prostate cancer using intra-prostatic fiducial markers for computed tomography co-registration. *Radiother Oncol.* 2003;66(2):217–224.

20. McLaughlin PW, Evans C, Feng M, et al. Radiographic and anatomic basis for prostate contouring errors and methods to improve prostate contouring accuracy. *Int J Radiat Oncol Biol Phys.* 2010;76(2):369–378.

21. Rasch C, Barillot I, Remeijer P, et al. Definition of the prostate in CT and MRI: a multi-observer study. *Int J Radiat Oncol Biol Phys.* 1999;43(1):57–66.

22. Roach M, Faillace-Akazawa P, Malfatti C, et al. Prostate volumes defined by magnetic resonance imaging and computerized tomographic scans for three-dimensional conformal radiotherapy. *Int J Radiat Oncol Biol Phys.* 1996;35(5):1011–1018.

23. Roberson P, McLaughlin PW, Narayana V, et al. Use and uncertainties of mutual information for computed tomography/magnetic resonance (CT/MR) registration post permanent implant of the prostate. *Med Phys.* 2005;32(2):473–482.

24. Soffen EM, Hanks GE, Hwang CC, et al. Conformal static field therapy for low volume low grade prostate cancer with rigid immobilization. *Int J Radiat Oncol Biol Phys.* 1991;20(1):141–146.

25. Rosenthal SA, Roach M, Goldsmith BJ, et al. Immobilization improves the reproducibility of patient positioning during six-field conformal radiation therapy for prostate carcinoma. *Int J Radiat Oncol Biol Phys.* 1993;27(4):921–926.

26. Bentel GC, Marks LB, Sherouse GW, et al. The effectiveness of immobilization during prostate irradiation. *Int J Radiat Oncol Biol Phys.* 1995;31(1):143–148.

27. Rattray G, Hopley S, Mason N, et al. Assessment of pelvic stabilization devices for improved field reproducibility. *Austr Radiol.* 1998;42(2):118–125.

28. Fiorino C, Reni M, Bolognesi A, et al. Set-up error in supine-positioned patients immobilized with two different modalities during conformal radiotherapy of prostate cancer. *Radiother Oncol.* 1998;49(2):133–141.

29. Nutting CM, Khoo VS, Walker V, et al. A randomised study of the use of a customised immobilisation system in the treatment of prostate cancer with conformal radiotherapy. *Radiother Oncol.* 2000;54(1):1–9.

30. Ten Haken RK, Forman JD, Heimburger DK, et al. Treatment planning issues related to prostate movement in response to differential filling of the rectum and bladder. *Int J Radiat Oncol Biol Phys.* 1991;20(6):1317–1324.

31. Balter JM, Sandler HM, Lam K, et al. Measurement of prostate movement over the course of routine radiotherapy using implanted markers. *Int J Radiat Oncol Biol Phys.* 1995;31(1):113–118.

32. Dawson LA, Mah K, Franssen E, et al. Target position variability throughout prostate radiotherapy. *Int J Radiat Oncol Biol Phys.* 1998;42(5):1155–1161.

33. Schallenkamp JM, Herman MG, Kruse JJ, et al. Prostate position relative to pelvic bony anatomy based on intraprostatic gold markers and electronic portal imaging. *Int J Radiat Oncol Biol Phys.* 2005;63(3):800–811.

34. Wu J, Haycocks T, Alasti H, et al. Positioning errors and prostate motion during conformal prostate radiotherapy using on-line isocentre set-up verification and implanted prostate markers. *Radiother Oncol.* 2001;61(2):127–133.

35. Ghilezan MJ, Jaffray DA, Siewerdsen JH, et al. Prostate gland motion assessed with cine-magnetic resonance imaging (cine-MRI). *Int J Radiat Oncol Biol Phys.* 2005;62(2):406–417.

36. Dawson LA, Litzenberg DW, Brock KK, et al. A comparison of ventilatory prostate movement in four treatment positions. *Int J Radiat Oncol Biol Phys.* 2000;48(2):319–323.

37. Crook JM, Raymond Y, Salhani D, et al. Prostate motion during standard radiotherapy as assessed by fiducial markers. *Radiother Oncol.* 1995;37(1):35–42.

38. Kupelian PA, Langen KM, Zeidan OA, et al. Daily variations in delivered doses in patients treated with radiotherapy for localized prostate cancer. *Int J Radiat Oncol Biol Phys.* 2006;66(3):876–882.

39. Nederveen AJ, Heide UAvd, Dehnad H, et al. Measurements and clinical consequences of prostate motion during a radiotherapy fraction. *Int J Radiat Oncol Biol Phys.* 2002;53(1):206–214.

40. Padhani AR, Khoo VS, Suckling J, et al. Evaluating the effect of rectal distension and rectal movement on prostate gland position using cine MRI. *Int J Radiat Oncol Biol Phys.* 1999;44(3):525–533.

41. Mah D, Freedman G, Milestone B, et al. Measurement of intrafractional prostate motion using magnetic resonance imaging. *Int J Radiat Oncol Biol Phys.* 2002;54(2):568–575.

42. Kupelian P, Willoughby T, Mahadevan A, et al. Multi-institutional clinical experience with the Calypso System in localization and continuous, real-time monitoring of the prostate gland during external radiotherapy. *Int J Radiat Oncol Biol Phys.* 2007;67(4):1088–1098.

43. Noel C, Parikh PJ, Roy M, et al. Prediction of intrafraction prostate motion: accuracy of pre- and post-treatment imaging and intermittent imaging. *Int J Radiat Oncol Biol Phys.* 2009;73(3):692–698.

44. Kerkhof EM, van der Put RW, Raaymakers BW, et al. Variation in target and rectum dose due to prostate deformation: an assessment by repeated MR imaging and treatment planning. *Phys Med Biol.* 2008;53(20):5623–5634.

45. Nichol AM, Brock KK, Lockwood GA, et al. A magnetic resonance imaging study of prostate deformation relative to implanted gold fiducial markers. *Int J Radiat Oncol Biol Phys.* 2007;67(1):48–56.

46. Booth J, Zavgorodni S. Modelling the variation in rectal dose due to inter-fraction rectal wall deformation in external beam prostate treatments. *Phys Med Biol.* 2005;50(21):5055–5074.

47. van der Wielen GJ, Mutanga TF, Incrocci L, et al. Deformation of prostate and seminal vesicles relative to intraprostatic fiducial markers. *Int J Radiat Oncol Biol Phys.* 2008;72(5):1604–1611.

48. Noel CE, Santanam L, Olsen JR, et al. An automated method for adaptive radiation therapy for prostate cancer patients using continuous fiducial-based tracking. *Phys Med Biol;*55(1):65–82.

49. Thongphiew D, Wu QJ, Lee WR, et al. Comparison of online IGRT techniques for prostate IMRT treatment: adaptive vs repositioning correction. *Med Phys.* 2009;36(5):1651–1662.

50. Godley A, Ahunbay E, Peng C, et al. Automated registration of large deformations for adaptive radiation therapy of prostate cancer. *Med Phys.* 2009;36(4):1433–1441.

51. van Herk M, Remeijer P, Rasch C, et al. The probability of correct target dosage: dose-population histograms for deriving treatment margins in radiotherapy. *Int J Radiat Oncol Biol Phys.* 2000;47(4):1121–1135.

52. Yan D, Wong J, Vicini F, et al. Adaptive modification of treatment planning to minimize the deleterious effects of treatment setup errors. *Int J Radiat Oncol Biol Phys.* 1997;38(1):197–206.

53. Yan D, Lockman D, Brabbins D, et al. An off-line strategy for constructing a patient-specific planning target volume in adaptive treatment process for prostate cancer. *Int J Radiat Oncol Biol Phys.* 2000;48(1):289–302.

54. Nuver TT, Hoogeman MS, Remeijer P, et al. An adaptive off-line procedure for radiotherapy of prostate cancer. *Int J Radiat Oncol Biol Phys.* 2007;67(5):1559–1567.

55. Litzenberg DW, Balter JM, Lam KL, et al. Retrospective analysis of prostate cancer patients with implanted gold markers using off-line and adaptive therapy protocols. *Int J Radiat Oncol Biol Phys.* 2005;63(1):123–133.

56. Litzenberg DW, Willoughby T, Kupelian P, et al. Prostate margins for real-time monitoring and correction strategies. *Int J Radiat Oncol Biol Phys.* 2007;69(3 suppl 1):S676–S677.

57. Ronson BB, Yonemoto LT, Rossi CJ, et al. Patient tolerance of rectal balloons in conformal radiation treatment of prostate cancer. *Int J Radiat Oncol Biol Phys.* 2006;64(5):1367–1370.

58. D'Amico AV, Manola J, Loffredo M, et al. A practical method to achieve prostate gland immobilization and target verification for daily treatment. *Int J Radiat Oncol Biol Phys.* 2001;51(5):1431–1436.

59. Wachter S, Gerstner N, Dorner D, et al. The influence of a rectal balloon tube as internal immobilization device on variations of volumes and dose-volume histograms during treatment course of conformal radiotherapy for prostate cancer. *Int J Radiat Oncol Biol Phys.* 2002;52(1):91–100.

60. van Lin ENJT, van der Vight LP, Witjes JA, et al. The effect of an endorectal balloon and off-line correction on the interfraction systematic and random prostate position variations: A comparative study. *Int J Radiat Oncol Biol Phys.* 2005;61(1):278–288.

61. Patel R, Orton N, Tom W, et al. Rectal dose sparing with a balloon catheter and ultrasound localization in conformal radiation therapy for prostate cancer. *Radiother Oncol.* 2003;67(3):285–294.

62. Sanghani M, Ching J, Schultz D, et al. Impact on rectal dose from the use of a prostate immobilization and rectal localization device for patients receiving dose escalated 3D conformal radiation therapy. *Urologic oncology.* 2004;22(3):165–168.

63. van Lin ENJT, Kristinsson J, Philippens MEP, et al. Reduced late rectal mucosal changes after prostate three-dimensional conformal radiotherapy with endorectal balloon as observed in repeated endoscopy. *Int J Radiat Oncol Biol Phys.* 2007;67(3):799–811.

64. Lattanzi J, McNeeley S, Pinover W, et al. A comparison of daily CT localization to a daily ultrasound-based system in prostate cancer. *Int J Radiat Oncol Biol Phys.* 1999;43(4):719–725.

65. Langen KM, Pouliot J, Anezinos C, et al. Evaluation of ultrasound-based prostate localization for image-guided radiotherapy. *Int J Radiat Oncol Biol Phys.* 2003;57(3):635–644.

66. Scarbrough TJ, Golden NM, Ting JY, et al. Comparison of ultrasound and implanted seed marker prostate localization methods: Implications for image-guided radiotherapy. *Int J Radiat Oncol Biol Phys.* 2006;65(2):378–387.

67. McNair HA, Mangar SA, Coffey J, et al. A comparison of CT- and ultrasound-based imaging to localize the prostate for external beam radiotherapy. *Int J Radiat Oncol Biol Phys.* 2006;65(3):678–687.

68. Kupelian PA, Willoughby TR, Meeks SL, et al. Intraprostatic fiducials for localization of the prostate gland: Monitoring intermarker distances during radiation therapy to test for marker stability. *Int J Radiat Oncol Biol Phys.* 2005;62(5):1291–1296.

69. Pouliot J, Aubin M, Langen KM, et al. (Non)-migration of radiopaque markers used for on-line localization of the prostate with an electronic portal imaging device. *Int J Radiat Oncol Biol Phys.* 2003;56(3):862–866.

70. Poggi MM, Gant DA, Sewchand W, et al. Marker seed migration in prostate localization. *Int J Radiat Oncol Biol Phys.* 2003;56(5):1248–1251.

71. Moseley DJ, White EA, Wiltshire KL, et al. Comparison of localization performance with implanted fiducial markers and cone-beam computed tomography for on-line image-guided radiotherapy of the prostate. *Int J Radiat Oncol Biol Phys.* 2007;67(3):942–953.

72. Kudchadker RJ, Lee AK, Yu ZH, et al. Effectiveness of using fewer implanted fiducial markers for prostate target alignment. *Int J Radiat Oncol Biol Phys.* 2009;74(4):1283–1289.

73. Willoughby TR, Kupelian PA, Pouliot J, et al. Target localization and real-time tracking using the Calypso 4D localization system in patients with localized prostate cancer. *Int J Radiat Oncol Biol Phys.* 2006;65(2):528–534.

74. Balter JM, Wright JN, Newell LJ, et al. Accuracy of a wireless localization system for radiotherapy. *Int J Radiat Oncol Biol Phys.* 2005;61(3):933–937.

75. Litzenberg DW, Balter JM, Hadley SW, et al. Influence of intrafraction motion on margins for prostate radiotherapy. *Int J Radiat Oncol Biol Phys.* 2006;65(2):548–553.

76. Bittner N, Butler WM, Reed JL, et al. Electromagnetic tracking of intrafraction prostate displacement in patients externally immobilized in the prone position. *Int J Radiat Oncol Biol Phys;*77(2):490–495.

77. Langen KM, Zhang Y, Andrews RD, et al. Initial experience with megavoltage (MV) CT guidance for daily prostate alignments. *Int J Radiat Oncol Biol Phys.* 2005;62(5):1517–1524.

78. Wang K, Wu X, Bossart E, et al. The uncertainties in target localization for prostate and prostate-bed radiotherapy with Calypso 4D. *Int J Radiat Oncol Biol Phys.* 2009;75(3):S594.

79. Schiffner DC, Gottschalk AR, Lometti M, et al. Daily electronic portal imaging of implanted gold seed fiducials in patients undergoing radiotherapy after radical prostatectomy. *Int J Radiat Oncol Biol Phys.* 2007;67(2):610–619.

80. Chinnaiyan P, Tomee W, Patel R, et al. 3D-ultrasound guided radiation therapy in the post-prostatectomy setting. *Technol Cancer Res Treat.* 2003;2(5):455–458.

81. Nath SK, Sandhu AP, Rose BS, et al. Toxicity analysis of postoperative image-guided intensity-modulated radiotherapy for prostate cancer. *Int J Radiat Oncol Biol Phys.* 2009;78(2):435–441.

82. King CR, Kapp DS. Radiotherapy after prostatectomy: is the evidence for dose escalation out there? *Int J Radiat Oncol Biol Phys.* 2008;71(2):346–350.

83. Zelefsky MJ, Fuks Z, Hunt M, et al. High-dose intensity modulated radiation therapy for prostate cancer: early toxicity and biochemical outcome in 772 patients. *Int J Radiat Oncol Biol Phys.* 2002;53(5):1111–1116.

84. Sanda MG, Dunn RL, Michalski J, et al. Quality of life and satisfaction with outcome among prostate-cancer survivors. *New Engl J Med.* 2008;358(12):1250–1261.

85. Sandler HM, Liu P-Y, Dunn RL, et al. Reduction in patient-reported acute morbidity in prostate cancer patients treated with 81-Gy intensity-modulated radiotherapy using reduced planning target volume margins and electromagnetic tracking: assessing the impact of margin reduction study. *Urology.* 2010;75(5):1004–1008.

86. Engels B, Soete G, Verellen D, et al. Conformal arc radiotherapy for prostate cancer: increased biochemical failure in patients with distended rectum on the planning computed tomogram despite image guidance by implanted markers. *Int J Radiat Oncol Biol Phys.* 2009;74(2):388–391.

Treatment of Intermediate-Risk Prostate Cancer

John A. Kalapurakal*

Northwestern University Feinberg School of Medicine, Chicago, IL

■ ABSTRACT

This chapter will describe the clinical presentation, diagnostic work-up, and current risk-stratification for patients with prostate cancer. The modern advances in radiation therapy such as IMRT, IGRT, low- or high-dose-rate brachytherapy, and proton therapy will be discussed. The clinical basis for the treatment of these patients with either higher doses of radiation therapy or a combination of radiation therapy and androgen-suppression therapy will be described. The acute and delayed toxicities associated with these treatments and their management will also be summarized.

Keywords: prostate cancer, radiation therapy, protons, brachytherapy, androgen suppression

Prostate cancer is the most common cancer in males and the second most common cause of cancer death behind lung cancer. It is estimated that 217,730 men will be diagnosed and 32,050 men will die of prostate cancer in 2010 (1). Based on the data from 2005 to 2007, it has been estimated that approximately 16.2% or 1 in 6 men will be diagnosed with prostate cancer during their lifetime. This chapter will focus on the current role of radiation therapy in the treatment of intermediate-risk prostate cancer.

■ PROGNOSTIC CLASSIFICATION

The common prognostic factors that are considered for prostate cancer risk stratification include serum prostate-specific antigen (PSA) level, clinical tumor (T) stage and biopsy Gleason score. There are several risk-stratification schemes that have been proposed based on these factors (2,3). The most widely utilized scheme and that recommended by the National Comprehensive Cancer Network (NCCN) stratifies clinically localized prostate cancer patients into three risk groups. Low-risk group includes patients with all of the following factors: stage T1c to T2a tumors and PSA ≤ 10 ng/mL and Gleason score ≤6. Intermediate-risk group includes patients with any of the following factors: stage T2b to T2c tumors or PSA >10 but ≤20 ng/mL or Gleason score 7. High-risk group includes patients with any of the following factors: stage T3-T4 or PSA >20 ng/mL or Gleason score 8–10. The other prognostic factors that are presently being used to further refine this risk-stratification scheme include percentage of positive prostate biopsy cores and pretreatment PSA velocity (4,5).

*Corresponding author, Northwestern University Feinberg School of Medicine, Chicago, IL

E-mail address: j-kalapurakal@northwestern.edu

Radiation Medicine Rounds 2:1 (2011) 131–144.
DOI: 10.5003/2151–4208.2.1.131

■ CLINICAL PRESENTATION

The routine use of PSA screening has resulted in an increase in the overall number of prostate cancer patients diagnosed with early stage disease. The majority of patients with intermediate-risk prostate cancer are asymptomatic and present with a history of an elevated serum PSA. In symptomatic patients the complaints are mostly urinary and may include narrow urinary stream, nocturia, urgency, frequency and urinary hesitancy. It would be uncommon for these patients to present with rectal symptoms.

■ DIAGNOSTIC WORK-UP

The diagnostic work-up includes a routine history and physical examination including a digital rectal examination. The laboratory tests that may be obtained include a complete blood count, blood chemistry, serum PSA, and serum testosterone. Radiographic imaging tests for the evaluation of extent of primary disease and metastatic work up may include a CT scan of the abdomen and pelvis or preferably an MRI, and a bone scan.

CT scans were the mainstay for the primary and metastatic work-up of prostate cancer. The main disadvantage of CT scans is its lack of soft tissue resolution that is needed to detect disease within the prostate gland and seminal vesicles. CT scans rely predominantly on size criteria and is also suboptimal for detection of nodal metastasis (6,7). MRI has several advantages over CT scans including better visualization of the zonal anatomy of the prostate gland, demarcation of the prostate apex from the pelvic floor musculature, better detection of extracapsular, seminal vesicle or nodal disease extension, and localization of the neurovascular bundles (8,9). Recent advances in MRI technology such as the use of endorectal coil and MR spectroscopy have improved the diagnostic accuracy of MRI in staging prostate cancer (10,11). MRI scans are also useful for radiation treatment planning. Studies using CT-MRI fusion have shown that MRI will improve the ability of the radiation oncologist to contour the prostate gland, prostate apex, seminal vesicles, penile bulb and rectum while planning definitive radiation therapy. The use of MRI has resulted in a reduction in volume of the irradiated normal tissues and this would likely reduce the normal tissue complications following

high dose radiation therapy (12,13). MRI and MRS have also been shown to be useful in evaluating the tumor response following external beam radiation and prostate brachytherapy (14).

■ RANDOMIZED TRIALS

Several phase II trials have shown that a higher total dose of radiation therapy (78–81Gy) is associated with improved freedom from biochemical failure and acceptable toxicity in intermediate-risk prostate cancer (15–18). A summary of the randomized clinical trials that have established the modern day standard of care for intermediate-risk prostate cancer are summarized below.

Harvard Trial

A total of 206 patients with clinically localized prostate cancer were randomized to receive 70 Gy 3D-conformal radiation therapy (CRT) alone or in combination with 6 months of androgen suppression therapy (AST). Eligible patients included those with stage T1b-T2cNXM0 adenocarcinoma of the prostate with a Gleason score of at least 7 (5–10), a serum PSA of at least 10 ng/mL, and in low-risk patients MRI evidence of extraprostatic disease or seminal vesicle invasion. All patients received a total dosage of 70.35 Gy (67 Gy normalized to 95%) to the prostate plus a 1.5-cm margin using a four-field 3D-CRT technique. The initial 45 Gy was delivered to the prostate and the seminal vesicles using a 1.5-cm margin. AST consisted of a combination of a luteinizing hormone–releasing hormone (LHRH) agonist (leuprolide acetate) or goserelin and a non-steroidal anti-androgen (flutamide). After a median follow-up of 4.52 years, patients randomized to receive 3DCRT plus AST had a significantly higher survival, lower prostate cancer–specific mortality and higher survival free of salvage AST. The 5-year survival rates were 88% in the 3D-CRT plus AST group versus 78% in the 3D-CRT group (19). After a median follow-up of 7.6 years, a significant increase in the risk of all-cause mortality was observed in men randomized to radiation therapy, compared with radiation and AST. However, the increased risk in all-cause mortality appeared to apply only to men randomized to radiation therapy with no or minimal co-morbidity (20).

MD Anderson Trial

A total of 305 Stage T1–T3 patients were randomized to receive either 70 Gy or 78 Gy to the prostate gland. A conventional four-field box was used for the initial 46 Gy in all patients. Dose was specified to the isocenter and was delivered at 2 Gy per fraction per day. The anterior-posterior fields were typically 11 × 11 cm and the laterals were 11 × 9 cm. After 46 Gy, the two treatment groups received a 3D-CRT boost of 24 Gy using a four-field technique in the 70 Gy arm and a 32 Gy boost using a six field technique in the 78 Gy arm, respectively. The freedom from biochemical failure rates for the 70 and 78 Gy arms at 6 years were 64% and 70%, respectively ($P = .03$). Dose escalation to 78 Gy preferentially benefited those with a pretreatment PSA >10 ng/mL; the biochemical control rates were 62% for the 78 Gy arm versus 43% for those who received 70 Gy ($P = .01$). For patients with a pretreatment PSA <10 ng/mL, no significant dosage response was found, with an average 6-year biochemical control rate of about 75%. Rectal side effects were also significantly greater in the 78 Gy group. Grade 2 or higher toxicity rates at 6 years were 12% and 26% for the 70 Gy and 78 Gy arms, respectively ($P = .001$). Grade 2 or higher bladder complications were similar at 10%. For patients in the 78 Gy arm, grade 2 or higher rectal toxicity correlated highly with the proportion of the rectum treated to >70 Gy (21,22). After a median follow-up of 9 years, patients with pretreatment PSA >10 ng/mL or high-risk disease who were treated to 70 Gy continued to have a higher biochemical and clinical failures rate and a higher risk of dying of prostate cancer compared to the higher dose arm (23).

Proton Radiation Oncology Group (PROG) 95–09

Three hundred and ninety three patients with stage T1b through T2b prostate cancer and PSA levels <15 ng/mL were randomized to receive external beam radiation to a total dose of either 70.2 Gy (conventional dose) or 79.2 Gy (high dose). This was delivered using a combination of conformal photon and protons. The initial 50.4 Gy was delivered to the prostate gland and seminal vesicles, with a 10 mm margin, using a conformal four-field technique with 10 to 23 MV X-rays. The conformal prostate boost was delivered with protons to a clinical target volume

that included the prostate gland with a 5 mm margin, with an additional 7 to 10 mm being added for a planning target volume. The boost dose was either 19.8 GyE or 28.8 GyE in 11or 16 fractions (1.8-GyE fractions). After a median follow-up was 5.5 years, the 5-year freedom from biochemical failure rate was 61.4% for conventional dose and 80.4% for high-dose therapy ($P = .001$). The advantage to high-dose therapy was observed in both the low-risk and the higher-risk subgroups. There was no difference in overall survival rates between the treatment groups. The acute and late RTOG grade 3 or higher morbidity rates ranged from 1% to 2% and were similar in the two groups at 1% to 2% (24). After a median follow-up was 8.9 years, the 10-year biochemical failure rates were 32.4% for 70.2 Gy and 16.7% for the 79.2 Gy arm ($P = .0001$). This difference held when only those with low-risk disease ($n = 227$; 58% of total) were examined: 28.2% for conventional and 7.1% for high dose ($P = .0001$). There was a strong trend in the same direction for the intermediate-risk patients ($n = 144$; 37% of total; 42.1% vs. 30.4%, $P = .06$). There remained no difference in overall survival and toxicity rates between the two treatment arms (25). After a median follow up of 9.4 years, the use of higher dose radiation was not associated with an increase in patient-reported prostate cancer symptoms (26).

Dutch Trial

Six hundred and sixty nine patients with stage T1b-4 prostate cancer patients were enrolled onto a multicenter randomized trial comparing 68 Gy and 78 Gy delivered with 3D-CRT. Patients were stratified by institution, age, (neo)adjuvant hormonal therapy (HT), and treatment group. The planning target volume (PTV) for radiation included the prostate with or without the SV with a margin of 10 mm during the first 68 Gy and 5 mm (except towards the rectum, 0 mm) for the last 10 Gy in the high-dose arm. Neo-adjuvant hormone therapy was prescribed in two institutions, predominantly to high-risk patients. After a median follow-up of 51 months, the freedom from biochemical failure was significantly better in the 78-Gy arm compared with the 68-Gy arm: 64% versus 54%, respectively ($P = .02$). There was no significant difference in overall survival between the treatment arms. There was no difference in late grade 2 or more genitourinary toxicity in the two arms. There was a slightly higher non-significant incidence of late gastrointestinal toxicity of grade 2 or more in the 78 Gy arm (27). After a median follow-up of 70 months, the 7-year biochemical control rates were still significantly better in the 78-Gy arm than in the 68-Gy arm (56% versus 45%, P = .03). However, the cumulative incidence of late Grade 2 or greater gastrointestinal toxicity was increased in the 78-Gy arm compared with the 68-Gy arm (35% versus 25% at 7 years; P = .04) (28,29).

MRC R01 Trial

The MRC RT01 trial is the largest randomized radiation dose-escalation trial and is the only one to study the effects of neo-adjuvant AST for 3 to 6 months for low-risk, intermediate and high-risk patients. Eight hundred and forty three men with stage T1b-T3a, N0, M0 prostate cancer, with serum PSA of <50 ng/mL were randomized to receive either 64 Gy in 32 fractions (standard group) or 74 Gy in 37 fractions (escalated group). The gross tumor volume for all patients included the prostate gland and the base of the seminal vesicles for low-risk patients, and all of the seminal vesicles for medium-to-high-risk patients. The clinical target volume added a 0.5 cm margin and the PTV added another 0.5 to 1 cm margin to the gross tumor volume. At the time of analysis, median follow-up was 63 months. The biochemical progression free survival rate was significantly higher in the 74 Gy arm (71%) compared to the 64 Gy arm (60%). There was no difference in the local control rate or overall survival. Similar improvement in biochemical control rates were observed with dose escalated treatment in the low, intermediate and high-risk patients. The biochemical progression free survival at 5 years for the standard and escalated groups were 79% and 85% in the low-risk group, 70% and 79% in the intermediate-risk group, and 43% and 57% in the high-risk group, respectively. There was an increased incidence of late gastrointestinal toxicity in the 74 Gy arm. Late genitourinary toxicity was also slightly increased in the escalated group (30).

Trans-Tasman Trial (TROG 96.01)

Eight hundred and eighteen men with clinical stage T2b, T2c, T3, or T4 N0M0 adenocarcinoma of the prostate were randomly assigned to: no AST (radiotherapy alone: 66 Gy in 33 fractions of 2 Gy per day

to the prostate and seminal vesicles); 3 months of AST with 3 to 6 mg goserelin given subcutaneously every month and 250 mg flutamide given orally three times a day starting 2 months before radiotherapy (66 Gy in 33 fractions); or 6 months of AST, with the same regimen, starting 5 months before radiotherapy (66Gy in 33 fractions). Median follow-up was 5.9 years (range 0.1–8.5). Compared with patients assigned no androgen deprivation, those assigned 3 months treatment had significantly improved local control (P = .001), biochemical failure-free survival (P = .002), disease-free survival (P = .0001), and freedom from salvage treatment (P = .025). Six months of androgen deprivation significantly improved local failure (P = .0001), biochemical failure-free survival (P = .0001), disease-free survival (P = .0001), freedom from salvage treatment (P = .0001), distant failure (P = .046) and prostate-cancer-specific survival (P = .04) compared with no androgen deprivation. This study demonstrated that six months of androgen deprivation with radiation therapy improves outcomes in patients with locally advanced prostate cancer (31).

Canadian Trial

Three hundred and seventy eight patients were randomized to either 3 or 8 months of AST with flutamide and goserelin, before conventional-dose RT (66 Gy), for clinically localized prostate cancer. Among these patients, 26% were low risk, 43% were intermediate risk and 31% were high risk. The median follow-up was 44 months. The freedom from biochemical failure rate for the 3-month versus 8-month arms was 66% versus 68% at 3 years, and by 5 years was 61% versus 62% respectively (P = .36). There was no significant difference in the biochemical, local and distant metastasis rates between the two arms. In the 8-month arm high-risk patients had a non-significant improvement in disease-free survival (39% versus 52%) (32). After a median follow-up of 6.6 years there was no difference in the 5-year rate of freedom from any failure for the 3-month arm versus the 8-month arm (72% versus 75%) (33).

Ontario Clinical Oncology Group

In a randomized trial from Ontario, 51 patients were randomly assigned to receive interstitial Iridium implant plus radiation therapy, and 53 patients were randomly assigned to receive radiation therapy alone in stage T2 and T3 prostate cancer. All patients underwent a staging lymphadenectomy initially. Patients in the combined modality arm received Iridium implant (35 Gy) followed by radiation therapy to 40 Gy in 20 fractions. Patients in the external radiation therapy only group received 66 Gy in 33 fractions to the prostate gland and seminal vesicles. After a median follow-up was 8.2 years, the biochemical control rate in the implant plus radiation therapy was significantly higher than radiation therapy alone (71% versus 39%). There was no difference in the overall survival rate between the two arms (34).

Modern Advances in External Beam Radiation Therapy and Brachytherapy

The retrospective and prospective clinical trials described above have shown that a higher dose of radiation therapy between 75 and 79 Gy is recommended for most patients with intermediate-risk prostate cancer. A number advances in the field of radiation oncology such as the use of IMRT, proton therapy and IGRT have enabled the safer delivery of such higher doses of radiation, thus increasing the likelihood of cure with lower rates of radiation-induced toxicity.

IMRT has been in clinical use since the mid 1990s. IMRT uses inverse treatment planning techniques and uses multiple photon beams with non-uniform intensity to achieve a very conformal dose distribution around the prostate gland with superior sparing of the urinary bladder and rectum. Presently IMRT is used in most centers in the US for the treatment of prostate cancer (18,35–37).

There has been a renewed interest in the use of proton therapy for prostate cancer with many new proton centers opening across the country. The main advantage of protons over photons: its unique physical depth-dose profile that results a low entrance dose, peak dose deposition at the end of its trajectory at the Bragg peak with no exit dose. The proton energy and the spread-out Bragg peak (SOBP) are selected to uniformly treat the prostate gland resulting in a homogeneous dose distribution within the target and a sharp dose falloff beyond the target (38). The use of pencil beam scanning and Intensity modulated proton therapy (IMPT) may provide further advantages over scattered proton beams. However, there are many

problems associated with protons. The presence of tissue heterogeneity such as the presence of bone, variable filling of bladder and rectum can cause uncertainties in the range of protons in tissues that can result in over or under-treatment of normal tissues (39). Proton beams also have a significant penumbra at depth compromising their ability to spare adjacent tissues (40). In a dosimetric comparison of IMRT with proton beam therapy, IMRT resulted in better dose conformity to the prostate and better sparing of the urinary bladder at a higher dose range, while protons achieved higher dose homogeneity and better sparing of the rectum and bladder at the low dose range. Proton therapy also resulted in a significantly lower total-body dose while IMRT resulted in irradiation of a larger volume of normal tissues to low doses (41). Another area of considerable controversy is the cost-effectiveness of proton therapy compared to IMRT (42).

Image Guided Radiation Therapy (IGRT) refers to the use of daily imaging of the prostate gland to enable both accurate and precise radiation therapy delivery to the target tissues thereby increasing the likelihood of tumor control and reducing the risk of complications. Daily external rigid immobilization of the pelvis and legs has been shown to reduce overall set up errors (43,44). A number of studies have shown that there could be significant movement and deformation of the prostate gland based on the volume changes of the rectum and bladder. The range of inter-fractional movement of the prostate gland is most pronounced in the antero-posterior (±1.5–1.7 cm) and supero-inferior axes (±1–1.6 cm) compared to the right-left axis (±2–6 mm) (45–47). Intra-fractional movement of the prostate gland due to respiratory movement, bladder filling or transit of gas through the rectum has also been reported of up to 3 to 5 mm in the antero-posterior axis (48,49). IGRT is designed to optimize accuracy of treatment and minimize uncertainties due to patient or target motion. The currently available IGRT systems include kV radiographs on implanted fiducial markers, kV or MV tomography, Cone beam CT (CBCT), trans-abdominal ultrasound, implantable sensors and optical imaging (50–52).

Unlike most cancers, it is estimated that prostate cancer cells may have a low alpha/beta ratio (1–2 Gy). The alpha/beta ratio for rectal damage is estimated to be around 4 to 6 Gy. The higher alpha/beta ratio for the rectum compared to the prostate gland would suggest that hypofractionated treatment regiments would result in larger clinical gains without any increase in late toxicity (53,54). This is the basis of many hypofractionated regimens that are currently being studied in the treatment of early and intermediate-risk prostate cancer. The most widely reported regimen from the Cleveland Clinic delivered 70 Gy in 28 fractions using IMRT in 770 patients. With a median follow-up of 45 months, the results were excellent with biochemical control rates of 94% in low-risk, 83% with intermediate-risk and 72% with high-risk disease. There was no increase in acute or late gastrointestinal or genitourinary toxicity (55). Preliminary reports following the use of Stereotactic Body Radiotherapy (SBRT) that delivers the total dose 33 to 36 Gy in approximately five fractions are encouraging. However further follow-up is required to establish its safety and efficacy. The main advantage of hypofractionated and SBRT regimens is the significant reduction in cost and overall treatment time (56).

In modern day practice, the incorporation of all of these novel technologic innovations, including IGRT with IMRT or protons and better prostate target definition with CT-MRI fusion, will enable the safe delivery of dose-escalated radiation therapy for intermediate-risk prostate cancer.

External Beam Radiation Therapy Localization, Simulation, and Immobilization

All patients should have a CT simulation with or without intravenous contrast. If MRI scans were preformed they could be registered with the CT images to facilitate accurate target definition. A urethrogram may aid in the definition of the prostate gland apex. Typically, patients are positioned in a supine position with an external immobilization cast. CT images should be acquired at 2 to 3 mm slice thickness.

Whole Pelvis Irradiation

The actual incidence of lymph node metastasis and the location of the lymphatic drainage sites from prostate cancer is not yet well defined. Compared to the incidence rates observed after standard pelvic node dissection, a significantly higher incidence of pelvic lymph node metastasis has been reported after extended pelvic lymph node dissection. These nodes are often found in the internal iliac and presacral nodes that are not explored during standard node dissection (57,58). In a report using

SPECT after injection of technetium nanocolloid the most common sites of sentinel nodes were the external iliac 34%, followed by internal iliac 18%, common iliac 13%, sacral 9%, perirectal 6%, and 5% each in the right and left para-aortic nodes. Among these patients 66% had sentinel node locations that would not have been treated adequately with conventional pelvic radiation therapy portals. The lymph node regions associated with the highest probability of a geographic miss were the ventral external iliac, perirectal, para-aortic and sacral lymph nodes (59). Presently, the risk for lymph node metastases is estimated by using the Roach formula and those with a risk of >15% receive whole pelvis irradiation. It should be noted that as the Roach formula does not incorporate T stage, patients with T2c-T4 tumors with a Gleason score of ≥6 may also receive whole pelvis irradiation even if their risk of lymph node metastasis was <15%. The RTOG 94–13 trial showed that irradiation of the pelvic lymph nodes results in improvement in progression-free survival in patients with >15% risk of lymph node involvement (60). Whole pelvis irradiation (45–50 Gy in 25–28 fractions) may be delivered using the standard four-field technique with 3D conformal irradiation or by using IMRT. The use of pelvic nodal IMRT has been shown to improve the dose to the pelvic nodal groups while reducing the dose to the normal tissues like urinary bladder and rectum (61).

Brachytherapy Boost

The excellent biochemical control rates and minimal toxicity associated with modern prostate brachytherapy using I-125 or Pd-103seeds has resulted in a dramatic increase in the use of this technique for patients with early and intermediate-risk prostate cancer (3,62). In addition to delivering a high dose of radiation directly in the tumor with good conformality, there is no effect of inter or intrafraction prostate movement or set up errors on generating the PTV. Thus minimal margins may be used with better protection of normal tissues. The technical advances in brachytherapy such as the use of transrectal ultrasound for treatment planning, template-based transperineal implantation and the routine use of CT-based post-implant dosimetry have largely been responsible for the excellent results associated with this treatment technique.

In patients with intermediate-risk prostate cancer, prostate brachytherapy is used in conjunction with external beam irradiation. Typically a dose of 45 Gy is delivered to the pelvis and this is followed by a I-125 or Pd-103 boost with prostate brachytherapy (63). In a report from the Seattle Prostate Institute, 223 patients with clinically localized (stage T1-T3) prostate cancer were treated with I-125 or Pd-103 brachytherapy at a median interval of 4 weeks after 45-Gy neoadjuvant EBRT that included the prostate gland and seminal vesicles. The dose for Pd-103 boost was 100 Gy (NIST 99) and the I-125 boost dose was 108 Gy (TG-43).The majority of these patients had intermediate-risk prostate cancer. The Fifteen-year biochemical relapse free survival for low-risk, intermediate-risk and high-risk patients was 88%, 80%, and 53%, respectively (62).

High Dose Rate (HDR) Brachytherapy Boost

The advantages to HDR brachytherapy include elimination of radiation exposure to personnel and family members, shorter treatment times and superior radiation dose distribution and optimization by varying the source dwell times at various dwell positions within the target volume. From a radiobiologic perspective, the low alpha/beta ratio for prostate cancer will favor a superior response with higher dose per fraction. The higher alpha/beta ratio of the rectum and the use of higher dose/fraction will also increase the therapeutic window and limit the rectal toxicity from large dose per fraction in terms of cancer (53,54). A variety of dose-fractionation schemes have been used with HDR brachytherapy in conjunction with external beam radiation therapy for intermediate-risk prostate cancer (64,65). Long-term data from the California Endocurietherapy Cancer Center have shown excellent biochemical progression free survival of 90%, 87%, and 69% for the low-, intermediate-, and high-risk patients, respectively, at 10 years following external beam RT (36 Gy) and ^{192}Ir HDR brachytherapy with (22–24 Gy in four fractions) (64). A prospective dose-escalation study in intermediate and high-risk prostate cancer from William Beaumont Hospital showed significantly superior biochemical control and overall survival in the high dose HDR group (8.75 Gy × 2 to 11.5 Gy × 2) compared to the low-dose HDR (5.5Gy × 3 to 8.25Gy × 2) group. All of these patients received pelvic radiation to 46 Gy (65).

Radiation Therapy Dose-Prescription Guidelines

Most institutions have varying criteria to define target volumes, margins for treatment planning, and dose-volume normal tissue constraints for 3D conformal EBRT, IMRT or proton therapy. RTOG 0815 is a currently open prospective randomized trial of dose escalated radiation therapy, with or without short-term AST, in intermediate-risk prostate cancer. The external beam and brachytherapy dose prescription guidelines used in this protocol represents a consensus of most radiation oncologists and will be described below.

External Beam Radiation Therapy

RTOG 0815 recommends a dose of 79.2 Gy in 1.8 Gy fractions on this protocol. The Gross Tumor Volume (GTV) is defined by the planning CT, urethrogram, and clinical information. If a urethrogram is used, the GTV should encompass a volume inferiorly 5 mm superior to the tip of the dye. The Clinical Target Volume (CTV) is defined as the prostate gland plus areas at risk for microscopic disease extension plus the proximal 1 cm of bilateral seminal vesicles. The PTV should provide a margin ranging from 5 to 10 mm around the CTV to compensate for the variability of treatment set up and internal organ motion. The ICRU Reference Point is in the central part of the PTV typically located at the intersection of the beam axes. The dose should be normalized such that exactly 98% of the PTV receives the prescription dose. The minimum and maximum range of dose within the PTV is >95 to 107%. The urinary bladder maximum dose constraints for 15%, 25%, 35% and 50% of its volume are 80 Gy, 75 Gy, 70 Gy, and 65 Gy, respectively. The rectum maximum dose constraints for 15%, 25%, 35%, and 50% of its volume are 75 Gy, 70 Gy, 65 Gy, and 60 Gy, respectively. A dose reduction to 75.6 Gy minimum PTV dose is permitted if the above constraints cannot be met at the planned dose level of 79.2 Gy.

Low Dose Rate Permanent Seed Brachytherapy

There are certain specific selection criteria for patients undergoing permanent seed brachytherapy. They include a prostate volume of 50 to 55 mL on transrectal ultrasound (TRUS) volume study, AUA score of <15. Patients with a history of TURP, catheter dependence are not suitable candidates for brachytherapy given their higher rates of complications. The implant may be performed under either general or spinal anesthesia. Treatment planning may be performed preoperatively or intra-operatively using TRUS. The prostate volume is defined from base to apex in the axial plane at 5 mm slice intervals. The CTV is defined as the prostate gland only. For the PTV a margin of 2 to 3 mm is added anteriorly and laterally, 5 mm margin inferiorly and no margin is given posteriorly. Iodine-125 or Palladium-103 seeds may be used. For I-125, the allowable source strength for each seed is 0.277 U to 0.650 U (NIST 99 or later). For Pd-103 sources, this range is 1.29 U to 2.61 U (NIST 99 or later). The prescription dose for permanent seed interstitial boost will be 110 Gy for I-125 and 100 Gy for Pd-103. Doses should be prescribed as minimal peripheral dose to the PTV. Post-implant Imaging with a pelvic CT scan for post-implant dosimetry should be obtained following implant completion. DVH based D90 for prostate gland should be approximately >80 to 90% of the prescription dose but less than 130% of the prescription dose.

HDR Brachytherapy

The same patient selection criteria for low dose permanent seed brachytherapy described above should be used for HDR brachytherapy also. The implant may be performed during the EBRT portion of the treatment or within 1 week prior to its initiation or following its completion. All implants are performed under transrectal ultrasound guidance. Epidural, spinal, or general anesthesia may be used. At least 14 treatment catheters should be used to ensure adequate target coverage with acceptable dose heterogeneity. Fiducial markers identifying the prostatic base and apex should be placed at the time of the implant. Intra-operative cystoscopy should be used to ensure the absence of treatment catheters within the urethra or bladder and to confirm adequate coverage at the prostatic base. Two treatment fractions with a minimum inter-fraction interval of 6 hours may be delivered within a single 24-hour period. Implant dosimetry is performed using a planning CT scan with a Foley catheter in place. The CTV is the prostate gland plus any visualized extracapsular extension of the tumor. The PTV is equivalent to the CTV. A dwell time optimization program based on implant geometry or an inverse planning algorithm may be used. Manual optimization may also be used. The prescription dose of 21 Gy is to be delivered to the PTV in two equal fractions of 10.5 Gy. Ninety-five percent coverage of the PTV with the prescription dose is considered per protocol, ≥90% but <95% is considered acceptable. Attempts should be made to limit the volume of urethra receiving ≥115% of the prescription dose to ≤5%. The dose at the anterior rectal wall should not exceed 75% of the prescription dose. The volume of bladder and rectum receiving 75% of the prescription dose must be kept to less than 1 mL and the volume of urethra receiving 125% of the prescription dose must be kept to less than 1 mL.

Toxicity of Radiation Therapy and Hormone Therapy

Radiation therapy is well tolerated by most patients. The complication rates depend on a number of factors that may include among others prior TURP, presence of obstructive urinary symptoms, anticoagulant use, history of inflammatory bowel disease, total radiation dose and radiation field size. A significant proportion may have acute irritative urinary or rectal symptoms such as urinary frequency, urgency, nocturia, diarrhea and tenesmus that typically begin about 2 to 3 weeks into treatment. These symptoms are usually well controlled with supportive care, alpha blockers, loperamide and steroid suppositories and they disappear a few weeks after completing therapy. The late urinary (urethral strictures, bleeding) and rectal (bleeding, ulcers, incontinence) complications typically appear 1 to 3 years after completing therapy. The management of these late complications may include among others urethral dilatation, argon plasma laser coagulation, formalin therapy and hyperbaric oxygen (66,67). In a report from RTOG 7506 and 7706 with over a thousand patients followed for a minimum of 7 years, the incidence of ≥ grade 3 bowel complications was 3.3% with 0.6% of patients experiencing bowel obstruction or perforation. Grade 3 or more urinary complications were seen in 7.7% of patients with only 0.5% experiencing toxicity that would require a major surgical intervention (68). RTOG 9406 was a 3D-CRT dose escalation trial of five dose levels from 68.4 to 79.2Gy that accrued over a thousand patients. The primary endpoint was the development of grade 3 or greater GI or GU toxicity. Elective pelvic nodal irradiation was not allowed. Group 1 patients had no elective seminal vesicle irradiation. Group 2 patients received treatment initially to the PTV1 that encompassed the prostate and seminal vesicles (54–55.8Gy) followed by a boost that excluded the seminal vesicles. Because of the low rates of grade 3 toxicity, the rates of grade 2 or greater toxicity was analyzed. The grade 2 or greater GI toxicity rates were 9%, 7%, 11%, 10%, and 25% for group 1 and 13%, 9%, 14%, 16%, and 26% for group 2 at dose levels I through V. The incidence rates of grade 2 or greater GU toxicity were 24%, 22%, 18%, 29%, and 23% for group 1 and 19%, 16%, 21%, 21%, and 28% for group 2. There was significantly more grade 2 or greater toxicity with a dose of 78 Gy at 2 Gy/fraction. Compared to earlier non-conformal therapy trials, this trial showed that there was a significant reduction in grade 3 or greater toxicity, despite radiation doses that were more than 10 Gy higher (69). The use of IMRT has resulted in a significant reduction in grade 2 and grade 3 urinary and rectal complications in spite of delivering equivalent or higher doses. In a report from Memorial Sloan Kettering Cancer Center, among 561 patients treated with IMRT to 81 Gy, the 8-year likelihood of developing grade 2 and grade 3 rectal bleeding was 1.6% and 0.1%. The 8-year grade 2 or 3 urinary toxicity rates were 9% and 3% respectively (18). The impotence rates after external beam radiation therapy range from 35% to 70% (70). The use of drugs like sildenafil improved erectile function in >70% of patients (71).

The most common symptoms after prostate brachytherapy are urinary obstructive symptoms due to the swelling of the prostate gland caused by procedure-related bleeding and radiation from the seeds. These symptoms peak around 1 to 4 months after brachytherapy and improve thereafter depending on the half-life of the isotope used. Most patients are placed on alpha-blockers which is effective in the vast majority of patients. The risk of acute urinary retention ranges from 5% to 15%. Patients with high urinary symptom scores and larger prostate volumes are more likely to have urinary retention (72). Urethral strictures may be seen in 2% to 12% of patients following prostate brachytherapy. Grade 2 rectal toxicity may be observed in 2% to 10% of patients. The incidence of other grade 3–4 urinary or rectal toxicity is <2% (73,74). The impotence rates after brachytherapy range are believed to lower compared to external beam radiation therapy and range

from 40% to 50%. Approximately 80% of patients with post-brachytherapy impotence respond to sildenafil citrate (75). Urinary incontinence is rare after brachytherapy except in patients with a prior history of a TURP (76).

The most common side effects following androgen suppression therapy include fatigue, hot flashes, osteoporosis, weight gain, loss of libido, gynecomastia, erectile dysfunction and anemia. The other side effects include loss of muscle mass, reduction in penile and testicular size, hyperlipidemia, hyperglycemia, cardiac events such as myocardial infarction, coronary artery disease, sudden cardiac death, deep vein thrombosis and depression (77–79). Patients on androgen suppression therapy should be counseled about these adverse events and discussions with the patient's internist or cardiologist regarding periodic monitoring of the blood sugar, lipids, liver enzymes, hypertension and other risk factors is very important. Supplemental vitamin D and calcium, a healthy diet and exercise regimen is beneficial for these patients. In spite of these significant risks, long-term data from randomized trials have not shown an increase in cardiovascular mortality rates among patients receiving short-term (4–6 months) or long-term (2–3 years) AST with radiation therapy (80–83).

■ CONCLUSIONS

Based on the available data patients with intermediate-risk prostate cancer may be treated with any of the following options: 1) Radical prostatectomy with adjuvant radiation therapy in high-risk patients. 2) External beam radiation therapy alone (daily IGRT with 3D conformal or IMRT) to total doses of 78–80 Gy. 3) Short-term AST (4–6 months) with external beam radiation therapy (daily IGRT with 3D conformal or IMRT) to total doses of 70–76 Gy. 4) External beam radiation therapy (45 Gy) followed by a) permanent seed brachytherapy boost with I-125 (110 Gy) or Pd-103 (100 Gy) or b) high dose rate brachytherapy boost (10.5 Gy × 2fractions). AST may be added in these patients.

RTOG 0126 will compare clinical outcomes after 70.2 Gy versus 79.2 Gy in patients with intermediate-risk prostate cancer. The EORTC trial 22991 will evaluate the addition of concomitant and adjuvant short-term AST to radiation therapy for patients with intermediate-risk prostate cancer. Both of these trials have been completed and their results will clarify the role of higher radiation doses and the addition of androgen suppression to radiation therapy in patients with intermediate-risk prostate cancer. The use of daily IGRT with IMRT or proton therapy will be very helpful in improving cure rates and reducing acute and late toxicities following the delivery of higher doses of radiation in these patients.

■ REFERENCES

1. Jemal A, Siegel R, Xu J, Ward E. Cancer statistics, 2010. *CA Cancer J Clin.* 2010;60(5):277–300.

2. D'Amico AV, Moul J, Carroll PR, Sun L, Lubeck D, Chen MH. Cancer-specific mortality after surgery or radiation for patients with clinically localized prostate cancer managed during the prostate-specific antigen era. *J Clin Oncol.* 2003;21(11):2163–2172.

3. Sylvester JE, Blasko JC, Grimm PD, Meier R, Malmgren JA. Ten-year biochemical relapse-free survival after external beam radiation and brachytherapy for localized prostate cancer: the Seattle experience. *Int J Radiat Oncol Biol Phys.* 2003;57(4):944–952.

4. D'Amico AV, Renshaw AA, Sussman B, Chen MH. Pretreatment PSA velocity and risk of death from prostate cancer following external beam radiation therapy. *JAMA.* 2005;294(4):440–447.

5. D'Amico AV, Schultz D, Silver B, et al. The clinical utility of the percent of positive prostate biopsies in predicting biochemical outcome following external-beam radiation therapy for patients with clinically localized prostate cancer. *Int J Radiat Oncol Biol Phys.* 2001;49(3):679–684.

6. Engeler CE, Wasserman NF, Zhang G. Preoperative assessment of prostatic carcinoma by computerized tomography. Weaknesses and new perspectives. *Urology.* 1992;40(4):346–350.

7. Flanigan RC, McKay TC, Olson M, Shankey TV, Pyle J, Waters WB. Limited efficacy of preoperative computed tomographic scanning for the evaluation of lymph node metastasis in patients before radical prostatectomy. *Urology.* 1996;48(3):428–432.

8. Wang L, Mullerad M, Chen HN, et al. Prostate cancer: incremental value of endorectal MR imaging findings for prediction of extracapsular extension. *Radiology.* 2004;232(1):133–139.

9. Cornud F, Flam T, Chauveinc L, et al. Extraprostatic spread of clinically localized prostate cancer: factors predictive of pT3 tumor and of positive endorectal MR imaging examination results. *Radiology.* 2002;224(1):203–210.

10. Scheidler J, Hricak H, Vigneron DB, et al. Prostate cancer: localization with three-dimensional proton MR spectroscopic imaging–clinicopathologic study. *Radiology.* 1999;213(2):473–480.

11. Yu KK, Scheidler J, Hricak H, et al. Prostate cancer: prediction of extracapsular extension with endorectal MR imaging and three-dimensional proton MR spectroscopic imaging. *Radiology.* 1999;213(2):481–488.

12. Kagawa K, Lee WR, Schultheiss TE, Hunt MA, Shaer AH, Hanks GE. Initial clinical assessment of CT-MRI image fusion software in localization of the prostate for 3D conformal radiation therapy. *Int J Radiat Oncol Biol Phys.* 1997;38(2):319–325.

13. Roach M 3rd, Faillace-Akazawa P, Malfatti C, Holland J, Hricak H. Prostate volumes defined by magnetic resonance imaging and computerized tomographic scans for three-dimensional conformal radiotherapy. *Int J Radiat Oncol Biol Phys.* 1996;35(5):1011–1018.

14. Pickett B, Kurhanewicz J, Coakley F, Shinohara K, Fein B, Roach M 3rd. Use of MRI and spectroscopy in evaluation of external beam radiotherapy for prostate cancer. *Int J Radiat Oncol Biol Phys.* 2004;60(4):1047–1055.

15. Michalski JM, Purdy JA, Winter K, et al. Preliminary report of toxicity following 3D radiation therapy for prostate cancer on 3DOG/RTOG 9406. *Int J Radiat Oncol Biol Phys.* 2000;46(2):391–402.

16. Leibel SA, Heimann R, Kutcher GJ, et al. Three-dimensional conformal radiation therapy in locally advanced carcinoma of the prostate: preliminary results of a phase I dose-escalation study. *Int J Radiat Oncol Biol Phys.* 1994;28(1):55–65.

17. Hanks GE, Schultheiss TE, Hanlon AL, et al. Optimization of conformal radiation treatment of prostate cancer: report of a dose escalation study. *Int J Radiat Oncol Biol Phys.* 1997;37(3):543–550.

18. Zelefsky MJ, Chan H, Hunt M, Yamada Y, Shippy AM, Amols H. Long-term outcome of high dose intensity modulated radiation therapy for patients with clinically localized prostate cancer. *J Urol.* 2006;176(4 Pt 1):1415–1419.

19. D'Amico AV, Manola J, Loffredo M, Renshaw AA, DellaCroce A, Kantoff PW. 6-month androgen suppression plus radiation therapy vs radiation therapy alone for patients with clinically localized prostate cancer: a randomized controlled trial. *JAMA.* 2004;292(7):821–827.

20. D'Amico AV, Chen MH, Renshaw AA, Loffredo M, Kantoff PW. Androgen suppression and radiation vs radiation alone for prostate cancer: a randomized trial. *JAMA.* 2008;299(3):289–295.

21. Pollack A, Zagars GK, Smith LG, et al. Preliminary results of a randomized radiotherapy dose-escalation study comparing 70 Gy with 78 Gy for prostate cancer. *J Clin Oncol.* 2000;18(23):3904–3911.

22. Pollack A, Zagars GK, Starkschall G, et al. Prostate cancer radiation dose response: results of the M. D. Anderson phase III randomized trial. *Int J Radiat Oncol Biol Phys.* 2002;53(5):1097–1105.

23 Kuban DA, Levy LB, Cheung MR et al. Long-term failure patterns and survival in a randomized dose-escalation trial for prostate cancer. Who dies of disease? *Int J Radiat Oncol Biol Phys.* 2010. Epub ahead of print.

24. Zietman AL, DeSilvio ML, Slater JD, et al. Comparison of conventional-dose vs high-dose conformal radiation therapy in clinically localized adenocarcinoma of the prostate: a randomized controlled trial. *JAMA.* 2005;294(10):1233–1239.

25. Zietman AL, Bae K, Slater JD, et al. Randomized trial comparing conventional-dose with high-dose conformal radiation therapy in early-stage adenocarcinoma of the prostate: long-term results from proton radiation oncology group/american college of radiology 95–09. *J Clin Oncol.* 2010;28(7):1106–1111.

26. Talcott JA, Rossi C, Shipley WU, et al. Patient-reported long-term outcomes after conventional and high-dose combined proton and photon radiation for early prostate cancer. *JAMA.* 2010;303(11):1046–1053.

27. Peeters ST, Heemsbergen WD, Koper PC, et al. Dose-response in radiotherapy for localized prostate cancer: results of the Dutch multicenter randomized phase III trial comparing 68 Gy of radiotherapy with 78 Gy. *J Clin Oncol.* 2006;24(13):1990–1996.

28. Al-Mamgani A, van Putten WL, Heemsbergen WD, et al. Update of Dutch multicenter dose-escalation trial of radiotherapy for localized prostate cancer. *Int J Radiat Oncol Biol Phys.* 2008;72(4):980–988.

29 Al-Mamgani, van Putten WLJ, van der Wielen GJ et al. Dose escalation and quality of life in patients with localized prostate cancer treated with radiotherapy: Long-term results of the Dutch randomized dose-escalation trial (CKTO 96–10 trial). *Int J Radiat Oncol Biol Phys.* 2011;79(4):1004–1012.

30. Dearnaley DP, Sydes MR, Graham JD, et al. Escalated-dose versus standard-dose conformal radiotherapy in prostate cancer: first results from the MRC RT01 randomised controlled trial. *Lancet Oncol.* 2007;8(6):475–487.

31. Denham JW, Steigler A, Lamb DS, et al. Short-term androgen deprivation and radiotherapy for locally advanced prostate cancer: results from the Trans-Tasman Radiation Oncology Group 96.01 randomised controlled trial. *Lancet Oncol.* 2005;6(11):841–850.

32. Crook J, Ludgate C, Malone S, et al. Report of a multicenter Canadian phase III randomized trial of 3 months vs. 8 months neoadjuvant androgen deprivation before standard-dose radiotherapy for clinically localized prostate cancer. *Int J Radiat Oncol Biol Phys.* 2004;60(1):15–23.

33. Crook J, Ludgate C, Malone S, et al. Final report of multicenter Canadian Phase III randomized trial of 3 versus 8 months of neoadjuvant androgen deprivation therapy before conventional-dose radiotherapy for clinically localized prostate cancer. *Int J Radiat Oncol Biol Phys.* 2009;73(2):327–333.

34. Sathya JR, Davis IR, Julian JA, et al. Randomized trial comparing iridium implant plus external-beam radiation therapy with external-beam radiation therapy alone in node-negative locally advanced cancer of the prostate. *J Clin Oncol.* 2005;23(6):1192–1199.

35. Burman C, Chui CS, Kutcher G, et al. Planning, delivery, and quality assurance of intensity-modulated radiotherapy using dynamic multileaf collimator: a strategy for large-scale implementation for the treatment of carcinoma of the prostate. *Int J Radiat Oncol Biol Phys.* 1997;39(4):863–873.

36. Price RA, Hanks GE, McNeeley SW, Horwitz EM, Pinover WH. Advantages of using noncoplanar vs. axial beam arrangements when treating prostate cancer with intensity-modulated radiation therapy and the step-and-shoot delivery method. *Int J Radiat Oncol Biol Phys.* 2002;53(1):236–243.

37. Spirou SV, Chui CS. A gradient inverse planning algorithm with dose-volume constraints. *Med Phys.* 1998;25(3):321–333.

38. WILSON RR. Radiological use of fast protons. *Radiology.* 1946;47(5):487–491.

39. Efstathiou JA, Trofimov AV, Zietman AL. Life, liberty, and the pursuit of protons: an evidence-based review of the role of particle therapy in the treatment of prostate cancer. *Cancer J.* 2009;15(4):312–318.

40. Zhang X, Dong L, Lee AK, et al. Effect of anatomic motion on proton therapy dose distributions in prostate cancer treatment. *Int J Radiat Oncol Biol Phys.* 2007;67(2):620–629.

41. Trofimov A, Nguyen PL, Coen JJ, et al. Radiotherapy treatment of early-stage prostate cancer with IMRT and protons: a treatment planning comparison. *Int J Radiat Oncol Biol Phys.* 2007;69(2):444–453.

42. Konski A, Speier W, Hanlon A, Beck JR, Pollack A. Is proton beam therapy cost effective in the treatment of adenocarcinoma of the prostate? *J Clin Oncol.* 2007;25(24):3603–3608.

43. Bentel GC, Marks LB, Sherouse GW, Spencer DP, Anscher MS. The effectiveness of immobilization during prostate irradiation. *Int J Radiat Oncol Biol Phys.* 1995;31(1):143–148.

44. Rosenthal SA, Roach M 3rd, Goldsmith BJ, et al. Immobilization improves the reproducibility of patient positioning during six-field conformal radiation therapy for prostate carcinoma. *Int J Radiat Oncol Biol Phys.* 1993;27(4):921–926.

45. Crook JM, Raymond Y, Salhani D, Yang H, Esche B. Prostate motion during standard radiotherapy as assessed by fiducial markers. *Radiother Oncol.* 1995;37(1):35–42.

46. Roeske JC, Forman JD, Mesina CF, et al. Evaluation of changes in the size and location of the prostate, seminal vesicles, bladder, and rectum during a course of external beam radiation therapy. *Int J Radiat Oncol Biol Phys.* 1995;33(5):1321–1329.

47. Dawson LA, Mah K, Franssen E, Morton G. Target position variability throughout prostate radiotherapy. *Int J Radiat Oncol Biol Phys.* 1998;42(5):1155–1161.

48. Ghilezan MJ, Jaffray DA, Siewerdsen JH, et al. Prostate gland motion assessed with cine-magnetic resonance imaging (cine-MRI). *Int J Radiat Oncol Biol Phys.* 2005;62(2):406–417.

49. Kupelian P, Willoughby T, Mahadevan A, et al. Multi-institutional clinical experience with the Calypso System in localization and continuous, real-time monitoring of the prostate gland during external radiotherapy. *Int J Radiat Oncol Biol Phys.* 2007;67(4):1088–1098.

50. McNair HA, Mangar SA, Coffey J, et al. A comparison of CT- and ultrasound-based imaging to localize the prostate for external beam radiotherapy. *Int J Radiat Oncol Biol Phys.* 2006;65(3):678–687.

51. Smitsmans MH, de Bois J, Sonke JJ, et al. Automatic prostate localization on cone-beam CT scans for high precision image-guided radiotherapy. *Int J Radiat Oncol Biol Phys.* 2005;63(4):975–984.

52. Langen KM, Zhang Y, Andrews RD, et al. Initial experience with megavoltage (MV) CT guidance for daily prostate alignments. *Int J Radiat Oncol Biol Phys.* 2005;62(5):1517–1524.

53. Brenner DJ, Martinez AA, Edmundson GK, Mitchell C, Thames HD, Armour EP. Direct evidence that prostate tumors show high sensitivity to fractionation (low alpha/beta ratio), similar to late-responding normal tissue. *Int J Radiat Oncol Biol Phys.* 2002;52(1):6–13.

54. Fowler JF, Ritter MA, Chappell RJ, Brenner DJ. What hypofractionated protocols should be tested for prostate cancer? *Int J Radiat Oncol Biol Phys.* 2003;56(4):1093–1104.

55. Kupelian PA, Thakkar VV, Khuntia D, Reddy CA, Klein EA, Mahadevan A. Hypofractionated intensity-modulated radiotherapy (70 gy at 2.5 Gy per fraction) for localized prostate cancer: long-term outcomes. *Int J Radiat Oncol Biol Phys.* 2005;63(5):1463–1468.

56. Buyyounouski MK, Price RA Jr, Harris EE, et al. Stereotactic body radiotherapy for primary management of early-stage, low- to intermediate-risk prostate cancer: report of the American Society for Therapeutic Radiology and Oncology Emerging Technology Committee. *Int J Radiat Oncol Biol Phys.* 2010;76(5):1297–1304.

57. Allaf ME, Palapattu GS, Trock BJ, Carter HB, Walsh PC. Anatomical extent of lymph node dissection: impact on men with clinically localized prostate cancer. *J Urol.* 2004;172(5 Pt 1):1840–1844.

58. Bader P, Burkhard FC, Markwalder R, Studer UE. Is a limited lymph node dissection an adequate staging procedure for prostate cancer? *J Urol.* 2002;168(2):514–8; discussion 518.

59 Ganswindt U, Schilling D, Muller AC et al. Distribution of prostate sentinel nodes: a SPECT-derived anatomic atlas. *Int J Radiat Oncol Biol Phys.* 2010. Epub ahead of print.

60. Roach M 3rd, DeSilvio M, Lawton C, et al. Phase III trial comparing whole-pelvic versus prostate-only radiotherapy and neoadjuvant versus adjuvant combined androgen suppression: Radiation Therapy Oncology Group 9413. *J Clin Oncol.* 2003;21(10):1904–1911.

61. Wang-Chesebro A, Xia P, Coleman J, Akazawa C, Roach M 3rd. Intensity-modulated radiotherapy improves lymph node coverage and dose to critical structures compared with three-dimensional conformal radiation therapy in clinically localized prostate cancer. *Int J Radiat Oncol Biol Phys.* 2006;66(3):654–662.

62. Sylvester JE, Grimm PD, Blasko JC, et al. 15-Year biochemical relapse free survival in clinical Stage T1-T3 prostate cancer following combined external beam radiotherapy and brachytherapy; Seattle experience. *Int J Radiat Oncol Biol Phys.* 2007;67(1):57–64.

63. Nag S, Beyer D, Friedland J, Grimm P, Nath R. American Brachytherapy Society (ABS) recommendations for transperineal permanent brachytherapy of prostate cancer. *Int J Radiat Oncol Biol Phys.* 1999;44(4):789–799.

64. Demanes DJ, Rodriguez RR, Schour L, Brandt D, Altieri G. High-dose-rate intensity-modulated brachytherapy with external beam radiotherapy for prostate cancer: California endocurietherapy's 10-year results. *Int J Radiat Oncol Biol Phys.* 2005;61(5):1306–1316.

65. Vargas CE, Martinez AA, Boike TP, et al. High-dose irradiation for prostate cancer via a high-dose-rate brachytherapy boost: results of a phase I to II study. *Int J Radiat Oncol Biol Phys.* 2006;66(2):416–423.

66 Villaviecencio RT, Rex DK, Rahmani E. Argon plasma coagulation as first line treatment for chronic radiation proctopathy. *J Gastroenterol Hepatol.* 2004;10: 1169.

67. Dall'Era MA, Hampson NB, Hsi RA, Madsen B, Corman JM. Hyperbaric oxygen therapy for radiation induced proctopathy in men treated for prostate cancer. *J Urol.* 2006;176(1):87–90.

68. Lawton CA, Won M, Pilepich MV, et al. Long-term treatment sequelae following external beam irradiation for adenocarcinoma of the prostate: analysis of RTOG studies 7506 and 7706. *Int J Radiat Oncol Biol Phys.* 1991;21(4):935–939.

69 Michalski JM, Kyounghwa B, Roach M et al. Long-term toxicity following 3D conformal radiation therapy for prostate cancer from the RTOG 9406 phase I/II dose escalation study. *Int J Radiat Oncol Biol Phys.* 2010;76:14–22.

70. van der Wielen GJ, Mulhall JP, Incrocci L. Erectile dysfunction after radiotherapy for prostate cancer and radiation dose to the penile structures: a critical review. *Radiother Oncol.* 2007;84(2):107–113.

71. Zelefsky MJ, McKee AB, Lee H, Leibel SA. Efficacy of oral sildenafil in patients with erectile dysfunction after radiotherapy for carcinoma of the prostate. *Urology.* 1999;53(4):775–778.

72. Crook J, McLean M, Catton C, Yeung I, Tsihlias J, Pintilie M. Factors influencing risk of acute urinary retention after TRUS-guided permanent prostate seed implantation. *Int J Radiat Oncol Biol Phys.* 2002;52(2): 453–460.

73. Merrick GS, Butler WM, Wallner KE, et al. Risk factors for the development of prostate brachytherapy related urethral strictures. *J Urol.* 2006;175(4):1376–1380; discussion 1381.

74. Gelblum DY, Potters L. Rectal complications associated with transperineal interstitial brachytherapy for prostate cancer. *Int J Radiat Oncol Biol Phys.* 2000;48(1): 119–124.

75. Merrick GS, Butler WM, Lief JH, Stipetich RL, Abel LJ, Dorsey AT. Efficacy of sildenafil citrate in prostate brachytherapy patients with erectile dysfunction. *Urology.* 1999;53(6):1112–1116.

76. Grimm PD, Blasko JC, Ragde H, Sylvester J, Clarke D. Does brachytherapy have a role in the treatment of prostate cancer? *Hematol Oncol Clin North Am.* 1996;10(3):653–673.

77. Keating NL, O'Malley AJ, Smith MR. Diabetes and cardiovascular disease during androgen deprivation therapy for prostate cancer. *J Clin Oncol.* 2006;24(27):4448–4456.

78. Holzbeierlein JM. Managing complications of androgen deprivation therapy for prostate cancer. *Urol Clin North Am.* 2006;33(2):181–190, vi.

79 Chen AC, Petrylak DP. Complications of androgen-deprivation therapy in men with prostate cancer. *Curr Urol Rep.* 2005;6:210.

80. Bolla M, Collette L, Blank L, et al. Long-term results with immediate androgen suppression and external irradiation in patients with locally advanced prostate cancer (an EORTC study): a phase III randomised trial. *Lancet.* 2002;360(9327):103–106.

81. Efstathiou JA, Bae K, Shipley WU, et al. Cardiovascular mortality after androgen deprivation therapy for locally advanced prostate cancer: RTOG 85–31. *J Clin Oncol.* 2009;27(1):92–99.

82. Efstathiou JA, Bae K, Shipley WU, et al. Cardiovascular mortality and duration of androgen deprivation for locally advanced prostate cancer: analysis of RTOG 92–02. *Eur Urol.* 2008;54(4):816–823.

83. Studer UE, Whelan P, Albrecht W, et al. Immediate or deferred androgen deprivation for patients with prostate cancer not suitable for local treatment with curative intent: European Organisation for Research and Treatment of Cancer (EORTC) Trial 30891. *J Clin Oncol.* 2006;24(12):1868–1876.

Chemoprevention in Prostate Cancer: Current Clinical Evidence

Jason M. Phillips[1] and Al Barqawi[2]*

[1]*The University of Texas, Houston, TX*
[2]*University of Colorado School of Medicine, Aurora, CO*

■ ABSTRACT

Prostate cancer continues to be the leading cause of newly diagnosed male cancer in the United States. Several large scale studies have evaluated the effects of chemoprevention on prostate cancer. We reviewed the current literature for randomized trials focusing on prostate chemoprevention including the PCPT, REDUCE, and SELECT trials. We evaluated the impact of these chemoprevention agents on prostate cancer including molecular effects, economic impact and future directions. Current evidence supports the use of 5-alpha reductase inhibitors (5-ARI) and micronutrients as possible inhibitors of prostate cancer. 5-ARIs are currently the only proven chemopreventative agents. 5-ARIs are not currently economically effective. Further cost benefit analyses are needed to better identify which populations will benefit from chemoprevention. Further analyses are needed to evaluate the overall effects of micronutrients and 5-ARIs on prostate cancer.

Keywords: prostate, prostate cancer, chemoprevention, REDUCE, PCPT, SELECT, finasteride, dutasteride

■ INTRODUCTION

Prostate cancer continues to be the leading cause of newly diagnosed male cancers in the United States. In 2010, the American Cancer Society estimates 217,730 new cases and 32,050 deaths from prostate cancer (1). The number of male deaths from prostate cancer is second only to lung cancer. Multiple treatment modalities such as surgery, radiation, chemotherapy and hormone therapies have had variable success treating prostate cancer. However, current therapies target only existing cancer and each carries a side effect profile.

Due to improved early detection, prostate cancer is now identified at an earlier stage and grade. These cancers are often organ confined and slow growing. However, strategies focused on surveillance are often not chosen by the patient. Treatment including radical prostatectomy or radiation has been shown to over treat prostate cancer in as many as 30% to 50% of patients (2). Morbidity, including incontinence and impotence can significantly affect a patient's quality of life. Given that the US male population faces a 16.7% lifetime risk of prostate cancer, prostate cancer is an ideal candidate for prevention strategies.

*Corresponding author, Division of Urology, University of Colorado School of Medicine, Academic Office One Bldg, 12631 East 17th Ave., Room L15–5602, Aurora, CO 80045
   E-mail address: Al.Barqawi@ucdenver.edu

Radiation Medicine Rounds 2:1 (2011) 145–152.
DOI: 10.5003/2151–4208.2.1.145

Chemoprevention focuses on the use of natural or synthetic agents that are used to suppress, delay, or prevent the development of cancer. 5-Alpha reductase inhibitors (5-ARI) and natural substances have been utilized with varying results for prostate cancer prevention. These substances have focused on both primary prevention and secondary prevention. Primary prevention focuses on deferring or preventing the presence of cancer prior to cancer formation. Secondary prevention focuses on preventing premalignant lesions from progressing to cancer. For prostate cancer, secondary prevention focuses on preventing the progression of high-grade prostate epithelial neoplasia (HGPIN). Tertiary prevention focuses on preventing a secondary malignancy in patients with known cancer.

■ CHEMOPREVENTION AGENTS IN QUESTION

Unlike cancer treatment which seeks to improve the condition of an already affected individual, cancer prevention requires patient compliance. The ideal chemopreventative agent should be minimally expensive and nontoxic. In addition, the agent in question is superior if it has multiple prevention benefits.

Both 5-ARI medications, finasteride and dutasteride, are used successfully to inhibit prostate growth with benign prostatic hypertrophy (BPH). Their effect on prostate cancer has been recently tested with multicenter, randomized, double blind, placebo controlled trials. 5-α-reductase has two isoenzymes. Finasteride inhibits the type 2 isoenzyme while dutasteride inhibits both the type 1 and type 2 isoenzymes. Dutasteride thus has more complete inhibition of DHT, roughly 90% as compared to finasteride's 70% reduction of DHT (3,4). It has been proposed that expression of the type 1 isoenzyme is increased with prostate cancer while the type 2 isoenzyme is unaffected with prostate cancer (5). 5-ARI medications focus on inhibiting androgen receptor (AR) activation. Research on BPH has shown that consistent use of 5-ARIs decrease prostatic volume 30% and reduce prostate-specific antigen (PSA) levels 50% to 60% (6).

Micronutrients have been found to correlate with an effect on the development or prevention of prostate cancer. The largest scale trial on micronutrients was for selenium. Antioxidants in vitro can inhibit cellular proliferation, induce apoptosis and modulate genes leading to the suppression of prostatic tumor (7,8). Similar to 5-ARIs, selenium targets the AR. Other molecular targets include nuclear factor-KB, AKt, Wnt, Hedgehog and Notch. Other chemopreventative micronutrients include vitamin-E, vitamin-D soy isoflavones, lycopene, green tea, DIM, and curcumin (9).

■ REVIEW OF RECENT CHEMOPREVENTION TRIALS

We reviewed the Prostate Cancer Prevention Trial (PCPT), the Reduction by Dutasteride of Prostate Cancer Events (REDUCE), and the Selenium and Vitamin E Cancer Prevention Trial (SELECT). Each of these trials was a multicenter randomized double blind evaluation of the chemopreventative agent in question versus placebo. Table 1 compares their study design.

Prostate Cancer Prevention Trial

The PCPT was the first large multicenter chemoprevention trial. In 2003, 18,882 men, 55 years or older with a PSA level less than 3.0 ng/mL and a normal digital rectal exam (DRE) were randomized on finasteride 5 mg daily or placebo for seven years.

The primary endpoint of the study was the prevalence of prostate cancer as diagnosed by biopsy for cause or end of study biopsies. Of the 18,882 men who participated, 48%, or 9,060 men were included in the final analysis. Enrollment criteria included men 55 years or older who were free of prostate cancer, no other significant co morbidities, and an American Urological Association symptom score (AUA-SS) of less than 20. Eligible participants were required to have a PSA less than 3.0 ng/mL, normal DRE, adherent to the study protocol and no side effects during placebo. Men were contacted every three months for medical event evaluation and were seen by the study site every six months for side effect evaluation and medication refills. Annual PSA and DRE were performed. Biopsy was recommended if the DRE was abnormal or PSA was greater than 4.0 ng/mL in the placebo arm or 2.0 times PSA (adjusted to 2.3× in year 4) in the finasteride arm. At the completion of the trial in year seven, all participants were recommended to undergo an end of study prostate biopsy

TABLE 1 Comparison of PCPT, REDUCE, SELECT trials

Trial	Population	Risk Category	Agent	Target	Reported
Prostate Cancer Prevention Trial (PCPT)	$n = 18,882$	PSA < 3.0 ng/mL; DRE Normal	Finasteride	Type 1: 5-ARI	2008
Selenium and Vitamin E Cancer Prevention Trial (SELECT)	$n = 32,400$	PSA < 4.0 ng/mL; DRE normal	Selenium, vitamin E	Oxidative stress	2008
Reduction by Dutasteride of Prostate Cancer Events Trial (REDUCE)	$n = 8,229$	PSA = 2.5–10 ng/mL; DRE normal	Dutasteride	Type 1, 2: 5-ARI	2009

with at least six cores. All biopsies were reviewed by a blinded pathologist.

Prostate cancer was found in 24.4% of the placebo group (1,147/4,692) and 18.4% of the finasteride group (803/4,368), representing a 24.8% risk reduction (confidence interval [CI] 19–31, $P < .001$). Finasteride's relative benefit was found across all groups including age, race/ethnicity, family history and entry PSA. In addition, Finasteride also reduced the risk of HGPIN compared to placebo

Paradoxically, tumors with a Gleason grade of 7–10, high-grade tumors, were found to be more prevalent in the finasteride group (37%), 280 of 757 graded tumors, as compared to the placebo group (22%), 237 of 1,068 graded tumors. This was statistically significant ($P < .001$). The increased prevalence of high-grade tumors in the treatment group has generated tremendous speculation and sub-analysis. Forty of the excess high-grade tumors were found in the "for cause" biopsies, clinically indicated due to increasing PSA or changes in the DRE. Only an excess of three tumors were found at the end of study biopsies. Because of disagreement on the clinical significance from the increase in high-grade tumors in the treatment arm, finasteride was not registered to the FDA for a new indication to prevent prostate cancer. However, secondary analyses based on prostatectomy actually demonstrated a small net reduction in high-grade cancers and a 53% decrease in low-grade tumors (10).

The Reduction by Dutasteride of Prostate Cancer Events

The REDUCE trial, recently published in the *New England Journal of Medicine* in April of 2010, was a 4-year multicenter, randomized, double-blind, placebo-controlled, parallel-group study. About 8,231 men were randomized equally to dutasteride 0.5 mg daily versus placebo. This trial was begun prior to the completion of the PCPT trial. Dutasteride was randomized to placebo only and not compared to finasteride.

The REDUCE trial evaluated the effects of dutasteride on prostate cancer. Similar to finasteride, dutasteride reduces dihydrotestosterone. Unlike finasteride, dutasteride affects the expression of both type 1 and type 2 isoenzymes of 5-ARIs. Animal studies demonstrate that compared to finasteride, dutasteride has an increased reduction in both DHT and tumor growth (11). The theory that if the type 1 isoenzyme affects cancer it would demonstrate a benefit.

The primary endpoint was the presence of prostate cancer detected on biopsy 2 or 4 years after treatment. Biopsies performed out of the protocol were considered protocol independent biopsies. Other important endpoints included Gleason score, tumor volume, percent of positive biopsy cores, presence of HGPIN, and presence of small acinar proliferation. BPH endpoints were also evaluated.

Eligibility participants were required to be 50 to 75 years old, have a serum PSA between 2.5 ng/mL and 10 mg/mL for men aged 50 to 60 years or 3.0 to 10 ng/mL for men aged >60 years, and had undergone a prostate biopsy within six months of enrollment. Men were excluded if they had more than one biopsy, had prostate cancer of any grade, HGPIN, atypical small acinar proliferation, or a prostate volume of more than 80 g, had previous prostate surgery of any kind, or had an international prostate symptom score (IPSS) of 25 or higher.

During the trial 6,726 men (82.6%) underwent at least one biopsy and 1,516 men (22.5%) were diagnosed with prostate cancer. The dutasteride arm represented an absolute risk reduction of 5% and a relative risk reduction of 23% (857 in the placebo arm vs. 659 in the dutasteride arm, $P < .001$). This benefit was across all subgroups including age, family history, PSA level, prostate volume, or body mass index. The odds ratio for prostate cancer, detected on biopsy, with dutasteride as compared with placebo was 0.60 for all tumors ($P < .001$) and 0.62 for Gleason scores of 7 to 10 ($P < .001$).

Low-grade tumors (Gleason 5, 6) were statistically higher in the placebo group (617 in placebo vs. 437 in dutasteride, $P < .001$). The evidence of premalignant lesions was also decreased. HGPIN had a relative risk reduction of 39% ($P < .001$) and small acinar proliferation (ASAP) had a relative risk reduction of 21% ($P = .04$).

Unlike the PCPT, REDUCE showed no significant overall increase in Gleason score 7 to 10, high-grade cancers. In aggregate, there were 220 tumors with a Gleason score of 7 to 10 among 3,299 men in the dutasteride group and 233 among 3,407 men in the placebo group ($P = .81$).

Looking specifically at the Gleason grade 8–10 tumors, there was no overall significant change, 19 in placebo versus 29 in dutasteride ($P = .15$). However, the second round of biopsies during years 3 and 4 of the study showed a statistical increase in high-grade tumors as compared to placebo. There were 12 tumors with a Gleason score of 8 to 10 in the dutasteride group, as compared with only 1 in the placebo group ($P = .003$) (12). The authors speculate that this was caused by more frequent early detection of low-grade tumors in the placebo group that might have progressed if left untreated. As expected, dutasteride also demonstrated improved outcomes with BPH. Prostate volume, acute urinary retention and BPH related surgery, and urinary tract infections were all significantly reduced in the dutasteride group.

The REDUCE trial demonstrated a significant effect on low-grade cancers (Gleason 5, 6), but did not appear to change the prevalence of high-grade cancers. Overall it was well tolerated but did have significant effects on libido, erectile dysfunction, and semen volume.

The Selenium and Vitamin E Cancer Prevention Trial

The SELECT trial, published in 2009, was a randomized, placebo controlled population based primary chemoprevention trial focused on the effects of selenium and vitamin E on preventing prostate cancer. SELECT randomized 35,533 men to four treatment arms: selenium with placebo, selenium with vitamin E, Vitamin E with placebo, placebo with placebo. Study supplements included 200 μg l-selenomethionine, 400 mg racemic α-tocopherol and an optional multivitamin containing no selenium or vitamin E. Eligible men were at least 50 years of age for African Americans, at least 55 for whites, negative DRE, PSA less than 4 ng/mL, and normal blood pressure.

The choice to use selenium and vitamin E was based on the Nutritional Prevention of Cancer Trial of oral selenium for nonmelanoma skin cancer in which men who were randomized to selenium versus placebo had a 65% reduction in prostate cancer incidence after a 4.5-year follow up. The choice to use Vitamin E was based on the Alpha-Tocopherol, Beta-Carotene Cancer Prevention Trial (ATBC) trial, which was a double blind randomized placebo controlled trial for lung cancer incidence and mortality. Incidentally, The ATBC trial demonstrated a statistically significant 32% reduction in prostate cancer for those taking Vitamin E.

The primary endpoint was the presence of prostate cancer found in the biopsy. The indications for biopsy were not indicated in the protocol and were at the discretion of the physician.

During the second interim analysis seven years after initiation of the trial, the independent Data and Safety Monitoring Committee recommended discontinuation of the SELECT because the data demonstrated no significant differences between groups. No statistically significant effects were reported on primary or secondary analyses of the data, suggesting no prostate cancer prevention benefits from selenium or vitamin E (13).

Other Chemoprevention Agents

No other chemoprevention agents have been tested on the scale of finasteride, dutasteride, vitamin-E or selenium. Other potential chemotherapeutic agents include lycopene, green tea, soy, statins, selective estrogen receptor modulators (SERMs), DIM, and curcumin. Molecular targets, these agents affect, include nuclear factor-KB, AKt, Wnt, Hedgehog, and Notch (9).

Lycopene is a biologically occurring carotenoid that is a potent antioxidant. It has been shown to be associated with lower prostate cancer risk in a number of epidemiologic studies (14). Using the preclinical TRAMP mouse model, prostate cancer was significantly decreased 60% versus 95% ($P = .01$). However, no correlation was found with prostate cancer in a PLCO trial examining 29,000 men.

Green tea contains several catechins believed to inhibit oncogenesis and provide antioxidants. Epidemiologic studies between Asian men with a high intake of green tea first suggested that green tea may provide a protective benefit against prostate cancer. Three clinical trials suggest a benefit (15). A small clinical trial ($n = 60$) using oral green tea catechins (GTC) found that patients with HGPIN randomized to GTC versus placebo had no change in PSA levels, but did have less progression of prostate cancer: 1 patient versus 9 patients progress (16).

Soy, like green tea, was also found to demonstrate lower prostate cancer in epidemiologic studies between diets high in soy versus western diets. The benefit is potentially a 70% reduction of prostate cancer (17). Soy affects signaling pathways, specifically Wnt and Hh signaling. Randomized studies are currently being performed.

Statins inhibit HMG-CoA, the rate limiting step of cholesterol synthesis. Statin use over 2 years has been associated with a decrease in PSA (18). By inhibiting prostatic cellular growth and promoting apoptosis, statins also decrease cellular growth. No large double blind study has evaluated the effect of statin use on prostate cancer but a meta analysis did find a protective effect (19). Further studies are needed to substantiate current evidence.

SERMs are best known for their effects on breast cancer. Toremifene has decreased prostate cancer in the TRAMP model. A phase 2b study found that 20 mg doses of toremifene resulted in a 48% decrease in prostate cancer at one year (20). A stage 3 study with 1,200 men is currently evaluating 20 mg toremifene on HGPIN. Results will be published in 2010.

DIM (the dimeric product of indole-3-carbinol) is found in a variety of plants and has been shown to inhibit α-reductase suggesting that it may have an inhibitory role in prostate cancer. Curcumin is a bioavailable agent in turmeric and is also an α-reductase inhibitor. Other regulators along the tumor pathway are inhibited by these two substances. Clinical trials are required to evaluate their effects.

Currently no biologically available agents have been proven to provide chemoprevention benefits of prostate cancer. As such, current patient recommendations are to eat healthy foods and pursue healthy lifestyle changes (21).

Controversy: Effects of Prevention on High-Grade Tumors

After the initial publication on the PCPT, the editorial authors concluded that the risk of finasteride on high-grade tumors was uncertain and recommended finasteride not be used as a chemopreventative agent (22). Different authors have since cited certain biases to account for the increase in high-grade tumors and secondary analyses have been performed. The REDUCE trial has since proven no overall difference for high-grade tumors between dutasteride and placebo. Secondary analyses have not yet been performed.

PSA, DRE, and prostate volume detection biases were initially described as contributing to the increase in high-grade tumors found in the "for cause" biopsies for the finasteride arm of the PCPT trial. Looking solely at the "end of study" biopsies performed, there was no increased risk of high-grade tumor (23). DRE has been shown to increase sensitivity for detecting cancer with finasteride. Detection increased from 16% to 21% ($P = .015$) (24). Similarly, 5-ARIs increase PSA sensitivity for detecting prostate cancer. 5-ARI medications decrease the PSA laboratory value by roughly half. As such, PSA is more sensitive in detecting high-grade tumors (10). For the PCPT, for cause biopsies from an increase in PSA levels artificially selected for more biopsies to be taken of the treatment group. Prostate volume decreases with finasteride use, allowing for a larger percentage of the surface area to be sampled with prostate needle biopsy as compared with large untreated glands. The PCPT did not stratify on prostate volume size.

When adjusting for prostate sampling density and baseline PSA levels, finasteride in the PCPT actually had a small net reduction in high-grade cancers and a 53% decrease in low-grade tumors (10). Reevaluation of the PCPT data using end point prostatectomy instead of prostate biopsy demonstrated a 16% reduction in high-grade tumor. Significant upstaging of cancer at the time of prostatectomy was detected in the placebo group but not in the treatment group. The misclassification rate of true high-grade disease (to low-grade disease on biopsy) was significantly lower for finasteride (34.6%) than for placebo (52.6%) (25). Another study looking at

500 patients who underwent prostatectomy demonstrated a high-grade cancer rates of 8.2% (placebo) versus 6.0% (finasteride), a 27% risk reduction (RR 0.73; 95% CI 0.56–0.96; $P = .02$) with finasteride (26). The increased sensitivity of the prostate biopsy after finasteride treatment will increase the detection of high-grade tumors but do not cause it.

Economic Impact of Prostate Chemoprevention

Chemoprevention for cancer should cost roughly $100,000 or less per life year (LY) saved. According to Laupacis et al., interventions that cost less than $20,000/year have a high adoption rate while interventions that cost greater than $100,000/year have a low adoption rate (27). Svatek et al. analyzed the cost-effectiveness of finasteride chemoprevention based on prevalence rates from the SEER data. Their findings found finasteride to be expensive $578,00 to $1,107,000 USD per LY saved (28).

Zeliadt et al. supported the expense per LY saved by estimating LY saved to be $1.6 million (29). However, an analysis on quality adjusted life-years (QALYs) based on PCPT prevalence rates showed a lower cost per LY due to higher PCPT prevalence rates. This analysis demonstrated $122,000 per QALY saved (30). If finasteride is assumed to not increase the incidence of high-grade cancers, then the analysis demonstrated $112,000 per QALY saved. Thus more patients benefit from chemoprevention. These analyses were based on the current price of finasteride at $66/month. If finasteride becomes less expensive, then the cost per QALY saved drops proportionally.

Currently, chemoprevention is not cost effective. A better understanding of which subgroups of men would benefit most from chemoprevention would decrease the cost to benefit ratio; thus making chemoprevention feasible from an economic standpoint.

■ DISCUSSION

5-ARIs are currently the only proven chemopreventative agents. Selenium and vitamin E are not recommended for prevention. Evidence from the PCPT and REDUCE trials demonstrate a ~24% reduction in prostate cancer with the use of either 5-ARI (24% PCPT, 23% REDUCE). The increased incidence of high-grade prostate cancer found in the PCPT was

initially alarming, but challenged with both the results from the REDUCE trial and with revaluation by Pinsky et al. and Redman et al. Reanalysis of the PCPT suggests that high-grade cancer is not associated with finasteride therapy (31). Prostatectomy is the only definitive diagnosis for the evaluation for prostate cancer. Patients should feel confident that the prostate biopsy performed during 5-ARI treatment will have a low risk of upstaging. The effects of PSA, DRE and prostate volume bias will continue to play a role in the detection and evaluation of high-grade and low-grade cancers (32).

Despite evidence from the PCPT and REDUCE trials, there does not appear to be a trend towards prescribing 5-ARIs for the prevention of prostate cancer. Approximately 64% of Urologists and 80% of PCPs never prescribe finasteride for prostate cancer chemoprevention with over half of Urologists reporting concerns for inducing high-grade tumors. Approximately half of the PCPs were not aware 5-ARIs could be used for chemoprevention (33).

5-ARIs are not currently economically effective. With the widely held belief that chemoprevention should cost less than $100K per life year saved, current costs fall well short of this goal. The high prevalence of prostate cancer makes it an ideal cancer to target with chemoprevention. However, its indolent and slow growing nature of prostate cancer makes the appropriate target population a difficult target to narrow down. In the current United States economic environment, prostate cancer prevention will likely have to cost far less than $100K per life year saved to be effective and accepted.

Further analyses are required to pinpoint the subgroup population that will benefit most and the timing that is required to be effective. The PCPT revealed a high prevalence of prostate cancer, but no reliable markers were available to determine who would benefit most from biopsy or treatment. REDUCE prospectively collected samples to retrospectively analyze potential biomarkers (34). Further analysis will hopefully make 5-ARIs economically available for at risk individuals.

In 2009, the American Urologic Association (AUA) and the American Society of Clinical Oncology (ASCO) published guidelines based on expert review stating that finasteride should be discussed with at risk patients (35). No current guideline makes a more definitive statement. With the recent findings from the REDUCE study and future analyses, the guidelines may be updated.

Current investigations into biomarkers, nutritional supplements and other pharmacologic agents may impact the success at primary prevention. No current literature supports the use of nutritional supplements for prostate cancer prevention. The PCPT and REDUCE provide evidence that finasteride and dutasteride may offer chemopreventative benefits. Further analyses are required to determine which cohorts of men will benefit most from chemoprevention

■ REFERENCES

1. Jemal A, Siegel R, Xu J, Ward E. Cancer statistics, 2010. *CA Cancer J Clin.* 2010;60(5):277–300.
2. Etzioni R, Penson DF, Legler JM, et al. Overdiagnosis due to prostate-specific antigen screening: lessons from U.S. prostate cancer incidence trends. *J Natl Cancer Inst.* 2002;94(13):981–990.
3. Titus MA, Gregory CW, Ford OH 3rd, Schell MJ, Maygarden SJ, Mohler JL. Steroid 5alpha-reductase isozymes I and II in recurrent prostate cancer. *Clin Cancer Res.* 2005;11(12):4365–4371.
4. Frye SV. Discovery and clinical development of dutasteride, a potent dual 5alpha-reductase inhibitor. *Curr Top Med Chem.* 2006;6(5):405–421.
5. Thomas LN, Lazier CB, Gupta R, et al. Differential alterations in 5alpha-reductase type 1 and type 2 levels during development and progression of prostate cancer. *Prostate.* 2005;63(3):231–239.
6. Marberger M. Drug insight: 5alpha-reductase inhibitors for the treatment of benign prostatic hyperplasia. *Nat Clin Pract Urol.* 2006;3(9):495–503.
7. Dong Y, Zhang H, Hawthorn L, Ganther HE, Ip C. Delineation of the molecular basis for selenium-induced growth arrest in human prostate cancer cells by oligonucleotide array. *Cancer Res.* 2003;63(1):52–59.
8. Zhao H, Dupont J, Yakar S, Karas M, LeRoith D. PTEN inhibits cell proliferation and induces apoptosis by downregulating cell surface IGF-IR expression in prostate cancer cells. *Oncogene.* 2004;23(3):786–794.
9. Sarkar FH, Li Y, Wang Z, Kong D. Novel targets for prostate cancer chemoprevention. *Endocr Relat Cancer.* 2010;17(3):R195–212.
10. Cohen YC, Liu KS, Heyden NL, et al. Detection bias due to the effect of finasteride on prostate volume: a modeling approach for analysis of the Prostate Cancer Prevention Trial. *J Natl Cancer Inst.* 2007;99(18):1366–1374.
11. Xu Y, Dalrymple SL, Becker RE, Denmeade SR, Isaacs JT. Pharmacologic basis for the enhanced efficacy of dutasteride against prostatic cancers. *Clin Cancer Res.* 2006;12(13):4072–4079.
12. Andriole GL, Bostwick DG, Brawley OW, et al. Effect of dutasteride on the risk of prostate cancer. *N Engl J Med.* 2010362(13):1192–1202.
13. Lippman SM, Klein EA, Goodman PJ, et al. Effect of selenium and vitamin E on risk of prostate cancer and other cancers: the Selenium and Vitamin E Cancer Prevention Trial (SELECT). *JAMA.* 2009;301(1):39–51.
14. Thompson IM. Chemoprevention of prostate cancer: agents and study designs. *J Urol.* 2007;178(3 Pt 2):S9–S13.
15. Johnson JJ, Bailey HH, Mukhtar H. Green tea polyphenols for prostate cancer chemoprevention: a translational perspective. *Phytomedicine.* 2010;17(1):3–13.
16. Bettuzzi S, Brausi M, Rizzi F, Castagnetti G, Peracchia G, Corti A. Chemoprevention of human prostate cancer by oral administration of green tea catechins in volunteers with high-grade prostate intraepithelial neoplasia: a preliminary report from a one-year proof-of-principle study. *Cancer Res.* 2006;66(2):1234–1240.
17. Jacobsen BK, Knutsen SF, Fraser GE. Does high soy milk intake reduce prostate cancer incidence? The Adventist Health Study (United States). *Cancer Causes Control.* 1998;9(6):553–557.
18. Mener DJ. Prostate specific antigen reduction following statin therapy: mechanism of action and review of the literature. *IUBMB Life.* 2010;62(8):584–590.
19. Bonovas S, Filioussi K, Sitaras NM. Statin use and the risk of prostate cancer: a metaanalysis of 6 randomized clinical trials and 13 observational studies. *Int J Cancer.* 2008;123(4):899–904.
20. Price D, Stein B, Sieber P, et al. Toremifene for the prevention of prostate cancer in men with high grade prostatic intraepithelial neoplasia: results of a double-blind, placebo controlled, phase IIB clinical trial. *J Urol.* 2006;176(3):965–970; discussion 970–961.
21. Venkateswaran V, Klotz LH. Diet and prostate cancer: mechanisms of action and implications for chemoprevention. *Nat Rev Urol.* 2010;7(8):442–453.
22. Scardino PT. The prevention of prostate cancer—the dilemma continues. *N Engl J Med.* 2003;349(3):297–299.
23. Roehrborn CG. Prevention of prostate cancer with finasteride. *N Engl J Med.* 2003;349(16):1569–1572; author reply 1569–1572.
24. Thompson IM, Tangen CM, Goodman PJ, et al. Finasteride improves the sensitivity of digital rectal examination for prostate cancer detection. *J Urol.* 2007;177(5):1749–1752.
25. Pinsky P, Parnes H, Ford L. Estimating rates of true high-grade disease in the Prostate Cancer Prevention Trial. *Cancer Prev Res (Phila).* 2008;1(3):182–186.
26. Redman MW, Tangen CM, Goodman PJ, Lucia MS, Coltman CA Jr, Thompson IM. Finasteride does not increase the risk of high-grade prostate cancer: a bias-adjusted modeling approach. *Cancer Prev Res (Phila).* 2008;1(3):174–181.
27. Laupacis A, Feeny D, Detsky AS, Tugwell PX. Tentative guidelines for using clinical and economic evaluations revisited. *CMAJ.* 1993;148(6):927–929.
28. Svatek RS, Lee JJ, Roehrborn CG, Lippman SM, Lotan Y. The cost of prostate cancer chemoprevention: a decision analysis model. *Cancer Epidemiol Biomarkers Prev.* 2006;15(8):1485–1489.

29. Zeliadt SB, Etzioni RD, Penson DF, Thompson IM, Ramsey SD. Lifetime implications and cost-effectiveness of using finasteride to prevent prostate cancer. *Am J Med.* 2005;118(8):850–857.

30. Svatek RS, Lee JJ, Roehrborn CG, Lippman SM, Lotan Y. Cost-effectiveness of prostate cancer chemo-prevention: a quality of life-years analysis. *Cancer.* 2008;112(5):1058–1065.

31. Strope SA, Andriole GL. Update on chemoprevention for prostate cancer. *Curr Opin Urol.* 2010;20(3):194–197.

32. Crawford ED, Andriole GL, Marberger M, Rittmaster RS. Reduction in the risk of prostate cancer: future directions after the Prostate Cancer Prevention Trial. *Urology.* 2010;75(3):502–509.

33. Hamilton RJ, Kahwati LC, Kinsinger LS. Knowl-edge and use of finasteride for the prevention of prostate cancer. *Cancer Epidemiol Biomarkers Prev.* 2010;19(9):2164–2171.

34. Andriole G, Bostwick D, Brawley O, et al. Chemopre-vention of prostate cancer in men at high risk: rationale and design of the reduction by dutasteride of prostate cancer events (REDUCE) trial. *J Urol.* 2004;172(4 Pt 1):1314–1317.

35. Kramer BS, Hagerty KL, Justman S, et al. Use of 5alpha-reductase inhibitors for prostate cancer chemoprevention: American Society of Clinical Oncology/American Uro-logical Association 2008 Clinical Practice Guideline. *J Urol.* 2009;181(4):1642–1657.

Quality-of-Life Issues in the Radiotherapeutic Management of Localized Prostate Cancer

Thomas J. Pugh* and Steven J. Frank

The University of Texas MD Anderson Cancer Center, Houston, TX

■ ABSTRACT

The process of deciding how best to treat localized prostate cancer is complicated. Surgery, external beam radiation therapy, and brachytherapy are all viable treatment options, with historical evidence indicating that each option has a comparable likelihood of cancer control in low risk patients. The optimal treatment, regardless of modality, will be one that maximizes disease-related outcomes while minimizing health-related risks. Several health-related quality of life (HRQOL) measurement scales have been developed to assess side effects from the patient's perspective and gauge their overall satisfaction with the treatment. Instruments such as these can allow physicians to inform patients about the likelihood of certain side effects associated with various treatment options for prostate cancer. Here we review the research done to date on HRQOL outcomes associated with radiation therapy for prostate cancer and address issues for future study.

Keywords: prostate cancer, health-related quality of life, radiation therapy

Nearly 200,000 men will be diagnosed with localized prostate cancer in the United States in 2010. As yet, no consensus has been reached regarding the optimal management strategy, and so these men will be presented with a variety of treatment options including active surveillance, brachytherapy, surgery, external beam radiation therapy (EBRT), androgen-deprivation therapy (ADT), or a combination of these modalities. Regardless of which modality is ultimately chosen, a small proportion of these men will die of prostate cancer, but virtually all will live at least several years after treatment (1,2). In this clinical setting, the oncologist is obligated to provide objective and accurate counseling regarding not only survival, disease control, and toxicity projections but also how the potential side effects of various types of therapy may affect overall quality of life (QOL) after treatment. This role is complicated by the fact that physicians' ratings of symptoms correlate poorly with patients' self-perception of their symptoms and their QOL (3).

Health-related quality of life (HRQOL) encompasses an array of variables that extend beyond traditional measures of treatment-related toxicity, including events related to social activity, cognition,

---

*Corresponding author, Division of Radiation Oncology, The University of Texas MD Anderson Cancer Center, Houston, TX

E-mail address: tpugh@mdanderson.org

Radiation Medicine Rounds 2:1 (2011) 153–162.
DOI: 10.5003/2151–4208.2.1.153

emotion, vitality, health perception, and general life satisfaction. Aspects of HRQOL after prostate cancer treatment have recently become defined endpoints in several clinical trials of various treatment options for localized prostate cancer. The ability to interpret and apply the findings from instruments that attempt to document HRQOL is important for treatment assessment, and use of these instruments provides a construct for patient counseling. This review is intended to familiarize the reader with the various tools for assessing HRQOL outcomes and to discuss the impact of HRQOL research for radiation oncologists treating localized prostate cancer.

■ HRQOL MEASUREMENT TOOLS

As is true for any type of questionnaire, questionnaires on HRQOL should be tested to determine if their measurements are consistent (reliability) and that the results accurately represent what the tool was intended to measure (validity) before such tools are put into broad use. The metric being assessed should also be meaningful rather than simply arbitrary. Ideally, development of these tools should be a cooperative effort that includes patient advocacy groups, health care practitioners, and experts in psychometric testing. After the questionnaire is developed, its applicability to current practice must be assessed continually to ensure that the elicited information actually aids medical decision-making. Because use of non-validated instruments or misapplication of

validated instruments may result in misappropriated conclusions, the use of validated instruments within their intended clinical context is paramount when assessing HRQOL in men with prostate cancer.

Several instruments have been developed, validated, and used during the evolution of HRQOL research (Table 1) (4–12). Familiarity with these instruments can be useful for interpreting the results and the reported conclusions of HRQOL studies. The Medical Outcomes Study 36-Item Short Form (SF-36) was one of the first tools used to measure HRQOL (4). The SF-36 includes questions in eight general 'domains': physical function, social function, bodily pain, emotional well-being, energy/fatigue, general health perceptions, role limitations due to physical problems, and role limitations due to emotional problems. Other cancer-specific HRQOL instruments have been developed that more specifically focus on areas of significance to patients with cancer. Two of the more commonly used cancer-related HRQOL instruments are the European Organization for Research and Treatment of Cancer (EORTC) Quality of Life Core Questionnaire (QLQ-C30) and the Functional Assessment of Cancer Therapy-General (FACT-G) (6,7). Each of these tools allows assessment of overall well-being across physical, emotional, social, and functional domains. Although these instruments have been invaluable in HRQOL research on various types of cancer, they lack the specificity to document and quantify the treatment-specific side effects and HRQOL outcomes relevant to localized prostate cancer (13).

TABLE 1 Some validated instruments that have been used for assessing health-related quality of life before and after treatment for localized prostate cancer

Type	Instrument	Reference
General	Medical Outcomes Study Short Form (SF-36)	Ware et al. (4)
	Profile of Mood States (POMS)	Lim et al. (5)
Cancer-specific	Functional Assessment of Cancer Therapy-General (FACT-G)	Cella et al. (6)
	European Organization for Reseacrch and Treatment of Cancer Quality of Life Questionnaire (EORTC-QLQ-30)	Aaronson et al. (7)
Prostate cancer–specific	UCLA Prostate Cancer Index	Litwin et al. (8)
	Expanded Prostate Cancer Index (EPIC-50/EPIC-26)	Wei et al. (9)
	Functional Assessment of Cancer Therapy-Prostate Module (FACT-P)	Esper et al. (10)
	Harvard Symptom Index	Talcott et al. (11)
	EORTC-QLQ-30 prostate module	Joly et al. (12)

Several prostate cancer–specific HRQOL instruments are currently being used to quantify HRQOL outcomes for men with prostate cancer. One of the first such instruments was reported in 1998 by Litwin et al., who described the psychometric properties of the 20-item UCLA Prostate Cancer Index (UCLA-PCI) for assessing HRQOL in men after surgery or radiation therapy for localized prostate cancer (8). The UCLA-PCI was designed to capture patients' perception of their urinary, bowel, and sexual function before and after treatment as well as the level of "bother" experienced over each of these domains. Use of the UCLA-PCI in different settings by other groups revealed its limitations in terms of its incomplete assessment of urinary irritative or obstructive symptoms and hormonal effects. Thus although the UCLA-PCI is appropriate for patients treated with surgery, it may underestimate the effects of radiation therapy on HRQOL. The UCLA-PCI was subsequently modified by several groups to accommodate changes in the therapies used for localized prostate cancer and the resulting effects on HRQOL. One such modification resulted in the development and subsequent validation of the 50-item Expanded Prostate Index Composite (EPIC-50), an instrument that measures a broad spectrum of urinary, bowel, sexual, and hormonal symptoms (9). The EPIC-50 divides the urinary domain into two independent subcategories (irritation versus incontinence) but preserves the key component of discerning functionality and level of bother. The EPIC-26, a truncated version of the EPIC-50, retains summary domain scores for urinary irritation/obstruction, urinary incontinence, bowel, sexual, and hormonal domains in a shorter and thus more efficient questionnaire that has led to improved patient participation (14). The EORTC and investigators from Harvard University have also developed prostate cancer–specific instruments (11,12).

■ LEVELS OF EVIDENCE

To date, no prospective, randomized clinical trials have been conducted to compare the commonly recommended treatments for localized prostate cancer, nor are such trials likely to be conducted in the future because of the difficulty of randomly assigning men to receive a particular kind of treatment. As a result, the highest level of evidence currently available for such comparisons is from prospective longitudinal studies. Because studies of this type have inherent selection biases, direct comparisons between various treatment modalities are problematic. However, the information obtained from studies such as these can be valuable for estimating how a particular HRQOL domain may be affected if one primary treatment were to be selected over another. Considering the potential impact of having this sort of information available on medical-decision making, familiarity with these longitudinal studies and the relative limitations of each study is paramount for physicians counseling men as to the choice of treatment for localized prostate cancer. Select longitudinal series are summarized in Table 2 including prospective series from hospitals in the Netherlands and the Harvard hospital system. Brief descriptions of the multicenter, longitudinal studies of HRQOL in men with localized prostate cancer are given in the sections that follow and are also summarized in Table 2.

Prostate Cancer Outcomes Study

The Prostate Cancer Outcomes Study (PCOS) was the first large, multicenter, prospective study to report HRQOL outcomes in men treated for localized prostate cancer (15,16). The cohort included 1,187 men with newly diagnosed, clinically localized prostate cancer from six geographic regions in the United States. The primary aim of the study was to compare HRQOL at 2 years and 5 years after prostate cancer treatment with baseline values obtained by using a modified version of the UCLA-PCI and SF-36. Although the PCOS introduced an innovative primary endpoint to prostate cancer clinical research, it had several shortcomings that make interpretation of its results problematic. First, no patients received brachytherapy, so outcomes after that treatment were not represented. Second, no patients were treated with other advanced forms of radiation therapy, such as three-dimensional conformal radiation therapy or intensity-modulated radiation therapy, treatments that have since been proven to produce better HRQOL outcomes (23,24). Third, the results of this study were subject to recall bias because the surveyed patients were asked to remember their baseline function either during treatment or after the treatment had been completed. Despite these limitations, the PCOS provided an important framework for subsequent HRQOL research in prostate cancer survivors.

TABLE 2 Multicenter longitudinal studies of health-related quality of life after treatment for localized prostate cancer

Study and References	Study Period	No. of Patients	HRQOL Instruments	Limitations
Prostate Cancer Outcomes Study (15,16)	1994–1995	1,187	UCLA-PCI, SF-36	Applicability to modern treatment; recall bias; selection bias
Cancer of the Prostate Strategic Urologic Research Endeavor (CaPSURE) (18,20–22)	1996–present	>13,000	UCLA-PCI, SF-36	Poor patient retention; coercion bias; selection bias
Madalinska et al. (19)	1996–1998	278	UCLA-PCI, SF-36	Applicability to modern treatment; selection bias; small sample size
Talcott et al. (11)	1994–2000	417	Harvard Symptom Index, SF-36	Poor patient retention; coercion bias; selection bias
Sanda et al. (17)	2003–2006	1201	EPIC, SCA	Selection bias

HRQOL, health-related quality of life; UCLA-PCI, University of California Los Angeles Prostate Cancer Index; SF-36, Medical Outcomes Study Short Form; EPIC, Expanded Prostate Cancer Index; SCA, Service Satisfaction Scale for Cancer Care.

CaPSURE: The Cancer of the Prostate Strategic Urologic Research Endeavor

The CaPSURE study is a prospective, longitudinal observational study of men with localized prostate cancer enrolled through multiple urology practices throughout the western United States. CaPSURE has been criticized for design flaws (potential coercion bias arising from the administration of the posttreatment questionnaire by the treating physician), lack of participation by radiation oncologists, and poor overall compliance with completing the questionnaire by the participants (25). Nevertheless, the CaPSURE findings represent one of the few comprehensive datasets that include men treated with brachytherapy, and it has provided important information regarding patterns of change in various aspects of HRQOL after prostate cancer treatment.

Another multi-institutional longitudinal study reported by Sanda and others involved 1,201 men with localized prostate cancer treated from 2003 through 2006 at one of nine university-affiliated institutions (17). The participants completed EPIC-26 questionnaires via a third-party phone survey before treatment and at regular intervals thereafter. Patients' partners were also surveyed using the EPIC partner model (EPIC-P). A relatively high proportion of patients (>90%) completed the required follow-up.

Eligible patients received surgery (retropubic, laparoscopic, or robot-assisted prostatectomy), EBRT (IMRT or 3D-conformal) with or without ADT, or brachytherapy. The aims of the study were to identify which QOL domains were affected over time by each type of treatment; to identify baseline factors that affected changes in QOL within study groups; to determine whether patient-reported changes in QOL were distressing to the spouses/partners; to assess the relative effects of various changes in QOL domains on overall outcome; and to identify baseline factors that affected satisfaction with outcome after treatment. Although this study, like all other studies of this design, was limited by selection bias, it was nevertheless an improvement over the methods of the preceding observational QOL studies, it addressed the impact of ADT on HRQOL, and it included men treated with modern radiation therapy and surgical techniques.

■ EFFECTS OF RADIATION TREATMENT ON SPECIFIC HRQOL DOMAINS

Urinary Domain

The anatomic proximity of the urethra and bladder to the prostate means that radiation therapy inevitably involves some toxicity to the urinary system that may or may not affect urinary function. Some have reported increases in the incidence of urinary incontinence after radiation treatment, although defining a clinically relevant measure of urinary incontinence has been historically problematic (14). The study by Sanda et al. involved the use of the EPIC-20 questionnaire, which includes measures to quantify urinary incontinence (i.e., leaking >1 time per day, frequent dribbling, or the need for urinary pads) and to assess the level of distress caused by urinary leakage after radiation therapy, delivered either as EBRT or brachytherapy (17). Men treated by either EBRT or brachytherapy both experienced significant detriments in urinary incontinence after treatment compared with baseline. In the brachytherapy group, urinary incontinence scores remained statistically different from baseline at 24 months of follow-up, whereas the urinary incontinence scores for men treated with EBRT had returned to baseline by 12 months of follow-up and remained stable thereafter. The actuarial percentage of men with urinary incontinence (defined as a moderate or big problem with urinary leaking) was low in both groups at 4% to 6%. These findings support results from previous studies characterizing urinary incontinence as uncommon after either EBRT or brachytherapy (11,15,18,19,26–29). More often, urinary function and bother scores in men who undergo radiation therapy are attributable to urinary irritation or obstruction symptoms such as frequency, weak stream, or dysuria (11,17,18). The impact of these urinary symptoms on domain-specific satisfaction scores seems to follow a predictable time course after EBRT or brachytherapy, with the greatest detriments occurring within the first several months after therapy, followed by a progressive return to baseline within approximately 12 months after treatment. This pattern of symptom onset and recovery has been reported by several other investigators (20,27,28,30,31), including the most recent analysis of the CaPSURE database (13). In that analysis, HRQOL scores of 1,269 men who had been treated with prostatectomy, brachytherapy, EBRT, or EBRT combined with brachytherapy or ADT, declined during the first year after radiation treatment and then either reached a plateau or improved by 2 years after treatment. Little to no changes in HRQOL scores were observed after that point. Another study by Roeloffzen et al., one of the few brachytherapy series that measured HRQOL with long-term follow-up (31), also found that HRQOL scores were no different at 6 years after treatment from scores obtained at 12 months of follow-up.

Bowel or Rectal Domain

HRQOL with regard to bowel or rectal function is also significantly influenced by treatment with EBRT or brachytherapy (11,15,17–19,21,32). The range of reported symptoms has included fecal incontinence, bloody stools, and rectal pain, but fecal urgency and frequency seem to be the most common symptoms affecting the bowel or rectal domain after radiation treatment (17). In the first few months after treatment, the time course of scores on bowel or rectal HRQOL surveys are similar to that of the urinary domain scores. However, unlike the urinary problems, difficulties in the bowel domain can persist for well after the first year after EBRT or brachytherapy. The study by Sanda et al. showed that the bowel or rectal scores obtained at 2 years after EBRT or brachytherapy were still significantly worse than scores obtained before treatment (17), A similar pattern of rapid early recovery followed by a sub-baseline plateau that persisted for more than a year after radiation therapy was also noted in another analysis of the CapSURE database (21). Unfortunately improvements in bowel or rectal function scores after the 2-year time-point are rare (13). The effect of elective radiation to the pelvic lymph nodes on HRQOL outcomes remains unclear at this time. Although the treatment volume might be expected to affect bowel or rectal HRQOL scores, having higher-risk disease, a potential surrogate for inclusion of the pelvic lymphatics in the radiation fields, has not been shown to correlate with bowel or rectal HRQOL scores (17,21). Nevertheless, despite the relative impairment of bowel function, the overall level of patient distress relative to bowel or rectal function seems to be low. For example, in the study reported by Sanda et al., 88% of the respondents treated with EBRT and 90% of the respondents treated with brachytherapy reported either "no problem" or "small problem" relative to bowel or rectal function at 1 year after treatment (17).

Sexual Domain

Erectile dysfunction after treatment for localized prostate cancer is the most common of the

HRQOL issues and the most likely to result in greater levels of distress for both patients and their partners (16,17). Several studies that have used patient-reported outcomes suggest that EBRT and brachytherapy can both have adverse effects on sexual HRQOL (17,22,33–37). Although the precise physiologic mechanism underlying erectile dysfunction after radiation therapy is not as clear as it is for men treated surgically, its full impact on HRQOL after radiation therapy can persist for years beyond the completion of treatment (16,19,33,38). Sexual function is an intricate interface between physiology and psychology. Potential confounders of proposed measures of sexual HRQOL include the natural progression toward impaired sexual function with age, subsequent or concurrent co-morbid illnesses or medications, concomitant ADT, the partner's sexual health status, or interdependence of sexual domain scores on other HRQOL domains (i.e., having high levels of distress associated with urinary/bowel function can impair sexual function) (39,40). Baseline erectile function is an important predictor of sexual HRQOL after radiation therapy. In the study by Sanda et al., approximately 1/3 of men electing to undergo EBRT or brachytherapy for localized prostate cancer reported having "erections not firm enough for intercourse" at baseline assessment (17). The complexity of erectile function along with the high incidence of baseline dysfunction in this population of men underscores the need for baseline adjustments and consideration of additional confounders (41,42).

In terms of temporal patterns, sexual HRQOL scores seem to decline within the first several months after radiation treatment, with minimal to no long-term recovery (17,22). The use of phosphodiesterase inhibitors or other pharmacologic/mechanical interventions intended to enhance erectile function may improve sexual HRQOL scores after prostate cancer treatment (43). Although all available treatments for prostate cancer adversely affect sexual HRQOL scores, some have suggested that brachytherapy may produce the smallest amount of decline after treatment (44–46). However, a matched-pair analysis comparing men treated with EBRT with those treated with brachytherapy showed no difference in EPIC-26 sexual domain scores when the men were matched according to age, prostate volume, anti-androgen use, and baseline erectile function (47). Randomized, prospective studies designed to account for confounding factors and baseline function will ultimately be necessary to resolve this question

Vitality/Hormonal Domain

The effect of prostate cancer treatment on vitality and hormonal function has been an underexplored aspect of HRQOL. The ability to measure patient-reported symptoms within this domain is becoming increasingly important with the emergence of androgen manipulation combined with local therapy. Early attempts to quantify the effect of ADT on HRQOL failed to independently assess symptoms associated with vitality or hormonal changes, ultimately underestimating the overall impact of treatment (48,49). Symptoms within this domain include the formation of breasts (gynecomastia), lack of energy, weight gain, hot flashes, and depression. The study by Sanda et al. was the first multicenter longitudinal study to prospectively assess patient-reported vitality/hormonal HRQOL outcomes (17). Even though a minority of patients received ADT with radiation in that study (31% of patients treated with EBRT and 7% treated with brachytherapy), significant declines in vitality/hormonal HRQOL scores were seen in men receiving ADT after treatment compared with the baseline assessment. On the other hand, men who had been treated with neoadjuvant ADT before brachytherapy experienced a gradual increase in vitality/hormonal HRQOL scores after the brachytherapy, with return to baseline at 12 months' follow-up. A similar effect of cytoreductive ADT before brachytherapy on HRQOL has been characterized in a single-institution series (50). In the study by Sanda et al., vitality scores for men treated with EBRT plus ADT had not returned to baseline levels at the time the final questionnaire was completed (24 months after treatment), but an insignificant trend toward baseline was evident. The incomplete return to baseline vitality scores in men treated with EBRT plus ADT may have been attributable to the sustained androgen suppression achieved with luteinizing hormone–releasing hormone therapy prescribed neoadjuvantly, concurrently, and adjuvantly in conjunction with EBRT for men with localized intermediate- to high-risk prostate cancer. Interestingly, no clinically relevant differences from baseline were apparent in men who had received only local therapy, without ADT. High-quality data with extended follow-up are needed to clarify the effect of ADT on HRQOL.

■ FUTURE DIRECTIONS

The effects of combining therapeutic modalities such as ADT with radiation therapy clearly require further research. Little high-quality evidence is also available on the effects of the combination of EBRT plus brachytherapy on HRQOL. Much of the data published to date are limited by small patient numbers and the use of HRQOL instruments that were not specifically designed for men with prostate cancer (51–54). Some investigators have suggested that supplemental EBRT has adverse effects on bowel or rectal HRQOL scores compared with brachytherapy alone (55,56), whereas others have suggested that the combination of EBRT plus brachytherapy has only minimal effects on EPIC-26 scores relative to baseline measurements (57). Treatment with more than one local modality may not necessarily result in additive negative effect on HRQOL For example, in a trial by the Southwestern Oncology Group that assigned men with localized high-risk disease to undergo surgery with or without adjuvant radiation therapy, men who received postoperative EBRT experienced worse urinary frequency and bowel dysfunction than those treated with surgery alone (58). However, by 5 years of follow-up, bowel dysfunction had returned to normal and EBRT did not affect erectile function. Clearly, practitioners considering the overall impact of combination therapy must weigh the established benefit in terms of disease control against the increased toxicity of the treatment and the resultant effect on the patient's QOL.

For the foreseeable future, the choice of treatment for newly diagnosed prostate cancer will remain challenging for both patients and practitioners. Given the relatively indolent natural history of localized prostate cancer, information on HRQOL after each of the various types of treatment will continue to be important when making management decisions. Therefore, the ability to assimilate, apply, and articulate the findings from HRQOL studies such as those described here is required for those practitioners responsible for counseling men with prostate cancer. Future studies should focus on the effects of combinations of prostate cancer treatments and quantifying the impact of dosimetric parameters and technologic advances such as proton therapy on HRQOL. The utility of current instruments should continue to be regularly assessed, with the goal of uniformity in reporting HRQOL outcomes. Moreover, these instruments must be modified as needed

to consider all of the management options available for these patients; one issue ongoing at this time is whether the full effects of active surveillance are adequately captured by currently available HRQOL questionnaires. Further initiatives should take advantage of advances in electronic information transfer and connectivity to improve data collection and analysis. We encourage all practitioners to prospectively gather information on HRQOL after treatment for prostate cancer so that they can appropriately gauge the experience of their particular patient population against that of published studies.

■ REFERENCES

1. Potters L, Klein EA, Kattan MW, et al. Monotherapy for stage T1-T2 prostate cancer: radical prostatectomy, external beam radiotherapy, or permanent seed implantation. *Radiother Oncol.* 2004;71(1):29–33.
2. Klotz L, Zhang L, Lam A, Nam R, Mamedov A, Loblaw A. Clinical results of long-term follow-up of a large, active surveillance cohort with localized prostate cancer. *J Clin Oncol.* 2010;28(1):126–131.
3. Sonn GA, Sadetsky N, Presti JC, Litwin MS. Differing perceptions of quality of life in patients with prostate cancer and their doctors. *J Urol.* 2009;182(5):2296–2302.
4. Ware JE Jr, Sherbourne CD. The MOS 36-item short-form health survey (SF-36). I. Conceptual framework and item selection. *Med Care.* 1992;30(6):473–483.
5. Lim AJ, Brandon AH, Fiedler J, et al. Quality of life: radical prostatectomy versus radiation therapy for prostate cancer. *J Urol.* 1995;154(4):1420–1425.
6. Cella DF, Tulsky DS, Gray G, et al. The Functional Assessment of Cancer Therapy scale: development and validation of the general measure. *J Clin Oncol.* 1993;11(3):570–579.
7. Aaronson NK, Ahmedzai S, Bergman B, et al. The European Organization for Research and Treatment of Cancer QLQ-C30: a quality-of-life instrument for use in international clinical trials in oncology. *J Natl Cancer Inst.* 1993;85(5):365–376.
8. Litwin MS HR, Fink A, Ganz PA, Leake B, Brook RH. The UCLA Prostate Cancer Index: development, reliability, and validity of a health-related quality of life measure. *Med Care.* 1998;36(7):1002–1012.
9. Wei JT, Dunn RL, Litwin MS, Sandler HM, Sanda MG. Development and validation of the expanded prostate cancer index composite (EPIC) for comprehensive assessment of health-related quality of life in men with prostate cancer. *Urology.* 2000;56(6):899–905.
10. Esper P, Mo F, Chodak G, Sinner M, Cella D, Pienta KJ. Measuring quality of life in men with prostate cancer using the functional assessment of cancer therapy-prostate instrument. *Urology.* 1997;50(6):920–928.

11. Talcott JA, Manola J, Clark JA, et al. Time course and predictors of symptoms after primary prostate cancer therapy. *J Clin Oncol*. 2003;21(21):3979–3986.

12. Joly F, Brune D, Couette JE, et al. Health-related quality of life and sequelae in patients treated with brachytherapy and external beam irradiation for localized prostate cancer. *Ann Oncol*. 1998;9(7):751–757.

13. Huang GJ, Sadetsky N, Penson DF. Health related quality of life for men treated for localized prostate cancer with long-term followup. *J Urol*. 2010;183(6):2206–2212.

14. Miller DC, Sanda MG, Dunn RL, et al. Long-term outcomes among localized prostate cancer survivors: health-related quality-of-life changes after radical prostatectomy, external radiation, and brachytherapy. *J Clin Oncol*. 2005;23(12):2772–2780.

15. Potosky AL, Davis WW, Hoffman RM, et al. Five-year outcomes after prostatectomy or radiotherapy for prostate cancer: the prostate cancer outcomes study. *J Natl Cancer Inst*. 2004;96(18):1358–1367.

16. Hamilton AS, Stanford JL, Gilliland FD, et al. Health outcomes after external-beam radiation therapy for clinically localized prostate cancer: results from the Prostate Cancer Outcomes Study. *J Clin Oncol*. 2001;19(9):2517–2526.

17. Sanda MG, Dunn RL, Michalski J, et al. Quality of life and satisfaction with outcome among prostate-cancer survivors. *N Engl J Med*. 2008;358(12):1250–1261.

18. Downs TM, Sadetsky N, Pasta DJ, et al. Health related quality of life patterns in patients treated with interstitial prostate brachytherapy for localized prostate cancer—data from CaPSURE. *J Urol*. 2003;170(5):1822–1827.

19. Madalinska JB, Essink-Bot ML, de Koning HJ, Kirkels WJ, van der Maas PJ, Schroder FH. Health-related quality-of-life effects of radical prostatectomy and primary radiotherapy for screen-detected or clinically diagnosed localized prostate cancer. *J Clin Oncol*. 2001;19(6):1619–1628.

20. Litwin MS, Pasta DJ, Yu J, Stoddard ML, Flanders SC. Urinary function and bother after radical prostatectomy or radiation for prostate cancer: a longitudinal, multivariate quality of life analysis from the Cancer of the Prostate Strategic Urologic Research Endeavor. *J Urol*. 2000;164(6):1973–1977.

21. Litwin MS, Sadetsky N, Pasta DJ, Lubeck DP. Bowel function and bother after treatment for early stage prostate cancer: a longitudinal quality of life analysis from CaPSURE. *J Urol*. 2004;172(2):515–519.

22. Litwin MS, Flanders SC, Pasta DJ, Stoddard ML, Lubeck DP, Henning JM. Sexual function and bother after radical prostatectomy or radiation for prostate cancer: multivariate quality-of-life analysis from CaPSURE. Cancer of the Prostate Strategic Urologic Research Endeavor. *Urology*. 1999;54(3):503–508.

23. Zelefsky MJ, Levin EJ, Hunt M, et al. Incidence of late rectal and urinary toxicities after three-dimensional conformal radiotherapy and intensity-modulated radiotherapy for localized prostate cancer. *Int J Radiat Oncol Biol Phys*. 2008;70(4):1124–1129.

24. Lips I, Dehnad H, Kruger AB, et al. Health-related quality of life in patients with locally advanced prostate cancer after 76 Gy intensity-modulated radiotherapy vs. 70 Gy conformal radiotherapy in a prospective and longitudinal study. *Int J Radiat Oncol Biol Phys*. 2007;69(3):656–661.

25. Dandapani SV, Sanda MG. Measuring health-related quality of life consequences from primary treatment for early-stage prostate cancer. *Semin Radiat Oncol*. 2008;18(1):67–72.

26. Frank SJ, Pisters LL, Davis J, Lee AK, Bassett R, Kuban DA. An assessment of quality of life following radical prostatectomy, high dose external beam radiation therapy and brachytherapy iodine implantation as monotherapies for localized prostate cancer. *J Urol*. 2007;177(6):2151–2156; discussion 2156.

27. Gore JL, Kwan L, Lee SP, Reiter RE, Litwin MS. Survivorship beyond convalescence: 48-month quality-of-life outcomes after treatment for localized prostate cancer. *J Natl Cancer Inst*. 2009;101(12):888–892.

28. Litwin MS, Gore JL, Kwan L, et al. Quality of life after surgery, external beam irradiation, or brachytherapy for early-stage prostate cancer. *Cancer*. 2007;109(11):2239–2247.

29. Grise P, Thurman S. Urinary incontinence following treatment of localized prostate cancer. *Cancer Control*. 2001;8(6):532–539.

30. Lee WR, McQuellon RP, Harris-Henderson K, Case LD, McCullough DL. A preliminary analysis of health-related quality of life in the first year after permanent source interstitial brachytherapy (PIB) for clinically localized prostate cancer. *Int J Radiat Oncol Biol Phys*. 2000;46(1):77–81.

31. Roeloffzen EM, Lips IM, van Gellekom MP, et al. Health-related quality of life up to six years after (125)I brachytherapy for early-stage prostate cancer. *Int J Radiat Oncol Biol Phys*. 2010;76(4):1054–1060.

32. Davis JW, Kuban DA, Lynch DF, Schellhammer PF. Quality of life after treatment for localized prostate cancer: differences based on treatment modality. *J Urol*. 2001;166(3):947–952.

33. Wei JT, Dunn RL, Sandler HM, et al. Comprehensive comparison of health-related quality of life after contemporary therapies for localized prostate cancer. *J Clin Oncol*. 2002;20(2):557–566.

34. Schover LR, Fouladi RT, Warneke CL, et al. Defining sexual outcomes after treatment for localized prostate carcinoma. *Cancer*. 2002;95(8):1773–1785.

35. Bacon CG, Giovannucci E, Testa M, Kawachi I. The impact of cancer treatment on quality of life outcomes for patients with localized prostate cancer. *J Urol*. 2001;166(5):1804–1810.

36. McCammon KA, Kolm P, Main B, Schellhammer PF. Comparative quality-of-life analysis after radical prostatectomy or external beam radiation for localized prostate cancer. *Urology*. 1999;54(3):509–516.

37. Smith DS, Carvalhal GF, Schneider K, Krygiel J, Yan Y, Catalona WJ. Quality-of-life outcomes for men with prostate carcinoma detected by screening. *Cancer*. 2000;88(6):1454–1463.

38. Beard CJ, Propert KJ, Rieker PP, et al. Complications after treatment with external-beam irradiation in early-stage prostate cancer patients: a prospective multiinstitutional outcomes study. *J Clin Oncol.* 1997;15(1):223–229.

39. Mantz CA, Nautiyal J, Awan A, et al. Potency preservation following conformal radiotherapy for localized prostate cancer: impact of neoadjuvant androgen blockade, treatment technique, and patient-related factors. *Cancer J Sci Am.* 1999;5(4):230–236.

40. Pinkawa M, Fischedick K, Gagel B, et al. Impact of age and comorbidities on health-related quality of life for patients with prostate cancer: evaluation before a curative treatment. *BMC Cancer.* 2009;9:296.

41. Chen RC, Clark JA, Talcott JA. Individualizing quality-of-life outcomes reporting: how localized prostate cancer treatments affect patients with different levels of baseline urinary, bowel, and sexual function. *J Clin Oncol.* 2009;27(24):3916–3922.

42. Staff I, Salner A, Bohannon R, Panatieri P, Maljanian R. Disease-specific symptoms and general quality of life of patients with prostate carcinoma before and after primary three-dimensional conformal radiotherapy. *Cancer.* 2003;98(11):2335–2343.

43. Lee IH, Sadetsky N, Carroll PR, Sandler HM. The impact of treatment choice for localized prostate cancer on response to phosphodiesterase inhibitors. *J Urol.* 2008;179(3):1072–1076; discussion 1076.

44. Mabjeesh N, Chen J, Beri A, Stenger A, Matzkin H. Sexual function after permanent 125I-brachytherapy for prostate cancer. *Int J Impot Res.* 2005;17(1):96–101.

45. Stock RG, Kao J, Stone NN. Penile erectile function after permanent radioactive seed implantation for treatment of prostate cancer. *J Urol.* 2001;165(2):436–439.

46. Taira AV, Merrick GS, Galbreath RW, et al. Erectile function durability following permanent prostate brachytherapy. *Int J Radiat Oncol Biol Phys.* 2009;75(3):639–648.

47. Pinkawa M, Asadpour B, Piroth MD, et al. Health-related quality of life after permanent I-125 brachytherapy and conformal external beam radiotherapy for prostate cancer—a matched-pair comparison. *Radiother Oncol.* 2009;91(2):225–231.

48. Hashine K, Azuma K, Koizumi T, Sumiyoshi Y. Health-related quality of life and treatment outcomes for men with prostate cancer treated by combined external-beam radiotherapy and hormone therapy. *Int J Clin Oncol.* 2005;10(1):45–50.

49. Lubeck DP, Grossfeld GD, Carroll PR. The effect of androgen deprivation therapy on health-related quality of life in men with prostate cancer. *Urology.* 2001;58(2 suppl 1):94–100.

50. Pinkawa M, Fischedick K, Gagel B, et al. Association of neoadjuvant hormonal therapy with adverse health-related quality of life after permanent iodine-125 brachytherapy for localized prostate cancer. *Urology.* 2006;68(1):104–109.

51. Egawa S, Shimura S, Irie A, et al. Toxicity and health-related quality of life during and after high dose rate brachytherapy followed by external beam radiotherapy for prostate cancer. *Jpn J Clin Oncol.* 2001;31(11):541–547.

52. Joseph KJ, Alvi R, Skarsgard D, et al. Analysis of health related quality of life (HRQoL) of patients with clinically localized prostate cancer, one year after treatment with external beam radiotherapy (EBRT) alone versus EBRT and high dose rate brachytherapy (HDRBT). *Radiat Oncol.* 2008;3:20.

53. Lev EL, Eller LS, Gejerman G, et al. Quality of life of men treated with brachytherapies for prostate cancer. *Health Qual Life Outcomes.* 2004;2:28.

54. Vordermark D, Wulf J, Markert K, et al. 3-D conformal treatment of prostate cancer to 74 Gy vs. high-dose-rate brachytherapy boost: a cross-sectional quality-of-life survey. *Acta Oncol.* 2006;45(6):708–716.

55. Merrick GS, Butler WM, Wallner KE, Hines AL, Allen Z. Late rectal function after prostate brachytherapy. *Int J Radiat Oncol Biol Phys.* 2003;57(1):42–48.

56. Brandeis JM, Litwin MS, Burnison CM, Reiter RE. Quality of life outcomes after brachytherapy for early stage prostate cancer. *J Urol.* 2000;163(3):851–857.

57. Morton GC, Loblaw DA, Sankreacha R, et al. Single-fraction high-dose-rate brachytherapy and hypofractionated external beam radiotherapy for men with intermediate-risk prostate cancer: analysis of short- and medium-term toxicity and quality of life. *Int J Radiat Oncol Biol Phys.* 2010;77(3):811–817.

58. Moinpour CM, Hayden KA, Unger JM, et al. Health-related quality of life results in pathologic stage C prostate cancer from a Southwest Oncology Group trial comparing radical prostatectomy alone with radical prostatectomy plus radiation therapy. *J Clin Oncol.* 2008;26(1):112–120.

Index

Note: Page numbers followed by "*f*" and "*t*" denote figures and tables, respectively.